SPECIAL
Delivery

Pregnancy during the Pandemic: Stories of 36 Women

MIRIAM SIVKIN, M.D, FACOG, MA, AASECT, CST, MSCP

ISBN

Paperback: 979-8-90190-339-1

Hardcover: 979-8-90190-340-7

Contents

Introduction

One day in 2025, I woke drenched in sweat. My mind was unexpectedly being pulled back to March of 2020, a time that many may wish to forget, but most may never. It was a moment destined for the history books, remembered as the beginning of the pandemic that brought the 21st-century world to a standstill. At that time, though, I believe that very few of us were sweating, at least not in anticipation or fear. We had been told that the lockdown would last two weeks. Seeing the strides made in medicine and technology, we believed that a cure would be found in no time. We trusted our governments, our scientists, and our doctors. But what we did not know was that the sheer magnitude of the pandemic would suspend our lives in limbo, leaving us waiting for a way to battle the virus and reclaim normalcy. Most of us had no idea what was about to unfold.

March 2020 marked an extraordinary turning point in our collective lives. Almost overnight, the world turned upside down. Confusion, fear, and uncertainty spread faster than the virus itself, leaving people unsure of what was happening or how to respond. Whether healthcare professionals, business owners, food service workers, or stay-at-home parents, every one of us felt our lives altered by the virus and the lockdown.

As an obstetrician and gynecologist, reflecting on this period inevitably brings my thoughts back to my patients and their growing families. How did they navigate the unprecedented reality of a world in lockdown? How did we, as healthcare providers, adapt to support them? Were their lives and plans completely uprooted when the seriousness of the virus set in, or did they accept, adapt, and persevere? Did COVID-19 cripple them, or did it empower them? Did expectant mothers discover new forms of community, even within their isolation?

Most importantly, I wanted to know what we could learn from those who prospered, those who, despite the odds, decided that they wanted to expand their families and cling to hope even in desperate times. I wanted to know what made mothers consciously plan to have babies during a period of global uncertainty. What sustained them, what gave them joy, and what reassured them that they and their children would remain safe and healthy despite the crisis?

Martin Luther King Jr. once said, “We must accept finite disappointment, but never lose infinite hope.” Nowhere was this more evident than among pregnant mothers during the pandemic, who saw hospitals overwhelmed, understaffed, and overcrowded, yet pressed forward with courage. These women understood they would face hurdles, especially given that women’s health has historically received little attention in medicine. And still, they chose resilience. I wanted to know what drove them, what gave them confidence, and what made them so certain that they could bring new life into a world so uncertain.

These questions inspired the foundation of this book.

I began speaking with women who had experienced pregnancy during this global crisis, documenting their stories, struggles, and resilience. Most were my patients, though some were acquaintances. Their voices form the heart of this work. By highlighting their experiences, I hope to illuminate not only the practical ways they found success but also the incredible strength of their spirit and the quiet power of the communities they built.

Birth Rates During COVID

Before presenting their narratives, it is important to first consider the broader cultural and demographic debate that arose early in the pandemic: would COVID-19 lead to a “baby bust” or a “baby boom”?

We all faced stay-at-home orders. Historically, pandemics have not sparked baby booms; instead, they have almost always led to a marked decline in births.[1] The event most comparable to COVID-19 was the 1918 Spanish Flu. That pandemic was particularly deadly for young adults between the ages of 20 and 40, which led to significant drops in birth rates across affected countries.[2]

---

[1] Aassve, Arnstein, Nicolò Cavalli, Letizia Mencarini, Samuel Plach, and Massimo Livi Bacci. "The COVID-19 pandemic and human fertility." *Science* 369, no. 6502 (2020): 370-371.
[2] Burke, Jessica L., Lisa A. Eargle, and Ashraf Esmail. "The Spanish Flu and its Effects on Population Growth." *Twenty-First Century Issues: Perspective on Climate Change, Pandemic, and Digital Transformation* (2025): 1.

Early data from the United States during COVID-19 reflected a similar pattern. In March and April 2020, individuals between the ages of 18 and 34 reported postponing or even abandoning plans for childbearing. By December 2020, when the effects of those decisions were evident, the fertility rate had dropped by 8%. Between October 2020 and February 2021, there were 60,000 fewer births than in the previous pre-pandemic years.[3]

Were people postponing or deciding not to have children because of health and money?

During the initial months of COVID, unemployment increased from 3.5% to 13.2%, and pregnancies declined the most in areas where unemployment was the highest.[4] Pregnancies also dropped significantly in regions experiencing the largest COVID outbreaks. The groups most affected by the decline in birth rates were women in their late 30s and early 40s, especially those who already had one child.[5] This suggests that multiple factors contributed to the decrease in birth rates during the pandemic, including health concerns, economic difficulties, childcare issues, and closures of healthcare services. Travel restrictions also played a role, as women born outside the United States, who accounted for nearly 23% of births in 2019, saw a sharp decrease in 2020.[6]

However, pregnancies did rebound. Looking at the data, we now know that the birth rates in the U.S. were initially a bust, followed by a boom, and then they resumed their historical downward trend.

In 2021, there was an unusually high number of babies born. The groups that experienced significant birth rate increases were first-time

---

[3] Anne Morse, "U.S. Births Declined During the Pandemic," *United States Census Bureau*, September 21, 2021, accessed August 20, 2025, https://www.census.gov/library/stories/2021/09/united-states-births-declined-during-the-pandemic.html.

[4] Smith, Sean M., Roxanna Edwards, and Hao C. Duong. "Unemployment rises in 2020, as the country battles the COVID-19 pandemic." *Monthly Lab. Rev.* 144 (2021): 1.

[5] Time. "How the COVID-19 Pandemic Affected U.S. Birth Rates." *Time*, published approximately 2.7 years ago, accessed August 20, 2025. https://time.com/6237576/covid-19-pandemic-us-birth-rates.

[6] Zorthian, Julia. 2022. "The Numbers Behind America's Quiet Pandemic Baby Surge." *Time*, updated October 21, 2022. Accessed August 20, 2025. https://time.com/6223625/covid-pandemic-birth-rates/

mothers and women under 25 years old. It was believed that this might be due to a decline in poverty during 2020 and an increase in net worth among higher-income families during the pandemic. Another important factor is that abortions declined because of reduced medical services. Additionally, women between 30 and 34 and college-educated women aged 25 to 44 saw increased birth rates, as many jobs became remote, which supported fertility by offering more flexibility. The decrease in spending on travel and social activities also played a role. Regions with the greatest improvements in the labor market saw the largest rise in pregnancies, while areas that experienced the biggest declines did not see similar increases. The baby boom in 2021 was also fueled by a decrease in pandemic-related anxiety in the summer and fall of 2020. By 2022, the U.S. birthrate returned to its long-term downward trend, which has been steady for the past 30 years.

The Effect of COVID on Pregnant Women

These fluctuations can be attributed to the fact that we did not have a clear understanding of what COVID-19 was and how it would impact us.

The first cases of COVID-19 were identified in December 2019, and it was declared a pandemic on March 11, 2020. As of July 2022, 90 million people in the United States had been infected, and over 1 million individuals had died from the disease. COVID-19 is an illness that affects the lungs and respiratory system. It is caused by the coronavirus. The symptoms of COVID-19 include fever, cough, sore throat, and myalgia. The initial variant that emerged in 2020 was named Alpha, followed by the Beta variant, then the Delta variant, and ultimately the Omicron variant. The Delta variant was linked to increased disease severity and placental dysfunction during pregnancy. The Omicron variant has been found to cause less severe symptoms but appears to spread more easily. As the coronavirus continued to mutate, new variants of COVID-19 have kept emerging. These variants display different rates of transmissibility and levels of symptom severity.

When COVID began, we had hardly any information about how this infection affected pregnancy and newborns. Therefore, for those pregnant at the start of the pandemic, it was challenging for everyone involved. The risks of pregnancy during COVID were real.

Maternal death rates were high during the pandemic, with 869 deaths per 100,000 infected pregnancies compared to 5.17 deaths per 100,000 in non-infected pregnancies. This difference is statistically significant. We learned that pregnant women did not become infected more often than non-pregnant women, but if infected, they faced higher risks of adverse effects. We found that pregnant women with COVID-19 were more likely to need ICU admission and ventilation support. They were also more likely to have cesarean births, preeclampsia or eclampsia, and blood clots. Preeclampsia was observed in 7% of infected pregnant women versus 4.5% in non-infected pregnant patients. Pregnant women with comorbidities such as obesity, diabetes, hypertension, or respiratory disease were at higher risk of severe illness. Newborns born to infected women were found to have an increased risk of needing NICU admission. It is believed that newborns contract the infection when in contact with an infected parent. However, COVID-19 does not seem to increase the risk of birth defects or growth retardation.

Being infected and pregnant was associated with a higher rate of miscarriage in the first trimester, with a 14% incidence in infected women compared to 8% in healthy pregnant women. Although the risk of stillbirth was low, it occurred in 13 out of 1000 infected pregnancies versus 6 out of 1000 healthy pregnancies. The risk of premature birth increased with infection when pregnancy was beyond 34 weeks of gestation. This increase is thought to be secondary to medical intervention. COVID-19 led to decreased rates of obstetrical intervention, which contributed to increased perinatal mortality. Obstetric visits shifted to virtual antenatal care appointments, and the use of ultrasounds was reduced. There was a decrease in clinician-initiated preterm births and overall preterm birth rates. Pandemic disruptions affected obstetrical surveillance, resulting in more macrosomic infants and a higher number of post-term pregnancies, as pregnancies were monitored without intervention for longer periods. At the onset of the pandemic, perinatal mortality rates increased, partly due to a decrease in clinician-initiated preterm births and other obstetrical concerns. Patients at high risk who required more intensive surveillance were most affected.

The effects of the pandemic on pregnancy and early motherhood were not limited to physical health outcomes. Beyond the risks of exposure to the virus itself, mothers faced heightened levels of stress, anxiety, and social isolation, while babies were born into an environment marked by uncertainty and disrupted support systems. Together, these challenges reshaped how many families experienced pregnancy, childbirth, and early infant care, leaving a lasting imprint that extended well beyond the immediate health concerns of COVID-19.

But statistics only tell part of the story. What I wanted to know was how this translated into the lived experience of mothers and families.

The Interview Process

To better understand these lived realities, thirty-six women who were pregnant and delivered during the pandemic, along with their Significant Others, were interviewed. Each participant was asked the same set of ten questions designed to capture not only their medical and logistical experiences but also the emotional, social, and relational dimensions of navigating pregnancy and new parenthood during COVID-19. The following questions were posed:

1. Was this a planned pregnancy?
2. If it was planned, what were your thoughts about COVID-19, and did it affect your opinion?
3. What preparations did you make in regards to your pregnancy and COVID-19?
4. What negative and positive experiences did you have during your pregnancy, keeping in mind COVID-19?
5. What negative and positive experiences did you have during your postpartum period?
6. What were your baby-care experiences during COVID-19?
7. What were your family's feelings about your pregnancy during the pandemic?
8. What were your experiences with antepartum visits with your OB/GYN, during delivery, and after your delivery?

9. What were your Significant Other's feelings about the pregnancy before, during, and after the baby was born?
10. If you look back on your decision to be pregnant during the pandemic, what are your thoughts now versus when you decided to have a baby?

The ten questions asked were chosen to capture the complexity of pregnancy during COVID-19, covering decision-making, preparation, emotional challenges, healthcare access, family dynamics, and reflections over time. Together, they provide a well-rounded understanding of how the pandemic shaped both the medical and personal sides of having a baby.

By covering medical, emotional, relational, and reflective dimensions, these questions aimed to provide a holistic view of how the pandemic influenced pregnancy, childbirth, and early parenting.

To protect the privacy of participants, all names and identifying details have been changed. The following sections adapt the interviews into real-life narrative stories rather than verbatim transcripts. This approach was chosen to preserve the authenticity of their experiences while presenting them in a way that is engaging, accessible, and respectful. By weaving their voices into story form, the goal is to highlight not only the facts of their experiences but also the emotions, challenges, and resilience that defined pregnancy and birth during the pandemic.

What follows are stories that remind us of the strength of mothers, the power of family, and the hope that endures even in the darkest times.

1
Laura

Laura Williams shuddered, knowing her due date was fast approaching. She looked down at her belly and then up at the television screen. In big, bold, red letters, the news banner read **"U.S. Cities Begin Lockdowns as COVID-19 Cases Surge."**

All the joy she had felt upon seeing those two lines on the pregnancy test strip turn red eight months prior had vanished, replaced by complete dread and confusion.

Not because the child who was now growing inside her was unwelcome. Not because she felt unprepared to bring new life into this world. But because a deadly virus was rampaging across the globe.

The year was 2020, and the coronavirus was spreading. Fast. Warnings, measures, rules, distancing, germs, spread, dead, infected, dying, tests, positive...These were the words that rang through her mind as she watched the news, as the reporter listed down the number of deaths in each state that week.

In just the last month, from February to March, the situation had escalated from a handful of confirmed COVID-19 cases to a national emergency and widespread shutdowns.

Laura was on her bed, safe in her home. But still, she clutched at her bedsheets with white knuckles.

She rushed to the bathroom feeling the need to throw up, but not from morning sickness. She looked at the mirror above her sink, staring back was the face of a woman who felt nothing but uncertainty. *How will I even get to the hospital?* She heaved into the sink.

Laura walked out of the bathroom in a daze. Her husband Matt had just come home for a grocery run. He stood in the doorway, a mask still on his face, and held up his recently washed hands. "I'm clean," he said. "I'll just hop into the shower now."

Oblivious to the terror that raged within his wife's mind, Matt went to the bathroom, and after a few seconds, Laura heard the faucet turn on.

Laura felt as if she was glued to the bed. The news had now moved on, covering the story of a teacher's dedication to educating her students despite the fact that she now had to figure out how to use Zoom.

Matt walked out minutes later, his hair wet. "Okay, I am fully clean and dressed now. Can I get a hug?" That was when he finally noticed how upset his wife was. "Honey?"

Then, the soon-to-be mother broke. "It...It's just...all of this...how will I...how will we?" Laura buried her face in her hands, overcome.

Matt whipped his head around and looked at the TV. He glared at it as if it were what had caused his wife such pain. Quickly grabbing the remote, he turned it off.

"Laura, listen," he said, turning to his wife. "We will do everything we possibly can to keep this baby safe. He will be safe. I will not let anything happen to you."

"But this virus has changed everything. I have no idea what things will be like in that delivery room."

"That much is true. But whatever it is, we will get through it. You can manage anything, sweetie. And I will be with you every step of the way." Matt urged Laura to sit on the bed. He grabbed a few tissues off the nightstand and handed them to her.

Wiping away her tears, Laura said, shaking, "Manhattan is the worst place for this! How are we supposed to get too East 98th Street from 56th? There's nothing closer. We don't even have a car."

"We will make it. We can get an Uber...or maybe our neighbor Jeff can give us a ride." Matt was now beginning to become uncertain himself. *Would Uber even be available and running?* he thought.

As if reading his mind, his wife said, "Not if they shut down too. Besides, how safe is it to travel in a car that 100s of people have sat in? With a driver who has interacted with so many? God. I don't even know what happens if you get COVID while you're pregnant."

Matt racked his brain for an answer. "What if we book a room? A hotel? One on 98th? We can walk to the hospital then. What do you say? It'll be comfy and clean; we can pack up our bags beforehand."

"…maybe," Laura replied in a small voice, rubbing her hair as she usually did when her nerves acted up. "That can be Plan B."

"Done." Matt pumped his fist in the air. "C'mon, honey. I know it's stressful, but just think about it. We are going to be parents!"

Laura let out a chuckle. "That is the one thing I'm not afraid of."

"You are going to be the best mom," he said. "Now let's just focus on getting you through this. I want my wife healthy and happy."

Laura took a deep breath. "Well then, I should probably make an appointment with my obstetrician again. Ask her about what to expect." Laura rubbed her belly.

Matt picked up Laura's phone from the side table and handed it to her.

"I'm famished." Laura scrolled through her contacts.

"I'll whip up something for you. Got some nice bagels. They were on sale. Go ahead and make the call."

Laura sat there while Matt was in the kitchen. She felt a bit better now, but concerns still floated in her mind. *At least I won't be alone,* she thought. After a few minutes, she made the call.

On the way to her appointment, Laura thought about her plans for the birth. She knew she wanted to have the baby on her own, naturally. A hospital birth was necessary in case of complications, but she had always envisioned a natural delivery. It was how her mother had given birth to her, and she wanted to experience the same. The only person she wanted in the delivery room was her husband. She needed Matt there. His presence would bring the calm she knew she would need in that moment.

As she neared the doctor's office, questions swirled in her mind. She knew she would have a clearer picture of what lay ahead after the appointment. The obstetrician had come highly recommended, and Laura trusted that she would help ease her nerves. She would offer both clarity and reassurance while also, of course, checking on the health of her baby.

Once she and Dr. Priya had settled in, completed the necessary health checks, and discussed recommendations, Dr. Priya asked if she had any further questions. That was when Laura shared her birth plan, asking about hospital arrangements, available resources, and the logistics of getting there when the time came. So much had changed since she had last met with Dr. Priya. It was as if she had to come up with a whole new plan.

Dr. Priya listened quietly, her hands folded on the table, her expression blank but concentrated. Then, in a soft, measured tone, she said, “Laura, many soon-to-be mothers have asked me the same questions. But I must be completely honest with you. There is not much certainty about what will happen with the pandemic. As you know, we’ve been given new sets of instructions to follow almost every week this month. I cannot say for certain what the situation will be when you give birth. From what scientists have found, we don’t expect the pandemic to end within the next week. It is more than likely that you will give birth while we are still in lockdown.”

Her words shattered the little hope Laura had been holding onto.

“Laura, look at me,” Dr. Priya said.

Only then did Laura realize she had been staring at the floor. She sniffed and looked up.

“Listen to me. No matter what happens, our people, our healthcare providers, our government…they will make sure that you are taken care of.”

“I know, but it’s just so strange. I don’t know what to expect.”

“Laura, women gave birth during the Great Plague. They gave birth during smallpox. Women have given birth in tubs, on the floor, in barns. Your body is made for this. You will be absolutely fine.”

Laura let out a small chuckle. “You aren’t wrong there.”

Dr. Priya smiled but then grew serious. “I do want to be honest with you, though.”

“Oh no,” Laura muttered.

"Yes. You said you wanted your husband with you in the delivery room. Is that correct?"

"It is."

"Well, I've heard rumors that they may not allow significant others or any family members to be present during labor."

"Oh."

"This is just something being discussed for now. Nothing is set in stone, and I'm not sure when or if it will be implemented. But if I hear anything more, I'll let you know. I have some friends at the hospital."

"Well, thank you, Doctor. I guess we'll cross that bridge when we get to it." Laura forced a weak smile.

But once her appointment was over and she was on her way home, there was little else she could do. The weight of it all was too much for her, and before she even reached her door, she broke down. It was many hours before she finally managed to stop crying.

A few days later, Dr. Priya told Laura that at 7 AM on March 24, 2020, the hospital would implement the no Significant Other allowed rule. The news had come in a rushed phone call, taken by Dr. Priya in between two appointments. Laura was so grateful for Dr. Priya and how much of a help she had been.

Laura called her mom and told her about the news.

"We got to get that baby out of you quick then," Mrs. Williams said.

Laura rolled her eyes. "I can't just will him to be ready, Mama."

The sound of a laugh came through the line. "You underestimate the power of the mind."

Laura twirled her hair.

"Anyway. How is the kid? Still kicking hard." Her mom sounded very chipper, which annoyed Laura.

Laura rolled her eyes. "He's going to be a soccer player one day, it seems. I am so sore."

"I wish I could be there with you, Laura. I'm sorry."

Laura's stomach dropped. "I know, Mom. It's been hard without family."

"I am sure. At least you have Matt."

Laura felt as if the ground had disappeared from beneath her. "Yes. Anyway, Mom, I'll talk to you later."

"Okay, love, I can't wait to see my grandbaby. Bye-bye then."

"Bye."

Laura lay there, unable to move. All she could think was that she wanted Matt to be with her. She knew she could have no one else. She knew she needed him.

That's when the idea formed in her mind. Out loud, she said, "I will do what I have to do to have my husband with me." There was only one way to achieve this, given the information she had and given the situation.

She needed to be induced.

On March 23, 2020, at night, Laura went to the hospital for her induction. The hospital was so short-staffed that after she was given medication and after her water broke, no one came to her room, not even to change the sheets.

When her pain became unbearable, she asked for an epidural. All plans for a natural birth went out the window.

Time passed in a blur as she became consumed by pain. Her husband was with her, urging her to stay calm and breathe. He was the only support she had, as no doctor or nurse stayed around for long. They had more pressing matters to attend to as more patients checked in, coughing, with masks on their faces, with fevers.

A few hours later, about 12 doctors and nurses walked in. All of them were covered head to toe in white and yellow. Hazmat suits.

Laura's own mask made it hard for her to breathe. But she would not…could not take it off.

"Please move into a different position, it will be better if you are on all fours," one of them said. The mask muffled his voice. It sounded as if it came from a speaker.

Laura obeyed.

The doctors gave information to each other in short bursts. "Heart rate slow…dropping…danger…cesarean section."

Laura was sweating, terrified, and in immense pain.

"What's happening?" she asked. "Why is no one telling me anything?"

"We are short-staffed, ma'am; I am very sorry." One of the other doctors had spoken. He sounded young. Too young.

Is a student really doing my delivery? thought Laura. The people before were young too.

Laura sat back down on the bed.

"Laura, you need to have an emergency delivery. The baby's heart rate is dangerously low. We must do a cesarean section."

Laura grunted in pain. "Do whatever you need to do. Save my baby."

Laura's baby was born at 06:56 AM. He was completely healthy. The policy to prohibit spouses from being in the hospital was scheduled to begin at 07:00 AM. After her delivery, Laura got to be with her baby and husband for exactly four minutes. Her husband was then asked to leave.

She had got what she wanted—her husband had been by her side while their baby was born—and for that, Laura was grateful.

Laura was brought into her room with her newborn baby. Being a new, first-time mom, she needed help. Laura looked around the room and pressed the call button. The baby was not crying and did not seem agitated. He had been fed about 30 minutes ago. But Laura was unsure about what needed to be done next. *Is he swaddled correctly? Is it too tight? Will he be hungry by now? Can he breathe in that position?* She had pressed the call button a few minutes ago, but no one had arrived yet.

Again, she pressed the button. Twice, it glowed red. She waited. A minute. Two. Still no one.

Laura felt lost. Her mother was not there to help her. No one was. The doctors seemed to be so understaffed, and the hospital was so full that they were not even able to send her a lactation consultant. Her stress became almost unbearable.

It was a whole hour before the nurse arrived.

After being discharged and returning home with her child, Laura noticed that the baby was losing weight rapidly. *Isn't he supposed to be gaining weight?* she thought.

Matt walked toward her and picked up the writhing infant.

"Doesn't he seem a bit too light?" Laura said in a shaky voice. "I have no idea what I'm doing. I don't know if I'm breastfeeding correctly."

The baby cooed, yawning and promptly falling asleep in his father's arms. "Seems okay to me. Why don't you ask your mom?"

"Her Wi-Fi has been down for the past couple of days. Can't get a call through."

"Let's try again soon."

"Alright."

Laura thought about her family and how she wanted them to be with her at this moment. No one had seen the baby in person yet. All they saw of him was from video calls and pictures. He had yet to be held by his grandparents, who longed to meet him but could not because they feared getting COVID-19. They didn't even know if the baby could get COVID, but either way, they would not risk the journey. Traveling from New Jersey to Manhattan would be incredibly difficult in any case. Laura could not go to them since she didn't have a car, and so, they decided it was best to wait for the lockdown to ease.

But soon enough, Laura and Matt were forced to make a long drive.

One afternoon, Laura noticed that the baby was tongue-tied. He was unable to lift his tongue, and upon inspecting it, Laura saw that it was almost fused to the flesh.

Matt was not home, and there was no one to ask about what was happening. Laura didn't even know if this was normal. She was hyperventilating, feeling guilty for not noticing it earlier. She did the first thing she could think of. She made an appointment with her baby's pediatrician. All doctors' visits were now online, something

Laura had yet to become accustomed to. It was strange not to have to wait outside an office, have an attendant call you in, and then sit before a doctor. Now the doctor seemed like a stranger, separated by screen and land, not just a table. All of her postpartum checkups had been virtual. Thankfully, the pediatrician was free and could slot her in within the next 30 minutes.

Guess there's some benefit to this telehealth thing, Laura thought.

But the appointment did nothing to calm her nerves. She was told that her baby needed surgery. It was a surgery he could not get in Manhattan. A trip to Long Island was in store.

On the day when the surgery was scheduled, Laura gripped the keys to her rented car tightly. She hadn't wanted this—had dreaded it, really—but there was no other way. The baby's tongue tie needed to be corrected, and the only available surgeon was on Long Island. Everyone else was occupied with other procedures because of COVID-19.

Matt adjusted the baby's car seat, making sure the straps were snug but not too tight. "You sure you're okay with this?" he asked, glancing at Laura.

"No," she admitted. "But what choice do we have?"

She opened the back door and carefully placed the baby inside. The thought of renting a car had been nerve-wracking enough, but now, every touch, every breath in a closed space felt like a risk. *Is the car truly clean? Had the last person who drove it been sick?* Her mind ran through the possibilities. Each felt unsettling.

Matt shut the door gently and stood beside her. "We'll be fine," he said, but she could hear the slight shake in his voice.

Laura nodded, more to convince herself than anything else. She slid into the driver's seat, took a deep breath, and turned the key. The engine rumbled to life. The road ahead was long, unfamiliar, and filled with unknowns, but they had to go. They had to keep moving.

Thankfully, all went well, and the baby was healthy once more. They managed to live happily as a little family in their small apartment.

Still, Laura felt burdened with the mounting stress and the isolation.

Laura sat on the edge of the bed, watching the baby sleep. The Night Nanny was supposed to arrive soon.

"I don't know about this," she said, rubbing her hands together. "She's a stranger, Matt. What if—"

"We talked about this," Matt interrupted gently, moving to sit beside her. "You need the help. You have been working too. It's a lot to handle for one person. It'll be fine."

Laura gave birth on a Tuesday and went straight back to work on the following Monday. She worked from home, though, which allowed her to be with her baby 24/7, something she was always grateful for. Still, holding the baby in one hand as he fed and typing an email with the other was getting difficult. Hearing the baby crying in the next room, knowing she would not leave the meeting to attend to him was soul-crushing. She barely even took her baby outside because of the virus and the risk involved. She could count on one hand the number of times they had gone for a walk together.

Laura nodded but didn't feel reassured. The thought of someone new in their space, around the baby, made her stomach twist.

Thankfully, the nanny was amazing and a great help.

Eventually, things began to get better. There were now clear guidelines and rules. COVID-19 testing was easy and accessible. Laura and her family became confident that they would be safe if they ventured outside.

In July, Laura finally saw her sister and mother. Three months. That's how long it had been. Her family had only seen the baby through a screen, had never held him, never kissed his cheek. When they finally managed to come to her house, her sister reached out instinctively, then stopped herself. She ran to the powder room and washed her hands. Laura's mother walked in and squealed, but Laura rubbed her hands together with a stern expression on her face, and her mother marched on to the restroom, following Laura's sister.

Her sister walked back in, now disinfected. "I can't believe it's been this long," she whispered. "I can't wait to hold this little tyke." She lifted the baby up onto her chest and put a firm hand under him to keep him steady.

“My Lord, he is so soft!” She inhaled the hypnotizing smell of the baby and held him close.

Laura couldn’t help but smile widely. Everything felt so perfect. Finally, her family could share in her joy.

Laura’s mother walked in and stood behind her sister, drying her own wet hands. She eyed her eldest daughter with jealousy, wishing she had made it to the baby first.

A few days later, after her family left, Laura traced a finger along the sleeping baby’s tiny hand, watching as it curled instinctively around hers. The past few months hadn’t been anything like she had imagined, but there was a silver lining.

“I got to be here for all of it,” she said, leaning against Matt on the couch. “Every milestone. Every little moment.”

She had seen her baby’s first smile, the first time the baby rolled over. She had been there for it all—something she never would have experienced if things had gone as planned, if there had been no lockdown, if she had not worked from home.

“I actually feel spoiled,” she admitted as Matt put his hand on her shoulder, looking at their baby. “I never thought I’d get this much time with him.”

Matt nodded. “Yeah. It’s not how we pictured it, but maybe it worked out the way it was supposed to.”

Laura thought about that. If she had to choose between the perfect delivery she had dreamed of and the uninterrupted time she had with her son, she knew which one she would pick.

“This,” she murmured to herself, pressing a kiss to the baby’s head. “I’d choose this every time.”

To Matt, she said, “It was truly a blessing in disguise.”

2
Ramona

Ramona Simone had planned her first pregnancy. She embraced the idea of motherhood and all that it brought with it, positive or negative. But what she hadn't planned for was carrying a child through the height of a global pandemic.

December 2019, the very month the pandemic first emerged, was the month she became pregnant. The world had changed almost overnight, and now, she had to think about the fact that she was bringing new life into an almost unrecognizable world. Ramona had hoped for baby showers and prenatal classes, but what she got instead were video calls with doctors whose faces she could not see, whose smiles or frowns she could not fully make out. What she remembered most from her pregnancy, though, were the long hours in emergency rooms. Alone.

In the early days of lockdown, she tried to focus on the good. COVID-19, in all its destruction, forced her to reevaluate her life. She cooked more than ever before, making sure to carefully choose nourishing ingredients. She did this to ensure that she and the baby growing inside her were both healthy. She thought more deeply about her time, her health, and her future, especially as a new mother. There were many concerns about how to maintain a work-life balance, how to keep her family healthy, and how to stay safe and socially distance effectively. Her husband was her biggest supporter through all of this. He was always willing to try new things, to make sure that his wife was well taken care of and comfortable.

Despite the state of the world, things seemed to be going well for Ramona. She was happy that her family was growing bigger, happy that she had now received a wake-up call to reflect on her life, and happy that she had her husband with her so much that they were able to bond well. All seemed to be close to perfect. That was until the visit with her obstetrician.

"You have a high-risk pregnancy."

The words shattered Ramona's world.

High risk? All I had was a fever. I just found it difficult to breathe for a moment. High risk?

Ramona's ears rang as the doctor continued, "You should go to the emergency room immediately. I cannot treat you for this over the phone. Go to the ER, then, we must make our visits more frequent so I can keep tabs on your condition."

All Ramona could do was nod. Her head had not even finished nodding the second time before the doctor ended the Zoom meeting. *I suppose there are other patients to attend to,* Ramona thought.

This was the second time she had been sent to the emergency room. The first visit was not needed. A result of poor communication. Now, though, she thought things might be serious. Either way, she wouldn't do anything to compromise the health of her child.

Ramona knew that she would have to go to the ER alone, as usual. No one could accompany her there; only essential persons, only serious cases, were allowed entry.

She drove to the hospital on her own, an N95 mask secured on her face, plastic gloves adorning her hands. She was careful to stay more than six feet away from other people. The doctors would have to approach her to examine her though—or so she thought.

Ramona waited for over an hour after being seated in the waiting room. Yet no one came to provide her medical care, to evaluate her. She called her husband in a panic, but all he could do was assure her that she was in the right place.

After waiting for five more hours, a doctor finally came to see her. He was quick with his evaluation. Too quick.

They did not even form full sentences when speaking to her.

"Testing."

A nurse whizzed past her.

"Examination."

A doctor put down his stethoscope.

"Elevated temperature."

A thermometer beeped.

"Difficulty breathing."

A group of students rushed past.

"Inconclusive."

A stressed Head Nurse barked out orders.

"We aren't sure what to do."

A doctor tried to console a critically ill patient from 6 feet away.

"You may go home."

The doctor coughed as he said it.

And so, she left.

Yet again, it was a case of poor communication, of inadequate care, of rushed treatment. The hospitals were obviously overburdened. The personnel were overworked and overloaded. Everyone feared for their lives. For their families' lives.

It was bad enough that she had to go to the ER alone. She had been muzzled by her mask for over 8 hours. She did not take it off even once to eat or drink. That in itself could not have been good for her or the baby. But to make things worse, many of the doctors themselves seemed sick. Ramona thought about the families these healthcare providers went back to. *Are their spouses sick? Are their kids safe? What if my doctor has a pregnant wife?*

I shouldn't think like this. It isn't my job to worry about these things.

The doctors in the emergency rooms seemed confused and on edge. They could not handle or understand the situation, and a lot of information regarding protocol and policies was being lost in translation. Although she knew the doctors were doing their best, she couldn't help but resent them and grieve over her situation.

Ramona drove back home in silence, sweat pooling beneath her mask. She knew that no one except her husband could console her now. Meeting with family or friends was out of the question, and Ramona was sick of Zoom calls with all their lagging, poor connections, and distorted voices. Often, Ramona did not feel like she was talking to people; she felt as if she was conversing with robots who wore masks resembling the faces of her loved ones. Nothing was going as planned.

At this point in her pregnancy, Ramona should have been getting regular lactation consultations and childbirth classes. This was especially needed since she was a first-time mother. *What does it matter, she thought. It's not like James was there with me for any ultrasounds or prenatal visits anyway. The beginning did not go well, so why would the end?*

She reached home, hoping that she would not have to go for any more unnecessary ER visits. But within a few weeks, she found herself back in the hospital.

The car had come out of nowhere and crashed right into the passenger-side door. Ramona remembered little of what happened next; all she knew was that she had woken up in the emergency room. I guess *they couldn't keep me waiting for six hours this time,* she thought wearily. *Or maybe I just slept through it.*

This time, the doctors were able to give her a real diagnosis: a broken rib and a concussion. But she also had a temperature of 103 degrees Fahrenheit. The baby was in distress and showed signs of fetal tachycardia. The doctors did not understand the etiology of these conditions, and they sent Ramona to an infectious disease specialist.

"You need a CT scan." He spoke to her plainly.

"Isn't that bad for the baby? Why can't I get an MRI?" Ramona was confused; she had always been told that radiation was bad for fetuses.

"It's the only option right now. Too many COVID cases. The hospital is at capacity, and many procedures are being delayed. You need to be tested as soon as possible."

"Will it be with contrast?"

"Yes."

"Then there is no way that I am doing it."

"Ramona. I am very sorry, but this is the only choice. We will do everything we can to make sure your baby is safe. Things could get worse if we don't figure out what the issue is."

Seeing no other option, Ramona went ahead with the CT scan with contrast. COVID made her have to make horrible and unacceptable decisions, decisions she would have never made in any other situation. Thankfully, the scan presented no complications, and she was followed on a cardiac monitor for the next six weeks as the diagnosis had still not been found.

As if things were not already bad enough, her car was then stolen. Her husband, James, called her one morning while she was still half asleep. He almost screamed into the phone, telling her that her car had been taken. Given the riots that had taken over the nation and the disruptions being caused despite the pandemic, this news did not surprise her. By this point, she was so accustomed to things going wrong that she continued going about her day without a hitch.

After that, the Uber took her to the hospital and back. She supported the BLM cause, but she wished they could have been more peaceful with their displays of resistance. Ramona started honing a new skill: sprinting to and from rented cars on dangerous streets. She also started becoming a master Google Maps user, finding routes through small alleys and backroads to reach her destination. She did all of these things so she could avoid the protests.

The moments when Ramona finally got a few wins were during labor. James was permitted into the room, and she was allowed to take off her mask while she pushed. These were small wins, true, but they made a big difference. She almost felt lucky, knowing that many mothers were not allowed the luxury of having a comforting spouse present as they delivered. Plus, now she had her beautiful baby girl, and she was worth every second of trouble.

But that was where her sense of peace ended. Postpartum was not the dream she had imagined. With no way to meet family and friends, Ramona found herself cooped up in her house with her husband and the baby. Postpartum doctors' appointments had to be taken over Zoom. The doctor could not figure out why her daughter was having severe stomach pain, and ultimately it turned out that she was lactose intolerant. This was something Ramona would have been taught to look out for if she had been able to access lactation consultations, and as a first-time mother, she felt extremely guilty that her baby had to suffer for so long because of her lack of knowledge and the pandemic.

Nothing was clear about the virus when her baby was born; in August 2020, there was still little information about how COVID-19 affected infants. Though she knew countless other new mothers were navigating the same storm, Ramona couldn't shake the helplessness of mothering in the dark, without a map, without a guide, and with everything she loved most at stake.

3
Kiara

The hospital room was quiet except for the soft hum of machines and Kiara's steady breathing. She gripped the side of the bed, her body slick with sweat and trembling from exertion. Her husband, Marcus, stood beside her, masked like everyone else, holding her hand and whispering, "You've got this, baby. You're doing amazing."

Kiara had been working from home for the last trimester of her pregnancy, which was, of course, a relief, but she wished the reason why she was allowed to do so had been different. Her only trips outside the safety of her home had been to the doctor's office. Today was one such rare excursion outside.

It was April 7, 2020, and their son was about to be born right in the heart of a pandemic.

She hadn't imagined it like this. No visitors. No cheerful waiting room filled with family. No mother at her bedside, brushing her sweat-soaked hair and telling her stories from her own deliveries. Her mother, whom she was so close to, hadn't even been allowed into the hospital.

It had taken her four hours to be given a room, as none were available in the hospital. Waiting had been nerve-wracking, surrounded by coughing patients and masked medical professionals. Now, it wasn't much better. Every person who entered the room was in what might as well have been a hazmat suit.

While these protocols and precautions did make her feel safe, Kiara couldn't help but wish that she could see an unobstructed smiling face. They had induced her so that the labor process could go by quickly, seeing as there were bigger fish to fry, sicker people who needed a bed. The first thing the doctors had done was make her take a COVID-19 test, saying, "If you're found to be positive, we will have to separate you from your child as soon as he is born for his safety." Those words had made her stomach drop. Marcus, her husband, had looked at her with a face that was only just managing to hide its sheer panic. He himself had also been tested. The thought that their baby may have to be separated from them as soon as he was born terrified them. That was a thought they could not bear, knowing it was crucial for an infant to feel their parents as much as possible for comfort. Because of the virus, Marcus had already let go of his hope to hold his newborn skin-to-skin, a moment he'd dreamed of. He was not prepared to give up being with his child for what could possibly be weeks. Thankfully, they were spared that trauma.

They had wheeled Kiara into her room, weeping, and so she remained until she laid eyes on her baby.

That day, a beautiful baby boy was born. He had soft tufts of brown hair, a pink, round face, tiny, delicate hands, and wide and curious eyes.

His parents decided to name him Kane.

Soon after the delivery and being moved to her hospital room, Kiara started calling the nurses, asking for a lactation consultation. As a new mother, she was anxious to make sure that she did everything correctly so that her baby remained healthy. While the nurses and other staff were sympathetic and helpful, giving her tips and suggestions, they said that a doctor was not available to speak to her. Instead, they encouraged her to leave the hospital as quickly as possible, given it was the height of the pandemic and the hospital was probably the least safe place for them to be with a newborn. Of course, this information had come to them through a fully masked individual standing at a distance.

"This doesn't feel real," she whispered to Marcus as she held their newborn to her chest. Marcus was already in the process of packing up their belongings, just hours after his wife gave birth. Still, the sooner they left, the better. Home life and one another would provide the comfort they needed. This they knew, for the two had forged a bond from the flames of chaos that the virus had brought them.

After having her baby, Kiara was able to stay home and continue to work from home. Marcus was home, too. The first two months of pumping had been hell for Kiara, as she never got the lactation consultation that she hoped for. Instead, all she had received was a few quick meetings over blurry, staticky Zoom calls, which did little to help her. Kiara found herself crying in frustration during pumping sessions. "This isn't how it's supposed to be," she murmured to herself at 3 a.m., watching the milk drip into a bottle as her son dozed nearby. Getting help from another mother was out of the question since they were not allowed to meet anymore. Kiara's own mother would have been her first choice, and it was only after numerous video calls, breakdowns, and setbacks that she was able to feed her son correctly while remaining out of pain and healthy.

On one of her walks, she had gone by the park, wishing she could take Kane there to enjoy the fresh air, mingle with other kids, and get some much-needed activity on the swings and slides. Kiara knew that if she did, she would be anxious every step of the way. In her mind, the very air was poisoned, and there was nothing her precious boy could touch. If she took him there, the swings and slides would have to be disinfected. She would have to bring cleaning rags and spray bottles, and a keen eye to make sure he'd stay safe. Plus, he wouldn't be able to interact with any of the kids. The park seemed almost deserted in any case, and there was not a single child in sight. She pocketed the hope of taking her son to the park, knowing that one day, it would all be over and he could have the life she had dreamed of for him.

And so, their life, which they could no longer recognize, moved forward. For a year and a half after their son was born, they lived in a cocoon with their son, learning the ropes of parenthood together. Her parents couldn't visit, and that absence weighed heavily on her. She believed it would have been better for everyone—her, Marcus, her son, and the grandparents—if they had been able to participate in those early days. Her child would have known them better, and their parents would have been able to spoil him (as well as her and Marcus by babysitting every once in a while).

They tried to make the most of it, FaceTiming her mom, celebrating milestones with homemade banners, taking walks around the block with masks on. But Kiara always felt the absence of something, of people, of help, of the joyful chaos she had dreamed would accompany her baby's first months.

One day, her mother had come to see her newborn grandson—not in the usual way, not with hugs and kisses and cooing. No. She brought a ladder.

The thud was what first alerted Kiara that something was amiss. It came from the windowsill and sent a shockwave through her body.

Kiara panicked. Burglars! she thought. She rushed to the bathroom to get Marcus. But then a head of curly white hair appeared just behind the glass, followed by a stocky hand with red-painted nails.

"Wait, Mom?" Kiara questioned, more to herself than anyone else.

Then her mother's grinning face was in the window, so lit up with joy, she eclipsed the light of the moon.

"MOM!" Kiara yelled out.

Her mother's eyes brimmed with tears as she looked down at her grandson. Then all of the answers clicked and Kiara knew that her mother had been driven by the insane desire to see her grandchild and had resorted to climbing a ladder in the dead of night to see him through a window.

Kiara moved to her baby just as Marcus exited the bathroom. "What in the—" He noticed his mother-in-law and froze, eyeing Kiara before shifting his focus back to the old lady in the window.

Kiara picked up Kane and brought him closer to the window to give her mother a better look. At this point, Marcus was laughing uncontrollably, even as tears streamed down his face.

That moment broke something open in Kiara. Her mother wanted to be a grandmother more than anything. Even a pandemic couldn't keep her away. She had found a way. A way for Kane to be safe and a way for her to be able to be a part of his infancy. Kiara knew this was a moment she would never forget and one that would be spoken about in all family gatherings for years to come. Here was her biggest supporter and the person who loved her the most, risking her own safety to be there for her grandson, if only just to see his face. It reminded her how much family mattered. How much connection mattered.

Later, when her mother was back in her own home, Kiara called her, not making a fuss, not saying it was dangerous, not saying she had scared her. Instead, she simply cried, thanked her mother, and told her she loved her and she was the best grandma in the world.

"Nothing on God's green earth can keep me from loving him," her mother had said. Then she went into her usual lecture about Kiara needing to have more kids and a big family, especially one with kids close in age. Kiara herself had always wanted this, but now, given the stress of the pandemic, she was not so sure. Her mother encouraged her gently. "You're strong enough," she told her over the phone. "You've always been strong. You can do this again. You should."

And Kiara believed her.

Though she knew that there was much that she could not do to have her family close, Kiara knew she wanted her own house to be filled with children.

That moment changed something for Kiara. The confidence she felt, the fact that she knew that the support she had from her mother and husband was never going to falter. It all made her have a much better outlook. Kiara was determined to look on the bright side and enjoy her baby's infancy, no matter how different the experience was from what she had imagined it to be.

She knew that there was much to be thankful for. They had more time. They cooked meals together, watched their son grow into his giggles and babbles, shared sleepless nights and early-morning grins. The world had slowed down, and in that stillness, Kiara found herself thinking, deciding.

"I want him to have a sibling close in age," she said to Marcus one evening as they sat on the couch, their son sleeping in his bassinet. "Not just because I want more kids, but because I want him to have someone. You know, like a partner in crime. We have always talked about having a big family, just like mine was growing up. I loved my sisters so much because we were only a year or two apart in age. There is nothing in the world that can compare to that kind of sibling relationship."

Marcus looked at her over the rim of his mug. "During a pandemic?"

She laughed softly. "I know it's crazy. But yes. I think I'm ready. Plus, no commute, and I am at home. I have all the time in the world to take care of myself and them. This pandemic isn't letting up. Why should we put our life on pause?"

Marcus knew that he was able to be more present with his wife and child. COVID had changed work schedules and forced the world to slow down. And because of that, he got to be there, really be there, for the feeding schedules, the late-night diaper changes, the cries that woke them up at night. Doing all of that again didn't seem that bad. In fact, it was ideal.

"Okay. I am in."

"Yes!" Kiara was ecstatic. "You have no idea how happy Mom is going to be. She's been hinting—wait, hinting isn't the right word. She's been basically demanding I give her another grandbaby. And after that stunt she pulled with the ladder, I think he deserves it."

"Well, if your mom is twisting your hands, who am I to say no?" Marcus chuckled.

"Yes, let's do it. Let's try. Let's really try. I know we will be up for it, and our relationship is stronger now than ever before."

"I agree. It is time."

A few months later, Kiara lay on the examination table, her heart thudding. The ultrasound technician moved the probe slowly, pausing more than once.

"This is taking longer than usual," she thought, frowning slightly. She was alone. Marcus was not allowed to be there for any antenatal visits since it was deemed unnecessary, and it was safer to have as few people present in the doctor's office. This was new for Kiara and not something she had expected. Marcus had been able to be present for almost every single antenatal visit for Kane, but now, with COVID, he hadn't even been allowed to come for one.

Her phone buzzed.

Marcus: "What's taking so long? Is it twins or something?"

Kiara stared at the screen, then looked at the technician, who was now quietly typing something into the monitor. The room felt colder suddenly.

"Well," the technician said finally, glancing at her with a raised brow, "it looks like you're having twins."

She blinked. "What?"

The technician turned the screen so she could see two little flickering heartbeats. Two.

Kiara's hands went cold. Her breath caught.

"Oh my God," she whispered. She grabbed her phone and texted Marcus back.

Kiara: "You better sit down."

She waited a minute, then texted again.

Kiara: "Yes. Twins."

His response came instantly.

Marcus: "YOU'RE JOKING."

Kiara: "Not joking."

For a moment, everything spun. Then, unexpectedly, she laughed.

"I had a dream," she told the technician. "A few nights ago. That I was pregnant with twins. We joked about it because…we don't have twins in either family."

The doctor laughed along with her and said, "Well, this one isn't a dream."

This was real. Two babies. Double the bottles. Double the diapers. Double the love.

Her phone started ringing, indicating that Marcus was calling. She wished he could have been there to share this new information with her, this milestone, this joy. She wanted to share it with him.

She answered her husband's video call, and the first thing she said was, "We need to talk about getting a new house and car."

The first part of Kiara's second pregnancy passed in a haze of logistics and nausea. Thankfully, she worked from home again—this time from the beginning. She was violently sick in the mornings and couldn't imagine commuting over an hour each way to work.

They started looking for a bigger car. A bigger house. She saved every ultrasound photo for Marcus, who still couldn't come to appointments. Instead, he joined on FaceTime when he could, and she'd bring home printed images of their two little miracles.

Her mom, thrilled at the news, was both excited and anxious. "I always knew you'd give me more grandbabies," she said through the screen one afternoon.

Her mother wanted to be involved so badly that it ached. She offered help from afar—researching twin strollers, sending her care packages, praying over her every phone call. Kiara knew that she had all the support she needed.

She and Marcus had decided that they would not dwell on COVID or the negative. They had learned how to parent together, and they already had one beautiful baby who brought them such joy. Now, they knew that no matter what happened, they would come out on top.

All seemed well. Then came the complications.

Iron deficiency. Her levels dropped dangerously low, and she was scheduled for an iron infusion. Alone. Hospitals still had visitor restrictions, so Marcus couldn't go with her.

She was terrified.

As the IV needle pierced her skin, she tried to calm herself. But halfway through the infusion, something went wrong. She felt hot, flushed, breathless—an allergic reaction. Nurses rushed to help. She couldn't speak, only blink.

When it was over, she lay there shaking. "I have to do this all by myself," she thought. "But I will. For them."

She never forgot how vulnerable she felt that day. And how strong she became because of it.

Her mom checked in constantly, worried about Kiara. Her daughter was growing a whole new world, and she was so proud. Kiara, though shaken and deeply petrified by her complication, was as determined as ever. She pushed through. She knew that she could.

The day of her delivery, August 26, 2021, was both terrifying and awe-inspiring.

But when she held her twins, both screaming and squirming in her arms, all of the negative thoughts faded.

"I did this," she said softly. "By myself. With support. With love. With faith."

Kiara was exhausted. But she was exactly where she was meant to be. She had gotten what her heart most desired, and she had grown stronger because of it.

Three children, all close in age. Her home is full of sound, life, and connection.

Everything was just as it was meant to be.

4
Blaire

Blaire sat in her hospital bed, doing breathing exercises. She inhaled for 4 seconds through her nose, held for 7 seconds, and then exhaled through her mouth for 8 seconds, just as her therapist had instructed her to do. She was not doing this to aid with the pushing process; she was attempting to calm her raging thoughts. They threatened to drown her in a sea of instability, but that was not how she wanted her birth to go; that was not the state she wanted to be in when she brought her daughter into the world.

Everything was fine just a few weeks ago, she thought. *My baby shower was perfect. That's what I wanted to feel throughout my pregnancy.*

Blaire touched the massager resting on her neck. It was one of the many gifts she had received at her shower. This gift had come from her mother, the only person who looked out for *her* baby, not just *the* baby. Blaire missed her mother dearly now, and she had always planned for her to be there while her grandchild was being born.

That dream was shattered by the pandemic, of course.

So now, she labored alone.

The world had closed down. Social distancing and remote work were the new normal. Leading up to her delivery, Blaire had had no idea what it would look like. Information changed every day, and so did her hopes.

Induction had never been part of the plan, and yet here she was. The hospital had suggested this as the best course of action. They said that her being there for longer than absolutely necessary was dangerous. They told her that she could not have her husband there either. It had to be in and out. As if a baby could pop out and they both be ready to face the unrecognizable world once again.

To be fair, it was the peak of the pandemic, and Blaire had also been diagnosed with gestational diabetes, which made induction even more important. Yet, she could not help but wish things could have been different.

She sat in her room alone, as they had no one to spare to watch over her as she waited for the induction medication to work. Blaire felt as if the walls were closing in on her. Before all of this, before COVID, she had never experienced anxiety issues. Now, she was having a panic attack almost every day. Her anxiety reached crippling levels after she found out about her father's cancer.

Now she thought of him. She hoped he would have the chance to be a grandfather and to enjoy all the beautiful moments that came with it. She had not even been able to visit him following his diagnosis, which was a fact she felt conflicted about. Did it mean she was a bad daughter, or did it mean that she was being a good mother by protecting her unborn child from the virus? The effects the virus could have on a baby were not yet apparent or studied. There was no telling what it would be like if she travelled the virus-ridden nation while pregnant and then later, while with an infant in tow.

She had put her baby in enough danger already. A month prior, Blaire had been found to be COVID positive.

Blaire felt a contraction and whipped her head around to glance at the call button. She had a similar one in her old hospital when she was COVID-positive. That one, they had said, should be pressed when she felt as if she could not breathe. Now, she wondered if it was the right time to press it. The contraction subsided, and she decided against pulling doctors away from other, perhaps more urgent, patients.

She thought of her last hospitalization. Of the feelings of dread she had, of how she was constantly worried for the life of her daughter. Her husband had been calm and collected through the whole ordeal. She never once doubted that everything would turn out okay in the end. That was something she tremulously envied him for. What was difficult for him was that he was a sociable person and came from a large family, so he craved human interaction. He felt upset about not being able to see his friends and family, rather than specifically due to being pregnant during the pandemic. That, he had no worries about, leaving Blaire to worry on her own.

Another contraction. Harder and longer this time.

Blaire pushed the call button.

Nolan, Blair's husband, was allowed to be in the hospital room after the delivery. He sat, rocking the baby in his arms and beaming for hours as Blaire slept and recovered.

Blaire had wanted to rush out of the hospital as soon as possible. As soon as the baby's tests were done and she was stabilized, she was determined to make her way back home, away from all the sick people surrounding her child.

When she woke up, a nurse was in the room. "Okay, we are all set, Blaire," she said. "We just need to check if you have the right equipment."

Blaire and Nolan nodded.

"Car seat?" The nurse read from her clipboard.

"Check," Nolan said.

"It's cover?"

"No, we don't have that." Nolan looked shocked.

Blaire sat up. "We don't? What do you mean we don't?"

"Okay. Where is the seat? I can check if it is up to standard here." The nurse set down her clipboard.

"Was I supposed to bring it in? It's in the car." Nolan was standing now.

"As per the hospital protocol, a baby cannot be moved without being in their car seat," the nurse stated.

"Nolan! What!" Blaire was furious. "I told you this!"

"I'll get it. Them… I'll go get the seat and the cover."

"Uhh…" The nurse raised her finger. "I'm not entirely sure if the hospital will let him back in after he leaves."

Blaire gave the nurse a look that could make a lion drop dead. She turned to her husband and said one simple word, "Go." And he left.

Three calls, two yelling matches, and a threat to sue later, Management allowed Blair's husband back into her room with the car seat and cover.

Blaire was ecstatic to be able to leave. But after just a few days, she found herself back in the hospital.

A blur of events later, she watched as nurses carried her baby to the NICU.

In the NICU, there was no specific protocol regarding who could visit their baby. Everyone they asked gave them a different answer. Questions arose about whether only one parent could visit at a time, how many visits per day were permitted, and whether both parents could visit together. Initially, they stated that both parents were allowed to enter, but later, only the mother was permitted to do so. Blaire had to be transported to the NICU in a wheelchair because of her own health complications after the birth, and she was not allowed into the hallway.

She frequently called for a nurse to take her to the NICU because she needed to breastfeed. Unfortunately, by the time she managed to get in, her baby had already been given formula. This was never something she wanted. Formula had always been out of the question. She tried to tell the nurses and doctors about her wishes, but still, this situation occurred multiple times, and her newborn began to prefer the ease of bottle feeding, making breastfeeding even more challenging for both of them.

Blaire was devastated. She wondered if her baby had COVID and what that might look like. No one had even taken the time to tell her what was going on.

After the baby was healthy again and Blaire was discharged. She did her best to block out those days from her memory.

Blaire's masked face stared down at her writhing infant. The child, who was lying comfortably in her stroller, had a quizzical look on her little face. Her brows were scrunched, and her mouth was slightly open, pouting.

'She doesn't know it's me,' Blaire thought. '*She's probably thinking, 'Where's Mama? She's not here for me.''*

Blaire was in their yard, taking her baby out for a stroll and some fresh air and sunshine. It was 2 PM. Her lunch break. Blaire had been working from home ever since the lockdown started, a month before Willow was born.

A neighbor walked by, also in a mask, and Blaire waved at her before walking back inside her home.

Inside, her husband Nolan sat in his plush office chair, typing away. “I have a meeting in 10. Think you can keep Willow quiet during it?”

“Yes, I already know the drill,” Blaire replied. She set Willow down on the couch beside Nolan and went to wash her hands in the powder room. “I saw Jenn by the way. She was on a walk or something.”

“I should say hi to her, too,” Nolan called back. “I miss having guests in our home. Used to be lively. Now Willow is our only company.” He turned and rubbed the baby’s tummy. “Aren’t you, little one?”

Willow giggled.

Blaire walked back in and picked Willow up. “I’m no hermit, but I have to say… It's been nice having the house to myself. I don’t have to worry about surprise visitors while I'm running on two hours of sleep because of this one.” She pointed an accusatory finger at Willow and then poked her on the cheek.

“No, no, I know, you're a hermit. You are living for this lockdown.”

Blaire chuckled. “I'm no hermit, but it's nice to have some peace. Now I have all the time in the world to spend with my baby girl. The biggest plus is not having to do piles upon piles of dishes. No hosting. No gathering. It's great.”

“You sure about that hermit thing?” Nolan raised an eyebrow as he put his headset on.

Blaire rolled her eyes and took Willow to her room. She breastfed the baby, and she fell asleep within a few minutes.

“Sure. Now you sleep,” Blaire muttered while smiling.

After setting the baby down in her bassinet, she called her father.

“Hey, Dad,” she said as the line clicked. “How are you?”

“The cancer is still there, so...” Her father laughed.

“Dad,” Blaire said as she rubbed her forehead, “I told you not to joke about these things.”

"Hey, you've got to have a positive attitude, right? There are studies that say being happy leads to a better prognosis."

"You aren't wrong."

"Don't worry about it, kiddo. How's the baby?"

"She's good. She's been gaining weight well, and she's sleeping soundly right now."

"That's great to hear. I want to see that girl looking like a big ol' bear when I see her."

When I see her, the words stuck with Blaire hard. Her father was dying, and yet, he could not see his own grandchild because of the restrictions.

"We will come to see you, Dad. As soon as we can."

"I know you will. Don't worry, I will hang on until then."

Blaire was crying now, but she was completely silent. She did not let her voice shake. "How about I video call you once she wakes up, huh. When will Mom be free?"

"Oh, in about two hours. She's been hard at work."

"Okay, I will talk to you then. Bye now."

"T.T.Y.L."

"Dad!"

"Oh, cheer up. Bye."

Blaire sat on her bed beside the baby, looking down at her. She couldn't stop her tears from falling. This task, this decision, felt like a burden she could not bear. How could she choose between the happiness of her father and the health of her baby?

"Babe! My meeting's done!" Nolan's voice rang out from the study.

Blaire wiped her tears, kissed her baby's forehead, and walked out of the room.

When Willow was three months old, they decided it was time to meet the family.

A new vaccine was introduced, and although it was highly effective for most, there was no information available on its impact on pregnancies. Her family was already vaccinated, and they had continued to quarantine up until the gathering day.

And so, at three months old, Willow finally experienced the feeling of being held in her grandparents' arms.

No more FaceTime. No more short calls. No more isolation. They were finally together.

From then on, when Blaire's parents wanted to see the baby, they would sit outside on porch chairs, and though they were not able to hold her, they wouldn't have it any other way.

Sitting on her porch, showing off Willow, Blaire turned to her husband.

"I want another baby," she stated.

"You sure? The pandemic hasn't ended yet." Nolan's tone was playful but had a hint of seriousness.

"Yes, I know, but it's been so fulfilling being able to be with her so much."

"That is true." Nolan held baby Willow on his knee, bouncing her.

"What other time can you think of when we would be allowed to work from home for so long? My job doesn't even give me maternity leave."

"Yeah. That much is true."

"If it lasts for a long time, as experts predict, then we might get enough time with our second baby too."

"I must say that sounds very enticing."

"You know I've always wanted our kids to be close in age. So that they can play together and be close when they grow up." Blaire imagined the scene: two toddlers in matching clothes, running around in a park, getting mud all over their pretty shoes.

"Then let's do it. I feel confident about this."

Blaire held out her hand, and Nolan took it.

"Our commute to work is usually an hour and a half. That's a whole ten hours a day that we get to spend with our kids," said Blaire.

"That is true. This pandemic baby thing is a blessing in the end. If anything happens to the baby while we are at work, it would be so long before we would be able to get to her. This work-from-home situation is much better."

"This time has been so precious to me." Blaire put her hand under her baby's chin and lifted up her face. "I want to experience this again. This is what I choose."

And so, with joy in their hearts and with a will that would not falter, Blaire and Nolan made their decision to have a second child.

Blaire gave birth to her second baby in September 2021, and although she contracted COVID while pregnant, which was something she had never in her wildest dreams imagined would happen, she felt blessed.

Blessed that this pregnancy was easier. Blessed that the care providers had made her feel safe. Blessed that her baby was completely healthy. Blessed that her parents could see her children whenever they desired. Blessed that she was able to spend every second of her kids' infancies with them. Blessed that her father was still with them and able to be a grandpa.

Blaire considered her blessings to be overwhelming, and she knew that if asked if she would do it all over again, her answer would be yes.

5
Serena

In March 2023, when COVID was considered over, Serena was in the park, sharing stories with her group, which consisted of women who had experienced pregnancy during the pandemic. This was a group built on support, built on listening and empathizing, built on shared experience. The women shared their stories, shared cakes and sandwiches, laughed and cried, and sang. They were a community now. They were friends.

Between the story of one woman who planned her induction just in time to have her husband by her side before a new policy shut partners out, and another whose world was turned upside down by both the pandemic and the surprise of twins, Serena shared her own tale.

In late February 2020, Serena contracted COVID. She was pregnant then, and although she had no symptoms, the positive test result was enough to change everything. She decided to start working from home. Going into the office no longer felt safe, not with a baby on the way.

Her first pregnancy had occurred at the start of the pandemic, before the world fully grasped what was to come. At that time, COVID hadn't really affected her pregnancy. But the second time around was different. This time, she and her partner made a conscious decision to expand their family, fully aware of the risks. They had educated themselves, followed every known precaution, and understood that the virus might always be part of their lives. But they also didn't want to wait. A vaccine was being developed. They didn't want their lives on hold indefinitely when the world was starting to move on.

Still, nothing could have prepared them for what it meant to bring a baby into a world gripped by uncertainty. The birth of their first child was not the joyous gathering of friends and family they had imagined. Instead, they were isolated. Groceries were delivered and disinfected. Diapers were counted with care, knowing that stores might run out. Serena's postpartum checkup was held online. It was supposed to be a huge milestone on her journey, but it ended up being an event that she only had a screen recording and a screenshot to show for.

They took care of the baby on their own, without the help they had once assumed would be there. Her mother 'visited' from a distance, standing outside their home with a mask on, peering toward her grandson in the bassinet through the window. No holding. No rocking. Her in-laws dropped off hot meals on the doorstep and waved from the sidewalk. No one entered. For the first three months of their son's life, no one saw him except his parents.

Even the baby's two-day checkup was not as she wished. The pediatrician's office tried to move the visit online. Serena refused. She wanted the doctor to examine her son in person, to look him over with trained eyes. She was a new mother. She didn't know what to look for, and she wasn't going to guess when it came to her child's health. She argued her way into the office, needing that reassurance. She would have made it happen, even if she had to fight to get inside, kicking and screaming.

Her anxiety during those early months was constant. It wasn't postpartum depression—she knew the difference—but it was something she couldn't shake. The world outside seemed to be falling apart. Crime rates were rising. The murder of George Floyd had shaken her to the core. She felt the pressure of raising a child in a society that suddenly felt unstable and unsafe. And yet, she found comfort in the things she could control. She had much to be thankful for. Her baby was healthy, well-fed, and loved.

She and her partner talked often about whether they should stop at one child. Maybe that was the safest choice. But they both longed for a sibling for their son, and they knew they wanted their children to be close in age. They also knew they weren't getting any younger. They weighed the risks and chose to move forward with a second pregnancy.

This time, no one knew she was pregnant, not until she was nearly seven months along. She hadn't shared the news with her employer or her coworkers. So much of life had shifted indoors, into private space, that the pregnancy felt quieter, more internal. Even so, the anxiety remained. But by then, their oldest child had been attending daycare for a few months with no major outbreaks, and that gave them some peace of mind.

They were still working from home, both of them, and that became a blessing they hadn't expected. They were together around the clock, parenting, supporting, and figuring things out. It wasn't always easy, but it brought them closer. They developed a rhythm. They leaned on each other more than ever before. Their bond deepened, and even through the stress, there was an increasing strength growing between them. They learned to appreciate the small things, to identify the things that they would not have had if her baby had been born a few years prior.

Breastfeeding was one area where the pandemic made things easier. Being home meant Serena could nurse longer than she ever imagined. She didn't have to pump frantically and build a freezer stash. That had always made her feel like a momma bear preparing for hibernation. There was no rush, no commute, no pressure to separate from her baby. If she had to leave a meeting or miss a call, no one gave her grief. Her coworkers and managers were supportive, understanding the weight of parenting during such an uncertain time.

But despite the positives, daycare brought new worries. They had to sign a clause agreeing to pay, even if the daycare closed due to an outbreak. Fees went up to cover cleaning and safety protocols. And the closures happened often, especially around the holidays, when COVID cases surged again. They never knew from week to week what to expect, and that unpredictability wore on them.

Still, through it all, they found reasons to be grateful. They watched their children grow up in front of them. They were there for every milestone, every smile, every late-night feeding, and every early-morning laugh. They built a cocoon around their little family, not perfect, not without cracks, but strong. Stronger than they ever imagined it could be.

Serena was a homebody by nature, and in some ways, that gave her a small advantage. She enjoyed being pregnant with her second child while staying at home for the most part. The quiet suited her. There were fewer obligations and fewer places to be, which gave her space to bond with the life growing inside her. Still, the public could be cruel. She remembers standing in line at the supermarket, heavily pregnant, when a woman behind her suddenly scolded her for being vaccinated. The woman claimed Serena had violated her unborn child's freedom of choice. The words hit her hard. No tests had been conducted on pregnant women, and no one knew if the vaccine had any serious side effects on babies.

"I felt that I had done the right thing for my pregnancy," she recalled. "But in that moment, I started to wonder—was I a bad mom? Had I already taken away my baby's autonomy?"

But after she thought about it, they also made her lament the stupidity of some of the American people. The vaccine had kept her safe, and a safe mother meant a safe baby.

Still, the pandemic blurred the line between personal decision and public debate. Even within her own extended family, COVID became a hot, highly debated topic. Vaccines? Masks? Outside or inside? Hug or don't hug? Allow someone to hold the baby, or not at all? Each and every conversation about COVID held the potential to spark drama. The very fabric of social interaction had changed, and with it, so had people's opinions.

Postpartum care, too, took on a unique shape during the COVID-19 pandemic. When she developed mastitis, a painful condition she had never even heard of before, she had to read the symptoms on Google, diagnose herself, and then wait for a provider to confirm her findings over video before prescribing treatment.

"I had never been pregnant before," she said. "And yet I was expected to just know that this was enough. That I was getting adequate care."

Her second pregnancy brought slightly different challenges. Her partner wasn't allowed to attend most of her early appointments. It fell on her to bear the emotional and informational weight, going to the doctor's office alone, asking their shared questions, taking mental notes, and then relaying everything back to him afterward. Even something as simple as touring the hospital unit, seeing the place where their child would be born, wasn't allowed. They had to imagine it all.

To give each other some sense of control, they decided to find out the baby's sex. This was something they had not opted for with their first. It was something concrete that helped her husband feel more involved in a process he was otherwise shut out from. They picked names together, built little stories about their future family life, and slowly became closer to this child they hadn't yet met. He packed the hospital bags carefully, making sure they would not face any last-minute surprises. It was his way of contributing, of being ready to act when the time came.

With that second pregnancy, something beautiful had formed in the silence. She and her husband figured things out. Together. They learned how to function, how to compromise, and how to share the work of parenting in real-time. The experience was far from ideal, but it brought them closer.

"Had the world been normal," she said, looking up at the strong women surrounding her. "My husband would have gone back to work within days, leaving me to manage the newborn alone. Instead, he was there for every feeding, every diaper change, every tear.

"Our relationship grew stronger. This was something we survived together." She looked down at the grass, smiling. "And not just survived, but grew through. It was never a loss. It was a gift. Now we are unshakable. We have built our foundation. It has been cemented. We know now that we can make it through anything."

6
Sofia

It was March 2020 when the news channels blasted with the news of the lockdown. Sofia's third trimester of her first pregnancy had just begun, and she was quite elated, yet concerned about it. The entire world was sealed off under lockdown following a massive and widespread outbreak of the coronavirus. The news was all about the new vaccines, variants of the coronavirus, instructions to follow the guidance issued by the government, and the daily death tolls around the world. All of this made Sofia's head spin, and it became harder for her to remain calm.

As her pregnancy was a hard-earned result of IVF, she was even more concerned. Even though they had wanted a baby and planned this pregnancy, she had not considered, even in her wildest thoughts, that she would have to deliver during a pandemic.

Her hands rubbing her protruding belly, she entered her bedroom after hearing a few horrific news reports on the TV. She picked up her phone with her mind brimming with worrying possibilities.

"Hello," she said when the beep ended, and her husband picked up the call.

"Hi, babe. How's the mood?" he answered with a chirpy, nonchalant tune.

"Did you see the news? The world has been turned upside down. We are all under a lockdown now. I don't know what we will do. Our baby is going to be delivered soon. What is going to happen? I am so worried." She blurted all that was running through her mind in one single minute while her husband listened on the other side with his eyes wide and mouth gaping. He couldn't process a single word.

"Honey, I need you to calm down. I will watch the news and call you back. Okay?" His tone transformed from chirpy to consoling in a second.

"Okay." Sofia agreed, even though the tears stuck in her throat as if she were about to cry.

She put the phone down and started pacing around the apartment. From the bedroom to the kitchen to the balcony to the living room and back to the bedroom, she must have achieved her daily step count. Then she sat down and thought about her circumstances. She belonged to the healthcare industry; she was a nurse; she needed to be in the hospital, but, above all, she needed to keep her baby safe.

The next day, she went to the hospital with her mind adamant. She was going to talk to Dr. Helman and request him to assign her to a floor without COVID patients.

"Sofia, there are thousands of patients coming in daily with cases like yours. Being in this field, you should be there for the people first. We can't shift you to that floor, as we are in need of more staff on the other floors, as there is an influx of COVID-19 patients."

Hearing her employer's response, she prioritized the safety of her child and quit her job on the spot. She came back home and spent the evening with her husband. They both lay on the big couch in their living room while the news reporter on the TV went on about that day's death toll caused by COVID-19. All the countries had shut down the flights, businesses were shutting down because of employees going remote, people were quitting jobs, families were losing their loved ones, hospitals were not big enough to admit the humongous number of patients, and so, different Airbnbs, hotels, and other centers were being turned into quarantine rooms to isolate the patients. The death toll in America only for that day was over a thousand.

"There is so much happening in the world right now. I don't even know how to process it all," she commented.

"You are right, vaccines are still being researched. I heard all the big countries are working on producing effective vaccines," Jonah replied.

"Leave it. You know what happened today at work?" she interrupted him, frustration audible in her voice.

Her head was on his lap, and he patted her head gently, listening to her attentively as she went on about her day and let him in on all the details of the conversation with Dr. Helman. He listened as she blabbered.

"So, I just quit. I couldn't jeopardize our baby's health, you know." Sofia moved her hands a lot while saying, and that's how he knew that she was more upset from inside than she let on.

As the days passed, with her husband on the job, Sofia started feeling the loneliness looming in on her. The pregnancy was becoming increasingly hectic as the delivery drew near. She visited her gynecologist wearing a mask, when it was already hard for her to maintain her pulse.

Doctor's appointments were tense and distant, conducted behind masks and plexiglass. On the first visit of her 8th month, she swiveled her way through the crowd of patients. *How many of them have COVID? What if I contract the virus? What if my baby is affected by this? What if I lose my baby?*

These and other million scary thoughts ran through her mind as she made her way to her gynecologist's room. She ran through a temperature test at every visit, and asked multiple questions to her doctor to make sure that she and the baby stayed safe.

"How's the baby? Is it fine? Is it moving? Do I need to be vaccinated again?" These were the questions repeatedly asked on every check-up visit. Dr. Bell was an immensely understanding and supportive gynecologist, and she routinely answered all these questions. She understood that this pandemic was a new and challenging experience, especially for first-time mothers. She made sure that Sofia felt calm and secure when she left her room.

After coming back home, she was pretty satisfied, but even she knew that she would have the same burning questions on her next gynecological visit.

With the passing days, her pregnancy took a toll on her physical and mental well-being. At eight months pregnant during the height of the COVID-19 lockdown, she faced each day as a test of endurance, physically, emotionally, and mentally. Her body was heavy and aching in almost every part; her feet were swollen, and her back protested even the simplest chores, such as bending to pick something up or standing too long at the sink. It had been days and she did not have a drop of sleep, it was disrupted not only by discomfort but by the constant hum of worry in her mind. The threat of the virus added a sharp layer of fear. She couldn't go outside to the grocery store or to run daily errands without worry and fear gripping her. Every delivery package had to be sanitized with care before being carried inside.

She had done her shopping for the arriving baby and had bought sufficient clothes and other essentials. However, with the shopping malls closed, she worried that she would run out of her baby's necessities. Additionally, her physical infirmity required assistance. She missed the comfort of her mother's presence, the simple reassurance of someone nearby to help without the looming anxiety of exposure, and the joy of pregnancy milestones had been stripped down—no baby showers, no friendly visits, just silence and caution.

As a part of her daily routine, she called her mother on Zoom. She laughed and cooed while looking at her daughter's belly bulging up as the baby kicked from inside. Whenever the baby kicked, she giggled, and a surge of warmth would run through her. It was moments like these that she yearned for someone to share with her. She missed her sisters, her mother, and her friends. She wanted to share this joy of pregnancy with all of them. The only option was to take them all on a Zoom conference call. The conversations would end with "I Miss Yous" and "I wish this would all end soon."

Eventually, the third trimester ended, and it was time for Sofia to be admitted into labor. It was the 21st of May 2020. The virus was still at its pinnacle; the daily death rate had increased. She was admitted to the hospital since morning because, before going into the labor room, Sofia was taken to run a COVID-19 test. They were still waiting for the results as Jonah veered her wheelchair into the labor room and was about to enter with his wife when he was told to wait outside because of the COVID precautions. No one except the medical staff was allowed to enter.

The hospital room buzzed with urgency and tension as she lay down on the bed. Soon, she was injected with some syringes and set up with an IV. Within an hour, a wave of excruciating pain surged through her pelvis. She gripped the bed rails and screamed through the mask, waves of labor pain crashing through her body. For the next hour or so, she continued to push. She was exhausted, drenched in sweat, her breath short and fast, and on top of that, the mask over her face made everything feel harder. Every gasp felt stifled, every contraction a battle not just against the pain, but against panic. Her

COVID test results were still pending, and until they arrived, eight long hours after being taken, she was required to remain masked, isolated, and surrounded by nurses in full protective gear. Their eyes were kind but distant behind goggles and face shields. Their voices came out muffled as they told her to breathe and push. No comforting touch, no visible smiles—only gloved hands and clinical efficiency. Her partner wasn't allowed in until the test came back negative, so she labored alone. The whole time, the sides of the bed were the only support as she cried in the sterile walls of the delivery room. The mask grew damp with tears and sweat, but she kept it on, knowing it was the only way to protect her baby. And when the moment finally came, and she pushed through the last surge of pain, it wasn't joy that filled the room first, it was relief. Relief that the baby cried, that she had made it through, that the masked silence had finally broken with the sound of new life.

The results came out to be negative as well, but that didn't matter when Jonah and Sofia came back home with their child after spending a day under supervision at the hospital. The couple was overwhelmed with a multitude of emotions: relief, happiness, excitement, all mixed up with the constant anxiety of taking care of their newborn during the pandemic.

A new phase began with a fresh bunch of problems for her to tackle. The postpartum period was nothing like she had imagined. There were no visits from family, no friends bringing over meals or holding the baby while she showered. The apartment was quiet except for the cries of her newborn and the steady whir of exhaustion in her bones. COVID restrictions kept her loved ones at a distance, and though they called and sent messages, the absence of physical presence was a sharp ache.

"Hi, Mom. Look! The baby's awake right now. You can talk to him," she would call her mother at random times of the day to wash away the gloom. Her mom would make weird, happy noises to make the baby smile.

However, in moments of silence, she found herself spiraling, her chest tightening, her thoughts racing, tears slipping down her cheeks for reasons she couldn't explain. There were nights she sat in the dark, nursing with trembling hands, feeling like the walls were closing in.

At one point, she was sure that she had postpartum depression. There was more exhaustion and desolation than contentment.

Anxiety came in waves: over the baby's breathing, the laundry piling up, the possibility of getting sick. Depression settled in quietly. Sometimes, she didn't recognize herself. But slowly, she began to piece together ways to cope. She began practicing mindfulness during feedings, grounding herself in her baby's warmth and the rise and fall of their breath.

Three months later, while she was still busy with her newborn, she found out that she was pregnant. Again. This time, it was completely unplanned and unexpected. Why would she want to go through the rollercoaster again when the pandemic was not over? If anything, it was worse now.

"Jonah, I don't think I can do this. I am barely holding onto my nerves right now. This would be too much." Sofia cried in the bathroom, nestled in Jonah's arms. He consoled her and told her that they had done it once, and they could surely do it again. He kept her rooted and strong when she was crumbling down.

"I am here with you. I can take off early from work and help you with the babies. We will do it together, don't worry." He kissed her forehead and hugged her tightly.

Contrary to her expectations, the second pregnancy was easier for Sofia. She knew what to do this time. She was armed and ready. She spent those months the same way she had during her previous pregnancy, however, this time it was a little hard for her to do mundane chores because of a newborn attached to her hip. Usually, Jonah helped her change diapers, cook meals, clean the house, all the mundane chores that had become a mountain-climbing challenge for Sofia. The months passed easily, and soon it was time for her to deliver her second angel.

Again, she was tested for COVID before going to the labor room. Luckily, this time the results came back in an hour, and she did not have to wear the mask. She had to go through all the precautionary steps as she did the first time, but this time, she was more ready, more prepared.

The baby was delivered with ease, and it was born as healthy as can be. Her two children, despite being born during a pandemic, were pretty healthy babies. Even though the pandemic was a tough time for her and everyone, it really unveiled the traumas of pregnancy and the importance of familial support during it.

During her second postpartum period, Jonah's parents came to stay with them and help with the babies. Hence, it was not at all lonely and depressing like the first. They helped her with house chores while Jonah was at work, and she was always grateful for extra helping hands. She would always be thankful to God, her husband, and her family for being there for her during her two pregnancies.

One weekend, while both the kids were sleeping soundly with their grandparents, she and Jonah sat together in the living room with cups of coffee in their hands. The TV was on, and even after a year, the news was the same, except the people were used to it now. Many were vaccinated and cured; the shopping malls, stores, and schools were all open again. This time, the world carried hope.

"Jonah, I am very grateful for Mom and Dad. Last year was a little crazy for us, no?"

"Yes, you are right. But you know, I am grateful that our babies are healthy. Even though it was tough, we made it through. We really did it," he paused in between and kissed her forehead, "but more than anything, I am proud of you."

Sofia smiled with warmth and gratitude in her eyes, "What can I say...When life gives you lemons, you make lemonade."

7
Margaret

At the vaccination center, Margaret Laney felt queasy. Wearing her mask had always made her feel as if she was constantly on the verge of throwing up. Regardless, she always made sure to keep it tightly fastened to her face.

Before the healthcare professional administered the shot, he asked her a few standard questions: Are you experiencing any COVID-19 symptoms, difficulty breathing, a fever, a sore throat? Do you have any other health conditions? Are you immunocompromised? Are you pregnant?

Margaret's answer to all of them was no. But at the time, she was unaware that one of her answers had been incorrect.

Later, once she was back home, Margaret scrolled through social media. TikTok, the newest, most popular platform, was filled with people talking about the global pandemic.

Margaret had spent the better part of the last half hour retching in her bathroom. She decided to test for pregnancy and the result was positive. She was both so excited and so nervous. Now, all she wanted was to sit down and relax for the rest of the day. The stress of knowing she had been in public, close to many other potentially sick people, was enough already. She realized that her knowledge about COVID and the vaccine was limited, and she preferred not to hear any more about the pandemic and its toll on lives.

But the video she had just scrolled down to caught her attention. It was a podcast, featuring two women debating. They spoke about their pregnancies and whether they would get the newly released vaccine or not. They cited others' experiences and concerns about the dangers of doing so. They also discussed the benefits of a vaccinated mother being safer, and how avoiding full-blown COVID could ultimately protect her fetus.

The woman on the left, a blonde, slender woman with a serious tone and wild eyes, was adamant that no matter what the government, the doctors, or the scientists said, she would never get the vaccine. Definitely not while pregnant and not even after.

Margaret looked down at the bandage still on her arm, her mind racing.

Only one sound came from her mouth. "Oh."

"You sure the baby won't be affected? I wouldn't have gotten that vaccine if I had known." Margaret sat on her sofa as her husband sprayed down the groceries with an antibacterial spray.

"I'm sure it won't. I haven't heard any official reports about adverse effects on pregnant women yet," Jimmy said.

"The vaccine hasn't even been around long enough for any studies to be conducted!" Margaret was becoming agitated. She was used to being the one who did the groceries, and right now, she saw that Jimmy had bought the wrong brand of peanut butter. "What? You think there's someone out there who got vaccinated yesterday and gave birth today? You really think they would have someone like her on the news by now?"

"Okay. There is no need to get upset. There is nothing we can do about it now. All we can do is hope for the best. I am sure our baby is going to be healthy." He finished spraying the peanut butter and then put the jar in the fridge, not in the cabinet, which made Margaret wince. She decided not to comment on it.

"Okay. But I do know that people are getting sick even after being vaccinated. In fact, some have gotten sick because of it. Maybe caught it from the center or the injection or the driver there, whatever," Margaret said.

"That's true. But you have been okay so far, other than the morning sickness. Plus, we have a good system. I'm the one who goes outside, and we've both been taking all the necessary precautions. I've stocked up on masks and gloves, and we've decided that you won't be leaving the house unless it's to go to the doctor's."

"Yeah." Margaret's voice was small. She did not much enjoy being cooped up at home. Neither did she like the fact that she was pretty obviously taking out her frustrations and fears on her husband. "I didn't even get to ask a doctor if it would be okay. If my baby would be safe."

Jimmy's shoulders slumped, his hands holding bags of vegetables. He knew he could not set them down and go hug his wife, whose face he could not even fully see as it was obscured by a mask. "I am sorry."

"I am too."

"Hey. At least we both get to work from home."

Margaret laughed. "Silver lining."

A few thuds could be heard from the direction of her daughter's room. "Looks like Lily is up," Jimmy said as he began washing the vegetables in the sink.

"I'll go see to her. Boy, a toddler, and a newborn. Going to be a handful."

"We have four hands together," Jimmy said, chuckling. "We will manage."

The next day, Margaret decided to call her mother and tell her the good news. But she didn't quite get a full sentence in before her mother launched into a rant about her own issues surrounding COVID.

"This young man at the grocery store had the nerve to tell me I couldn't come in without a mask," her mother huffed, as if personally offended by the concept of public health. "I told him, I've been breathing the good Lord's air for sixty-two years without a filter, and I'm not about to start now. He said it was company policy. Well, I said my personal freedom is not up for negotiation! Can you believe that? Like I'm some kind of criminal. Over a piece of cloth!"

Margaret rubbed her forehead. "Mom—"

"And then this other woman in line, nose all covered like a sheep, has the audacity to say I'm being selfish! Selfish? Me? I haven't been sick once yet. Heck, I haven't been sick for the last three years. They can keep their poison needles and muzzle mandates. I'm not putting that garbage in my body."

Margaret's stomach turned. She took a deep breath, clutched the edge of the kitchen counter, and shouted, "I'm pregnant!"

There was a long pause on the other end of the line. Then, her mother's voice returned.

"But… but you told me you got vaccinated just a few days ago," she said. She sounded panicked. "What will happen to the baby? Margaret, what were you thinking? You don't know what's in that stuff! They're saying it changes your DNA! What if it harms the baby? What if—"

"Mom!" Margaret snapped. "I called to tell you I'm having a baby, and all you can talk about is…" She flailed her free hand around. "…this. I don't need this right now."

"You don't understand, sweetie—"

"No, you don't understand," Margaret cut in. "I needed support. Not… this."

Without waiting for a response, she hung up the call. Her hands were shaking. Then the tears came, hot and sudden. She sank into the nearest chair, burying her face in her hands.

Following the call with her mom, Margaret paid close attention to the family group chat. Now that most of them knew she was pregnant, they had congratulated her and Jimmy. What shocked her was that many had also insisted they should be able to come visit her. The loudest out of these voices was that of her brother Todd.

Todd had been sending a lot of anti-vax, anti-mask, and anti-big pharma articles and posts on the family group chat. That did not surprise Margaret, especially after her conversation with her mother, with whom Todd still lived. What did surprise her was that most of the family seemed to feel the same. At least eighty percent of them. She had had private conversations with her cousin Trish about it, and they both shared their concerns regarding their conflicting viewpoints. Neither wished to have a fight with their families, but things seemed like they would soon get heated. One of the aunts, who was a nurse, had already stoked the flames, arguing against something her brother had claimed about the vaccines having tracking devices so the government could monitor you.

Most of the family refused to stay at home and social distance. They did not isolate themselves if they felt sick. They did not wear masks, and they certainly did not get vaccinated. This was in stark contrast with the way Margaret, Jimmy, and Lily were living. They didn't even go for walks around the neighborhood.

Every time Margaret opened up her chats, she was greeted by at least a hundred new texts on the group. Many times, she had managed to gather the strength to ignore them all. But sometimes, she would slip and open an article or two that discussed the vaccine's adverse effects. Any time any of these articles contained the word "pregnancy," she would feel her heart skip a beat. The sad part was that most of them did. It was the one aspect in the sea of misinformation about trackers, bio-weapons, and the deep state that actually made some sense. There was, in fact, no information about what the vaccine could do to pregnant women and their babies. Still, she was the only one in her family who was currently pregnant.

She knew there was no way she could meet any of her extended family, even after her baby was born. This was a fact that tore her up inside. She remembered the joy of having her mother rub her belly, of her friends around her, chatting and sharing their own experiences, of her father giving her words of wisdom and hugs, of her brother holding a newborn Lily.

Margaret had always considered those kinds of moments—the moments when she was able to share her joy with others—to be the most beautiful moments of pregnancy. Even all the chaos a new baby brought was missed. There would be no worried faces and praying hands when her baby was born. There would be no huge family dinners in celebration. No showing off the baby to the neighbors. No strangers making faces at the infant in a park. Those would all be things that Margaret and her unborn child would miss out on.

Feeling the weight of her emotions piling up, Margaret decided that no matter what her family believed about the pandemic, she would not be willing to lose her close connection with them.

She picked up her phone, opened up the group chat, and sent a short, simple text.

"Movie night on Friday at 7 PM. Join on Netflix Party! Let's get a new tradition going!"

That's how the family met every week. Watching movies online, sharing ideas, frustrations, and events. They all bonded together, and it made them feel closer to each other. The best thing was that, once distracted by the movie, any heated arguments about COVID were avoided.

In July 2020, Margaret gave birth to a beautiful baby boy. They decided to name him Logan.

Margaret was only allowed to remove her mask while pushing during childbirth. It broke her heart that her newborn's first sight of her was with her face covered. After being inside her for nine months, she wished he could have seen her real face instead. However, she took comfort in knowing that while he was in her womb, he was safe. Now that he was in the outside world, which was filled with viruses, he no longer had those protective walls around him.

Margaret was able to stay home throughout her pregnancy and even after her little baby boy was born. She had used her 16 weeks of maternity leave, and although offices had partly reopened after that, she asked her boss to let her continue working from home, as she needed her baby to be safe. Luckily, her boss agreed. This was something she was grateful for, as she remembered how it had been with Lily. She would have to rush home after work, enduring a forty-minute commute, and arrive home to an agitated infant who sorely missed her Mama.

After her boy was born, she, her husband, and his older sister were the only people the baby saw other than his doctors. Margaret's family was still not convinced that the virus was dangerous and required social distancing. They had continued to disregard all protocol and safety measures, and so, Margaret made the difficult decision to keep them from visiting her children.

Though she felt lonely and cooped up with a toddler and a colicky baby in her small house, she knew that this was the right thing to do to protect her family.

The person she missed the most was her brother. They had to completely shut him out and shut down any of his demands to see the baby. No one seemed to truly understand her concern for her family, and they began to portray her as a villain, but that was a title she was willing to accept if it meant that her children's health was not compromised.

Logan and Lily ended up becoming very attached, as they were the only friends the other had to play with during the pandemic. Even while on Zoom calls with the family, separated by miles and a screen, the two were as thick as thieves, Lily being able to understand what her little brother needed, despite the fact that all he could do was babble and cry. The family, however, was unable to interact with him. They had to make do with just seeing his little face on their phones and laptops.

The Laney family continued to follow the strict protocols they had established, which she and Jimmy had created together to manage their home. Although it was frustrating at times, it demonstrated that the two could work as a team, even in a world that had been turned upside down.

Through it all, Margaret was able to appreciate the positives of having a baby during COVID. They now had the ability to relax and spend time with their family. This would never have been possible with their old life, where they were constantly on the go. In addition to this, she realized the power of humanity. People seemed to genuinely want to help one another during the pandemic. There were food drives and clothing donations. Communities stepped up, even when everyone was scared.

She was part of a few Mom's Groups on Facebook, and those spaces became like little lifelines. Women she'd never met were checking in on each other, swapping advice, and offering help. Once, a mom posted that she was having a 'crappy' day; she was just completely overwhelmed. A stranger from across the country sent her a cup of coffee through Uber Eats, just like that. No questions asked. That story always stuck with Margaret. It reminded her that people really did care.

Of course, it wasn't all heartwarming moments. COVID made one thing painfully clear: we don't all see things eye to eye. And sometimes, those differences cut deep. Margaret had to trust her own instincts, her own moral compass. That meant following public health advice: wearing a mask, staying home, and getting vaccinated. Her kids didn't go to birthday parties or playgroups. For her daughter's birthday, she had friends and family send short video clips. Then she put them all together into a video montage. They watched it again and again. It became something special.

In the end, Margaret knew it had been a frightening time to be pregnant. But looking back, she also felt grateful. Her pregnancies went well. Her children were healthy. And the time they had together was quiet and uninterrupted. This was something she didn't take for granted. There were plenty of bumps along the way. But there was also love. Closeness. And a deeper kind of family connection that might not have been fostered if not for the lockdown.

8
Zoe

She picked up the grocery bags from the floor and locked the door behind her before paying the deliveryman. It had been more than a week since the pandemic began. All the grocery stores, markets, schools, and other institutions were shut down under a lockdown. Since she could not go anywhere, she just ordered the groceries online.

That day, she had been feeling extremely nauseated. She vomited violently as soon as she woke up. Her inner suspicion kicked in and she took out a pregnancy test strip from the bathroom drawer. While she was waiting for the results, she ordered the groceries and cleaned up the apartment a little. It had been more than three hours, and she decided to check the strip.

She went to the bathroom and held her breath. A whirlwind of anticipation circled in her stomach as she held the strip between her fingers. Two straight lines stared back at her with conviction. Before even a single tear could escape from her eyes, she picked up her phone and called Daniel.

"Hello, Zoe. What's up?"

"Dan, where are you? Can you come today?" Desperation dripped from her voice just as the tears fell from her eyes.

"Is everything good? You don't sound good to me?"

"I just did a pregnancy test and I think we are pregnant!" Zoe exclaimed.

She heard a pause on the other side of the line, and then a sniff. "What? Zoe, are you kidding? I am coming!"

After spending a week in quarantine, Dan took the first train leaving from his town. It was approximately a fifteen-hour journey. The whole way, he couldn't sleep a wink due to the excitement rushing through his blood. He would try to close his eyes, but to no avail. On the other hand, Zoe was also out of sorts. The whole week had been harsh on her. She would pace around the apartment anxiously. One minute her eyes would stare at the pregnancy test strip, and the other at the door in anticipation of Daniel. After a week of trepidation, it was finally the day when Dan was going to arrive. She talked to Dan on the phone, and he told her that he would come at night. She put her phone away and lay down on the couch watching TV. She did not realize when she fell asleep.

Around midnight that day, the knob turned, and Dan entered. He walked in and saw Zoe sleeping soundly on the couch. He spotted the pregnancy test strip in a tray glowing in the moonlight entering from the window. Zoe had not thrown it away. He stooped down and picked up the strip and finally looked at the first evidence of his baby. The two lines were prettier than anything in the world he had ever seen. He glanced at his sleeping wife; there were lines of uneasiness visible on her forehead. He placed the pregnancy test strip back on the table and put his briefcase aside. With slow and quiet steps, he walked toward Zoe and bent down to her level. He kissed the worry lines on her forehead, slowly taking away all her anxiety. He understood how hard that week must have been for her without anyone by her side.

The next day, they both went to the doctor's office to see the gynecologist. Zoe had gone alone the day she found out about her pregnancy. It was confirmed positive, and Zoe was also deemed to be COVID-free. However, now, after a week, the doctor had called in for another screening and for a regular check-up. Dan held Zoe's hand as they walked past the swarm of people. They both did not dare pull their masks down even for a second. Dan sanitized his hands and Zoe's and made sure both of them drank a lot of water. He was worried that they would catch COVID. Before entering the gynecologist's room, they had to go through a COVID-19 screening test.

"Dan, what if I turn out to be COVID positive? I don't want to spend this time without you."

"Don't worry. Nothing will happen. It's going to be fine."

After the screening test was done, they met the gynecologist, and after a quick check-up up, she asked Zoe some questions.

"So, Zoe. The baby seems fine. It hasn't developed much. It has been only 12 days since the fetus formed. How are you feeling, though? Are you good?"

"Yes, I am. As long as the baby is fine." Zoe smiled and looked at Dan.

"That's good to hear. We love a happy mama and a healthy baby." Dr. Samantha smiled. However, there was a little twitch in her eyes that Zoe did not catch.

Zoe's COVID-19 screening test turned out to be negative. They collected the reports and were on their way back in their car when Dan brought up what he had seen in the doctor's eyes.

"Zoe, you know that I am here to support you in any decision that you make. I also know that we planned this pregnancy. However, with all the pandemic and the virus in the air, if you feel like you know…"

"Feel like what, Dan?" Zoe cut him off.

"Do you feel like aborting the baby? It's only been 12 days. You can have a change of heart. I would totally support you. I know the pandemic situation is hard, and with the virus in the air, it will be hard for you to manage your health and the baby's."

"No, Dan. Never in a million years. Even if we were in the middle of a war right now, I would carry this baby. I know that you care for me, but I am fine. I have hope that it's just the beginning of this pandemic, but soon they will develop vaccines. It will all be good as before. Medicine has greatly advanced. I am sure the world will be fine." Zoe explained with conviction.

"I am happy as long as you are happy," Dan said with a big, satisfactory smile and kissed her hand.

Dan stayed with Zoe at their apartment before going back to his city. His firm still had not assigned work-from-home to its employees, but they said they would in a couple of months. The first two months of Zoe's pregnancy went pretty smoothly. She was isolated and had no worry of catching COVID-19. She was a medical student herself, and her university had gone completely online. They were only called for requirements, and even then, no students were allowed to go on the floors with COVID-19-positive patients. Everything was going smoothly, and Zoe was very grateful for her university's protocol.

Soon, the third month of pregnancy began, and she was going to university only once a week. By the end of the month, she started feeling a little queasy. The nausea had begun to hit her. The whole day, she would feel like throwing up whenever she stood up or raised her head. She also caught a little flu. The unease grew as a couple more days passed, and she decided to see the doctor. She went to the hospital out-patient location and had a COVID-19 screening test. After a couple of hours, the results came out to be negative. Instead of relief, a harrowing feeling took control of her. She booked her gynecologist's appointment for the next day.

If not COVID-19, then why was she feeling this way? Was her baby fine?

The next day, Dr. Samantha ran an ultrasound. Zoe lay on the recliner bed. Sweat dripped down her face as her eyes keenly watched the screen in which a little silhouette of her baby was being displayed. She gauged the doctor's expressions. Her eyebrows knit, lips bitten, and eyes narrowly watching the screen.

The horrible moments of anticipation finally passed, and the doctor put down the machine. She looked at Zoe and frowned a little, pressing her lips together.

Concern. Tension. Fear. She took Zoe's hands in hers. Her expression changed to condolence and hope.

"The reports will tell the truth, but from what I can see, the baby seems to have clubfeet," Dr. Samantha spoke in a low, concerned voice.

A little cry escaped from Zoe's throat, and she sat up. She put her hand on her little baby bump, and the tears gushed down in a waterfall. Dr. Samantha patted her back and consoled her the whole time, trying to give her hope.

"It's not something that can't be treated. We can't treat this now when the baby is still inside you, but after it's born, we will treat it. This is easily curable with a cast that will be tied to the baby's feet. It's going to be fine. The baby is fine otherwise; there are no internal problems to worry about. Relax, okay," she said before offering a glass of water to Zoe.

Zoe drove back home and called Dan, telling him about the misfortune. The earth moved from beneath Dan's feet, and the next second, he quickly dumped all his necessary belongings into a big duffel bag and sat in his car. Not having the patience to book the train tickets and then spend a week in quarantine, he sat in his car and drove for seventeen hours to be with the love of his life.

It was at the break of dawn when Dan rushed in through the apartment door. He ran straight to their bedroom and found Zoe sitting on the bed. Within three big strides, he was by her side, hugging her tightly.

"Don't worry. I am here. I am not going back again. I am going to stay with you, and we will go through this together."

Dan's office had finally shut down due to the strict order of lockdown. He was on work-from-home, and Zoe's university had also allowed her to stay at home because of her condition. They spent the rest of six months together in isolation. No one would visit them, and they would also refrain from going anywhere except the doctor's office or when it was very urgent.

Time passed quickly, and soon it was time for Zoe to go into labor. They both completed the screening test before Zoe was admitted to the labor room. Dan was not allowed inside, so he waited in the waiting room, his body tense with anticipation. He felt jittery and restless, pacing lightly and glancing repeatedly at the labor room door, behind which his wife was bringing their baby into the world.

For the first couple of hours, Zoe kept her mask on because the COVID results were not out. As soon as she was confirmed to be negative, she removed the mask, and then it was easier for her to push without being muzzled behind a mask. After long hours of excruciating pain, the baby was out. Her cries echoed through the labor room, and Zoe heaved a massive sigh of relief. The nurses cleaned the blood from the baby and handed her to Zoe. She cried when she first laid eyes on her healthy baby. She looked at the little miracle and kissed her head ever so gently. Within ten minutes, Dan was also brought in by one of the nurses. He walked inside with a big smile on his face and held his baby in his arms, cooing with warmth. Both of them looked at the clubfeet of their baby. Their faces fell. Their eyes locked, and a mix of worry and hope glistened in them.

Soon after Zoe was discharged, her mother came to visit, having completed her quarantine period. Her mother would cook and help Zoe with the baby. They were very careful with her in the initial weeks. Zoe's mother would visit often and take Evelyn on strolls to the parks. There were a few other kids as well, and all the adults made sure to carry sanitizers and masks with them. It was a lovely time when Zoe could raise her baby alongside her mother with no other things like a job or education to occupy her.

However, having no job was no fairy tale, especially if one had a newborn to care for. Sitting on the couch together, Dan and Zoe discussed how it was a little hard to manage everything with no job.

"You know, I am working from home, but they have reduced my salary to half. It's a little hard to manage everything with the baby, and then her medical needs," Dan expressed his concerns.

"I understand. But it's not that bad. Look. We are spending the most heavenly time together as a family. We are not miles apart anymore. Even though we are a little financially constrained, the brighter side is that we are together. That's all that matters," Zoe replied while rubbing his palms with her thumb.

After Evelyn turned eight weeks old, her treatment for the clubfeet began. Both Zoe and Dan were at the hospital the day Evelyn was supposed to undergo surgery. She was going to get a full cast attached to her feet and this was a restless and disconcerting time for her parents. Both Zoe and Dan attended all of Evelyn's check-ups together. The time passed, and Evelyn started to recover. Even though they missed the rest of their family, most of them had never met the baby in person because of the lockdown and airport closures. It was enough for Zoe and Dan to raise their child in isolation. It was enough that they were together throughout this period, and the pandemic came as a welcome blessing that united their family, giving them ample time to spend together and raise their baby with complete attention and relief.

9
Lana

Lana Grace had always imagined that her first pregnancy would be special, with people commenting on how radiant she looked, prenatal classes alongside other happy couples, family visits with everyone surrounding the baby, and the joyful chaos of baby showers. What she didn't expect was that the world would shut down just as her belly began to swell.

She and her husband, Timothy, had planned for their first baby long before the COVID-19 pandemic was even a concern. Now, stores were shutting down, borders were closing, and fears about the mysterious virus were growing. But for the couple, the pregnancy wasn't a surprise; it was a dream come true. So, when the test came back positive, Lana pressed it into Timothy's hand with a nervous laugh. He looked down, then up, then grabbed her by the waist and twirled her around their kitchen. For them, it was all perfect.

But as spring bled into summer and the virus held fast, Lana's joy came with an undercurrent of fear.

"I just… I didn't think it would look like this," she confessed one night, curled up on their living room couch, a hand on her belly. "It's like we're the only three people in the world."

Timothy kissed her forehead. "Maybe that's not such a bad thing."

As a NICU nurse, Lana knew too much to be comforted by sweet words. She saw the fragility of life every shift. She saw ventilators. She saw goodbyes that happened too soon, that weren't supposed to happen. And now she was carrying a baby of her own. One she had to protect.

While she could avoid restaurants, gatherings, and shops, she couldn't avoid work.

She and Timothy often discussed her work situation, and he even suggested that she quit her job for the safety of their baby. But Lana knew that now more than ever, the hospital needed her and others like her. She was an essential worker, and she realized she could do good for many people by continuing to go to work. So, they decided she would carry on. However, she did address her concerns with her manager.

Thankfully, her nurse manager had been kind and supportive, shielding her from known COVID-positive patients. But "unknown" cases still walked through the door. That could not be helped. It was difficult to determine who was COVID-19 positive, and so no matter how supportive her workplace was, Lana could not entirely avoid danger. She had learned to hold her breath behind her mask. Every shift felt like walking a tightrope.

Timothy noticed Lana was lost in thought and took her hand. "Hey, what are you thinking about?"

"Just the hospital," she said.

"Oh, your appointment?"

Lana hadn't even thought about her prenatal appointment planned for the next day. That was one aspect of her pregnancy journey she did not feel too stressed about. Annoyance and disappointment? Sure. But Lana had decided that she could put her skills to use and take charge of her own health. As a medical professional herself, Lana knew she was capable of keeping track of her own health and filling the gaps caused by the fact that she could not attend many in-person prenatal appointments. Her doctor had also instructed her to keep track of certain medical information for their records. Therefore, she turned their bedroom into a makeshift clinic. A Doppler rested beside her bed, its probe worn from daily use. She ran it slowly across her belly every evening until the rhythmic thump of her daughter's heart filled the room. *There you are,* she would whisper. *Still strong. Still safe.*

She weighed herself with a bathroom scale and recorded it in a little spiral notebook. Her blood pressure cuff beeped faithfully as she sat on the edge of their bed.

Ultrasounds were also reduced. She only had one. The rest were canceled in a flood of policies and precautions. Prenatal classes? Shifted to videos and Zoom calls. "Breathe in. Breathe out," a stranger's voice coached through tinny laptop speakers. It felt more like homework than preparation.

Despite it all, Lana knew that she was healthy, and so there was no need to worry excessively.

“Hello. Earth to Lana. You got lost again.” Timothy was growing a bit concerned now.

“I’m sorry. I’m just thinking too much, I want to get everything right.” Lana rubbed her temples.

“Alright, no worries. Do you have a headache or something?”

“No, no. I'm perfectly fine. I do miss Mom and Dad, though.”

Timothy’s face grew sad.

Her parents never got to see her bump in person. The border between the U.S. and Canada was closed. Once, just once, they met at a border crossing, masked and distanced, waving through a fog of longing. Lana had been safe in her clean car, crying as she watched her parents. They had spoken on the phone that day, whispering, as if that might make them feel like they were closer to each other.

“They’re so worried,” she told Timothy. “I keep telling them I’m being careful, but they can't help but be scared.”

“You’re doing everything right,” he reassured.

He meant it. Working from home, he saw her diligence every day. He watched as she changed out of her scrubs in the garage, wiped down her shoes, and sanitized her phone. He knew she was carrying more than just their baby; she was bearing the weight of doing everything right, even when the world was unrecognizable. The only place she went while pregnant was work, where they made sure to follow every precaution and protocol. All necessary steps had been taken, and there wasn’t a single moment when Lana allowed herself to grow lax and slip up.

“I know. I just hope it's enough.”

When labor finally arrived in late October 2020, Lana felt ready yet exhausted. So accustomed to hospitals, Lana was not afraid of her delivery. While many other women might be filled with nervous tension, Lana knew she would be in capable hands. Plus, she had her support system with her. Timothy drove her to the hospital in the early morning. The roads were quiet, and the air was damp and cold. She clutched his hand in the elevator and looked up at him.

"I'm glad you can be here."

"Wouldn't be anywhere else."

Because she tested negative for COVID, she was allowed to use nitrous oxide for pain management as planned. The relief was real. To her surprise, the delivery room was exactly what she needed: just her nurse, her midwife, and Timothy. No crowd. No interruptions. Peaceful.

The delivery went perfectly, and they welcomed a healthy baby girl.

"I couldn't imagine more people in here," she said to her husband as she rocked her baby girl in her arms. "It felt… sacred."

Isla was born with wide eyes and a strong cry. She was beautiful.

The joyful parents basked in their happiness, savoring every moment.

On her first day postpartum, three nursing students entered Lana's hospital room to check her blood pressure.

"Would prefer if only one of you stays," Lana said calmly.

"We're tested weekly," one of them replied. "It's completely safe."

"I understand. But still. Just one, please."

They hesitated, but Lana held her ground, knowing that she had to do everything possible to stay protected. Two of the students left the room.

Lana was discharged the next day, having met all her milestones. The young family made their way back home, excited to start their new life together.

But in those early days, Isla's weight dipped slightly. And so, they had to start doing weekly pediatric check-ins. Lana and Timothy sat in their car outside the pediatrician's office, masked and waiting for their name to be called. Sometimes they could go in together, sometimes only one was allowed. The rules changed with the tides of infection. Still, Lana was glad for all the rules; they helped her family stay healthy.

Back home, Lana longed to place Isla into her parents' arms. To let her siblings cradle their new niece. But all introductions were made through foggy glass and Zoom screens. Her friends dropped off food and waved from a distance. No one touched the baby. No one hugged her.

"I'm starting to forget what company feels like," Lana whispered one evening. Isla was asleep on her chest. Timothy rubbed her back gently.

"But she's healthy," he said. "We're safe. That's everything. Besides, my parents will be coming in tomorrow. Then things will get a bit more lively." He chuckled, knowing that the first thing his parents would do would be to rush to the baby and scream in joy.

Lana's parents-in-law did come for two weeks and helped with cooking and cleaning. This was a time filled with love, and Lana would not have traded it for anything. Yet, the time they could spend together was short. After those two weeks of rest and bliss, they did not see anyone else for approximately two months.

It was just the three of them. Lana sometimes felt like the world had shrunk into the square footage of their living room. But there was also a strange beauty in that closeness.

They split shifts. Cooked together. Watched Isla's every breath. Her first smile. The way her fingers curled around Timothy's thumb. Every moment, uninterrupted by visitors or noise. Their first taste of having a family was peaceful.

They didn't need daycare. They didn't need parties. They didn't even need a village. What they had was each other. And that, in the end, was more than enough.

10
Kiki

Kiki Abner left the nursery with a trolley full of baby bottles, discarded cotton pads, and syringes. She wheeled the trolley to the waste room to safely dispose of the items before going back to the staff room for a cup of coffee.

She entered the small staff room, which included a table with a coffee machine and stacks of disposable cups, two small, brown couches, and two chairs. Hannah was already there, going through some patient files. She readjusted her glasses and looked up at Kiki.

"Hi. How's the shift going?"

"Just about to end. I am done with my last round. Delilah will take my place after 20 minutes. The nursery is silent and peaceful as long as the babies are sleeping. I hope she comes before I leave." Kiki replied while making herself a cup of coffee.

"And how's your little baby doing?" Hannah asked, her eyes flicking toward Kiki's six-month-pregnant belly.

"She is also good. Has started to kick a lot. Do you want to feel?" Kiki asked Hannah with a big smile, even though she knew this was nothing new for both of them, being nurses in the pediatric unit.

"Sure, why not?"

They both talked a little more before Kiki packed her stuff and left for home.

She took the elevator down to the bustling ground floor filled with COVID-positive patients. She observed the emergency workers clad in protective gear moving hurriedly, families anxiously awaiting test results, and some weeping for loved ones lost to the deadly virus. Adjusting her own mask, she attempted to navigate through the crowd while minimizing human contact.

While in the pediatric unit, she did not encounter any COVID cases, and since she was pregnant, she was not permitted to go to the COVID floors, even during rotations. She was very grateful to the management for giving her such relief. Her last trimester was soon to start, and even though she knew that she wouldn't be going on

COVID rotations, she was still worried about herself and her unborn child. She wished to pass the last phase of her pregnancy without any added hassles.

Therefore, she wore the protective gear at all times in the hospital, made sure to wash and sanitize her hands regularly, and took a shower right after coming home. She also made sure that her husband followed the same instructions.

Showering was the moment she typically reflected on her day. Today was pretty normal, other than the unusual crowd of patients. She realized she might need to take a short break from work during her last month to ensure her and her baby's safety. She came out of the shower, picked up her iPad, and FaceTimed her mother for some advice.

"Kiki! My love. How are you? How's the little baby?" Kiki's mother's enthusiastic voice came through the speakers.

"Hi, Mom. We are both good. I am just worried about something. Need your two cents," Kiki replied in a little concerned tone.

"Yes, baby. Ask away,"

"Mom, I was thinking maybe I should go on a little break till my delivery. I don't think the hospital is a safe place anymore."

"Okay…,"

"I mean, the count of COVID patients is drastically increasing day by day. I don't want to sabotage mine and the baby's health, you know."

"I totally understand you, baby. You are constantly wearing your protective gear at work, right?"

"Yes, of course. No compromise on that. Still, I think I should stay at home to maintain safety."

"Do what you think is best. My prayers are with you and our little angel."

"Thanks, Mom. I wish you were here with me. Anyway, talk to you later. Theo will be here any minute."

"Okay, baby. Bye, and take care!"

With a quick glance at the clock, she put her iPad on the table and ran to the kitchen. It was already 6 PM. She had promised Theo that she would make his favorite chicken wings with buffalo sauce today. She needed to marinate the chicken at least and prepare the sauce before he came.

Within 15 minutes, she was done with her task, and Theo was also home. They ate dinner and washed it down with a homemade mocktail.

After a week at work and contemplating whether she should take leave, she finally went and talked to Dr. Gerard about maternity leave. After listening to her with great care and attention, he signed an excuse note for her and granted her the maternity leave one week before her third trimester began.

With an overwhelming feeling of gratitude, she ended her shift that day and went home with all her belongings, which she usually kept in her locker in the staffroom. She looked forward to spending the last months of her pregnancy completely focused on her baby's health and a great family time with her husband. She sat in the car and called Theo.

"Hello?"

"Theo! My maternity leave has been granted."

"I knew it, baby. Congratulations! You would still have to go to the doctor's office for the prenatal appointments, though."

"I know. But that would be only once a week. It won't be that much of a hassle, I guess. Also, I have the protective gear, and I will still follow all the hospital protocols."

"Okay, then. That's great news. I will come home early from work and I'll cook something for my girl. What do you feel like eating?" Theo spoke in a romantic voice that made Kiki giggle like a child.

"Okay! I don't know, surprise me!" With a light chuckle, she hung up.

That night, Theo prepared a delicious meal of mashed potatoes and steak for them both. As she was unable to drink, they enjoyed their favorite pineapple squash with the meal instead.

From the next week, regular follow-up appointments began. Since Theo was not allowed to accompany Kiki to the prenatal appointments every week, she would go to the doctor's office alone, leaving her with a sense of isolation in her heart. Theo also felt a crack in his connection with the baby. Kiki started to notice the shift too, and to mend that, she brought back pictures of ultrasounds of the baby for Theo. She hoped to bring back the feeling of connection within him, and it worked sometimes. Most times, she would overthink the worst-case scenarios if any of them failed to follow the precautionary procedures.

What if any of us catches COVID and we're not allowed to be near each other? What if he is not allowed to be with me during delivery? What if he is not allowed near the baby?

With all these concerns swirling through her brain, she thought that this brief period might be hard for Theo, but at least it was safe this way. Even when Theo came back from work, she made sure that he took a shower before even touching her. The COVID numbers were spiking on a day-to-day basis, and she did not want to jeopardize the possibility of him being with her in the delivery room if he caught COVID. Until the day of delivery, she took every precaution advised by the healthcare department.

Her family would often call to check that she and the baby were doing well. Her mother was still learning to make calls on Zoom, so she would just FaceTime her. However, when her siblings wanted to join the call too, they would all connect through a Zoom conference call.

"Hi, Kiki Freaky! How are you doing?" Her brother practically shouted from the other end.

"I am good," she laughed.

"I hope you are taking all the precautions? Taking your meds on time? Wearing a mask and sanitizing your hands? You need to be very careful." This time, it was her elder sister, the one who always looked out for her.

"Yes, I am. I wear a mask to all the appointments. Now that I am on leave, it is even safer. So, don't worry about me. What about you guys? What's up?"

Their conversations continued for hours, and her siblings would make sure that Kiki was feeling good by the end of it. They would call on a daily basis for the last months of pregnancy, and, sometimes, when Theo was home, he would join in too.

Slowly and surely, the last trimester also passed, and now it was time for Kiki to deliver the baby. One day before the delivery, they went to the hospital and got their COVID-19 screening tests done so they could have their results in time. Within 8 hours, the results came out. Negative. It brought the first wave of relief to the couple. That same night, Kiki was admitted to the labor floor, where she was prepared for the contractions with the help of an epidural. Since it was late June, the summer heat was at its apex. Even with their air-conditioning running at the minimum temperature, Kiki was feeling hot, and Theo kept fanning her and rubbing her back to comfort her. It was another relief that not many people were allowed to visit them because of the COVID-19 restrictions. It was just the two of them, and a couple of nurses going in and out, checking vital signs, all clad in their protective equipment. The doctor also visited and made sure that Kiki was doing well, until her water broke, and it was time for her to deliver the little angel into the world.

Kiki pushed with every ounce of strength left in her body. It took six hours of excruciating pain, and then, with a final relief of pain, she pushed for the last time. On the 29th of June, 2020, she gave birth to a beautiful daughter. Her cries bounced off the walls of the labor room, and it was filled with an mix of relief, wonderment, and disbelief.

Tears streamed down Kiki's face as the nurses rested the baby girl on her chest. She pulled her wonder close to her and looked at her in awe. Then she glanced at Theo's face. He was staring at his wife and daughter with the same feelings; his love for them was spilling through his eyes. They both clasped their hands together and prayed a silent word of gratitude to the Almighty.

"What should we name her?" After coming home, Theo asked Kiki while they were resting and their daughter was sleeping.

"Dorothy. It means "a gift from God". I had this name in mind for *months*," Kiki said.

"Dorothy, it is." Theo agreed with a smile.

The postpartum period was quite easy on Kiki, as it was summer and she could take Dorothy out. Her family also visited the baby and brought her gifts. All of them took great care in maintaining the COVID restrictions, and whenever anybody came to meet the baby, they made sure to wear masks and sanitize their hands. Kiki limited the number of people who could meet the baby. Only the most immediate family members came, and Kiki was grateful to spend the time with them. She would also take the baby out to the park in a stroller, taking all necessary protective measures. She made sure that everyone met the baby from a distance, and no unnecessary touching was allowed to ensure the utmost safety possible.

It was not easy for her to restrict everyone from holding her baby. Only she understood the depth of her desire for Dorothy to be cherished and embraced by her aunt and uncle. She wanted her daughter to experience physical love and to get familiarized with their touch when her senses were in their initial stage of development. On one hand, she had to restrict her baby, on the other, she was also happy to spend plenty of alone time with her. She spent all day with her daughter, noticed her small movements, and called her family whenever the baby reached any milestone. For the first time, when Dorothy held the bottle by herself without any support from Kiki, she immediately FaceTimed her mother to show her.

It would also hit Kiki sometimes that she could not share these small moments of bliss with anyone. She had dreamed about a grand baby shower when she got pregnant. It was heartbreaking that she could not do that because of the lockdown. Now, as her baby was growing, she wanted her family to be there with her and witness her daughter's milestones, but, unfortunately, none of that was possible.

Theo was very understanding of the bittersweet feelings bubbling inside of Kiki. After a month of delivery, he too was off work due to the shift to an online medium. He worked from home, allowing him to spend more time with his wife and daughter. Kiki was very thankful for the healthy family time they spent together. They would play with Dorothy and plan interactive activities for her.

Kiki would reminisce about her pregnancy and postpartum period and she would feel grateful for every part of it. Although there were pros and cons, for the most part, she was extremely grateful to have raised her child when she and Theo both could give their best without any distractions.

Now that Theo could be at home with Dorothy 24/7, Kiki decided to go back to work. Along with being a mother, she was also a dutiful nurse who knew that the hospital needed her. However, at work, she was mindful of the fact that her first priority was her daughter, so she would avoid any late shifts and go back home right after completing her shift. When she got home, Theo and Dorothy waited for her with big, welcoming smiles. However, before touching them, she would shower and clean herself. More than ever before, she followed the recommended protocols now and kept herself sanitized and clean at all times.

The pandemic was tough, but in retrospect, Kiki realized that it was a reward. Her daughter was a reward, and the safety and health measures that she was made to follow were also a blessing in disguise.

11
Jane

"Bye, Mrs. Scott! See you in two weeks," Ms. Dylan said to Jane as she left the teachers' staff room with all her belongings.

It was March 15, 2020, and the U.S. government had announced a shutdown due to the global outbreak of the COVID-19 virus. The teachers were informed that they would have to return once the curve of the virus flattened. Everyone hoped the world would return to normal in a couple of weeks. However, the virus had other plans.

Jane Scott, with all her belongings in a large carton balanced on her protruding belly, left the school halls and headed to the parking lot, where a couple of other teachers were preparing to leave. Everyone exchanged goodbyes and hopes to see each other again in two weeks.

Before switching on the ignition, Jane cleaned the steering wheel and the interior of the car with a sanitizing wipe. She sanitized her hands as well and then set off to pick up her toddler from daycare. Being a working mother was not an easy task for Jane. She used to drop her toddler at the daycare and then pick him up after work on a daily basis. However, now that the world was shut down, the daycare was closing down as well.

Jane was eight months pregnant at this point. She and her husband, after having a lovely son, had planned and wanted a second child. Throughout the pregnancy, Jane had been ecstatic; however, with the sudden emergence of the virus, the excitement was replaced with uncertainty. Her gynecologist had called her the other day and broken the news that her husband would not be able to accompany her to the rest of her prenatal visits.

Typically, her husband would go with her to the doctor's office for all of her check-ups, but today she was going alone while he stayed with their son at home. Her heart bubbled with questions and disquiet as she entered the ultrasound room.

After learning that the baby was fine, she decided to share her doubts with the doctor. The vague answers that she received in return did little to ease her nerves.

"Can my husband come with me to the next visit?"

"I'm afraid not. There are strict guidelines that the office has implemented to keep everyone safe."

"How long will this lockdown last?"

"We cannot say anything about that at the moment."

"Do you think I can catch the virus? Will it affect the baby?"

"I hope you don't. We will do our best to keep you and the baby safe."

"Would my husband be allowed to stay with me at the time of delivery?"

"That depends on the lockdown situation. We are hoping for the best."

That night, she went home and spent the rest of the evening in a state of unrest. She was grateful for the two-week break from work; however, with such anxiety occupying her mind, she really missed being busy at work and not having time to overthink.

After two more lonely visits to the doctor, her two weeks of break were about to be over. She was expecting to return to work and continue with her routine when the virus decided to disrupt everything. The news broadcast the wretched reports of increasing death tolls. Moreover, the first infant death was reported, which caused Jane and her husband to lose sleep.

The lockdown was extended indefinitely. The school decided to continue with online classes on Google Meet, and teachers were asked to assign easy, long-term projects; for example, students were encouraged to try to get outside for at least an hour a day and reflect on their experiences.

Jane's last days of pregnancy were a mix of relief and wariness. On one hand, she was at home, making it easy for her to care for her toddler while the daycare was closed. She could easily manage the household chores and give online classes simultaneously, while still having enough time to relax. On the other hand, she had lost all sense of routine and discipline. Even though she was entirely at home, she was still tired at the end of the day.

On top of everything, her delivery date was nearing. The news of the first infant death caused by COVID-19 had also made her restless. It was that last straw that broke the camel's back. She had begun feeling increasingly hopeless about the state of the U.S. medical situation. Her mind was constantly in a state of dilemma, and a big question mark was nagging her. She felt like no one had answers to the questions, and no one could understand her situation.

Her second child was born on April 10, 2020, and she remembered taking maternity leave a week prior. The day the baby was delivered was not an easy day for Jane. She was admitted to the labor floor at noon after doing a COVID-19 screening test. The sky outside was overcast, smudged with the dull gray of late afternoon as she pressed her hand against the cool hospital window. The hospital lights buzzed above her head, but even that sterile hum couldn't calm down the thrumming inside her chest. She was about to give birth during a global pandemic, and everything felt uncertain.

She was alone in the hospital room at that time. What she remembers most vividly now is the not knowing. For weeks leading up to her due date, one question gnawed at her: *Would her husband be allowed in the delivery room?* It seemed no one could give her a straight answer. Nurses offered different versions of the policy. Her Obstetrician wasn't sure if the hospital would change guidelines by the time she went into labor. Even online forums and hospital websites contradicted each other.

She had expressed her worry to the doctor many times before, and that uncertainty clung to her, growing heavier with each passing day.

And then, finally, it was time, and she still did not have a specific answer.

Before she was rushed to the labor room, a nurse handed her a surgical mask and a swab kit for the COVID test. The swab scratched the back of her nose with impersonal efficiency, and that was it. Done.

But then came another question that pulled her out of the fog: *Why wasn't her husband tested, too?*

He stood beside her with concern visible on his face, carrying her overnight bag. Yet no one swabbed him. No one even offered a test. He wasn't asked about symptoms. All he had to do was fill out a quick form and keep his mask on.

And even that didn't last.

By the time labor intensified, when Jane's world narrowed to the rhythms of her breathing and the contraction monitor's beeps, her husband had pulled his mask down below his chin. At first, she thought that he had done it by mistake and that he would fix it later upon reminder. But no one said anything. Nurses came and went, calm and unbothered.

Even between waves of pain, her mind spun with confusion. *Why did she have to be tested? Why was her mask mandatory while she labored, yet the man holding her hand was exempt?*

Then, at one point, he left the room altogether. She blinked up at the door as it closed behind him. The nurse didn't stop him. Jane lay there, stunned and sweating, until he returned over an hour later, carrying with him an overpowering scent of pizza with pepperoni.

He'd bought dinner for the nurses as a kind gesture. She later learned that all he needed to re-enter the room was a quick temperature check at the desk. No swab. No new mask. Just a nod from staff and back he came, as though everything was normal.

But it wasn't normal. Nothing about this was.

Jane lay there with her mask on. Her whole body was aching because of the contractions. The nurses told her to push while staring at the ceiling tiles, which would help distract her from the pain. Her muscles went weak by the time she thrust one last time. The labor room air became sacred all of a sudden, and the pain was mitigated by the joy of the birth of their second child.

Lying there with dried tears on her face, shaking hands and blood beneath her, she realized that she was bringing life into the world during a time when even the people in charge didn't seem to know what rules to follow, at a time when the whole world was in a frenzy.

The feeling of relief and bliss was mixed with a gnawing unease. The not knowing. The sense of being protected and unprotected all at once.

The school had asked her if she would like to give up her maternity leave and continue to teach remotely, to which she politely declined and decided to spend the maternity period focusing on her newborn. The time after the pregnancy brought both its positives and negatives. It was a plus that she had the opportunity to stay at home and spend time with her children; however, the uncertainty and constant anxiety about keeping the children safe weighed heavily on them. Scott was still working on-site, and he would make sure to take a shower right after coming back, even before touching anyone or anything in the house.

She was relieved that she had few visitors during her postpartum period. However, her parents had been a great blessing. In those early days after the birth, the house was quiet in a way that felt unnatural. Jane sat in the rocker in the nursery, her newborn curled against her chest, the weight of him acting as a comfort. The world outside was still locked down due to the pandemic. It was like time moved gently. Her once-busy days were now marked only by feedings, diaper changes, and the slow return of her strength.

Her parents didn't come right away.

Her mother had already made the hard decision to retire. After years of working in a nursing home, the virus had made her consider her growing age. Every day at the hospital brought more fear, more patients testing positive, more staff going home sick. She couldn't risk bringing it home to her older husband, so she made the hard decision to move into the trailer in their driveway.

That image stayed in Jane's mind for weeks. Her mother was living steps away from her own front door, waving at her husband through the window, leaving groceries on the porch, and eating dinner alone at a little folding table under dim overhead lights of the trailer. Her mother had always been the one to make everything better, to bring calm to the chaos. It broke Jane's heart to know she was distancing herself for the sake of everyone's safety.

Her father, on the other hand, didn't say much, nor did he care about the pandemic. He never really did.

He followed the news, certainly, but it held the same detached curiosity for him as the weather. He valued caution over fear. Above all, what he cherished and longed for the most were his grandchildren.

So, when the two weeks of self-imposed quarantine were up, he showed up on Jane's porch with a cloth mask in his pocket and his arms full of cinnamon rolls. He knew that Jane loved them. Jane was surprised and equally pleased to see him there.

"Dad! What a surprise. Are you not distancing yourself? You should know that the virus is not a friend to elderly people." She said as Scott held the door open and let him inside.

"I've been practicing social distancing for sixty years," he joked, stepping inside. "No one talks to me unless I go looking for 'em."

Jane laughed, even as her eyes filled. She hadn't seen him in months, and now here he was, standing in her living room like he'd just come in from the yard.

"Don't get up," he said gruffly, waving her back when she started to rise from the couch. "Let me see the baby."

However, before touching the baby, he went to the kitchen and washed his hands for twenty seconds, ensuring that he washed away all the germs before holding his grandchild. Jane handed over her son with gentle care, and her father, this quiet, stoic man, took him as if he were made of glass. He sat down heavily in the recliner, cradling the baby in the crook of his arm. His weathered hands, usually wrapped around tools or a newspaper, now held something softer, something fragile and miraculous.

Jane's father was a man of few words, and he barely expressed his emotions. He didn't say much, but his eyes said everything.

They sat like that for hours, the baby occasionally stirring in his sleep. Jane curled up on the sofa, watching her father as if she were seeing him for the first time. He wasn't one for big emotions or long speeches since Jane's childhood. He'd never been the hug-and-kiss type of dad. But in that quiet moment, Jane felt solidly safe as his presence filled the room.

Later, as the sky began to turn a peachy and violet hue with the approach of dusk, he finally spoke.

"I'm not good with babies," he murmured, eyes still on the tiny face in his lap.

Jane smiled. "You're doing just fine. You have raised one yourself. Look at me."

He looked up then, and for the first time that day, she saw the glimmer of tears in his eyes.

“Your mother says I shouldn’t be here yet,” he said. “But I couldn't wait. I just needed to see him. To know he’s real. That you’re okay.”

“We’re okay,” Jane whispered, her voice catching in her throat. “He’s here. And you’re here. That’s all that matters.”

Her father nodded, gently rocking his grandson, lost in the quiet that wasn’t so unnatural anymore.

The days following the birth created a lasting memory for Jane. The weather was warm, and the skies stayed mostly clear. Even with a newborn, Jane felt lucky.

They made the most of the outdoors with picnic dinners in the backyard and the sizzle of the barbecue, enjoying time with family and friends. There was laughter, and there were photos. Everyone kept their space, but the joy of seeing familiar faces, even six feet apart, was enough for her.

That season, however short, filled her life with calm and bliss.

But then September came, her maternity leave was over, and so was the summer break.

Returning to work was like stepping onto a tightrope with no safety net. The school building felt at once familiar and foreign. Bright posters still lined the walls, but the air was heavy with protocol and worry. She adjusted her mask over her nose and stepped into her classroom, where rows of desks stood awkwardly three feet apart.

There were rules everywhere. Indoors, masks stayed on. Outdoors, if students were closer than three feet, masks stayed on. The desks had been rearranged with military precision, and still, everything felt off-kilter. The classroom was no longer electrified with the easy chatter of kids. Instead, there were muffled voices behind fabric. The teachers needed to remind the students to follow the precautions constantly.

"Mask over your nose, please," she repeated at least twenty times a day. She said it gently, then firmly, then wearily.

Wednesdays were supposed to be a break, a day for deep cleaning the school and resetting. But for Jane, Wednesdays were anything but restful.

She perched at her kitchen table, laptop open, headset in, a stack of attendance sheets in one hand and a cup of cold coffee in the other. Her toddler colored underfoot, demanding snacks or climbing into her lap mid-lesson. Her infant cooed from the playpen or cried during her third-period Google Meet.

She never stopped moving. Lessons, grading, bottles, diapers, masks, reminders, nap times, and screen sharing. It all blended into one long, exhausting loop.

And then, there were the daycare closures.

After the summer, her children had gone back to daycare briefly. But closures were frequent. One exposure, one positive test, and the whole system would shut down. Sometimes for a day. Sometimes for a week.

Jane's stomach sank every time she got the call mid-morning: *"We're so sorry, but we've had a positive case. You'll need to come pick them up."*

She'd smile through the rest of the Zoom lesson, eyes darting to the clock, while already calculating how she'd finish the day's grading with two children at home, both needing her in different ways.

And still, somehow, she kept showing up. She realized that not only was it tough on her, but it was also tough on the students. She had seen students crying because they did not want to wear masks, or seen them struggling with setting up online classes.

As a teacher, she felt that COVID-19 highlighted the need for improved mental health care and helped identify the importance of addressing mental health issues, as well as the need for increased support for children and teachers.

12
Ivanna

Sunlight filtered through the clear glass windows of the living room. Ivanna Baker sat on a small couch by the window, soaking in the morning sun. She had a bowl of strawberries and yogurt balanced on her pregnant belly that she munched on while watching a new series on Netflix.

The pandemic had come as a blessing for her and Christopher. Both of them had been working remote jobs for almost a year now, and they embraced this new lifestyle with open arms. They got to stay at home with each other, and had recently moved into a new house. Last year, after the lockdown, when they both began working remotely, they decided to have a baby and made plans accordingly, considering the date they bought their new house. They wanted to start a family in a new, better place and begin with a fresh start.

Both Ivanna and Chris were risk-aware people who were not really afraid of the virus. They believed in vaccines and weren't overly concerned about the fact that they would be giving birth to their baby during a pandemic. If anything, they were happier than ever and awaited the arrival of their daughter.

Initially, Ivanna was overjoyed when she discovered her pregnancy. She had been waiting for this moment; she had planned it all, yet she had not made any special arrangements regarding the pandemic. She took it as a normal pregnancy, as it would have been in any normal time and place. It was only in her first trimester that she began to experience morning sickness and would spend her mornings puking in the toilet. At that time, she was grateful to be staying at home and not having to commute for two hours on the cramped metro just to get to work.

At the end of her first trimester, the morning sickness subsided, and she went back to enjoying her pregnancy until the prenatal visits started. Her Obstetrician told her that, according to the hospital's guidelines, her husband could not accompany her to the visits. She would have to come alone. That news really flustered Ivanna, but after a couple of visits, she came to accept the reality of the situation and grew accustomed to it.

Now, around eight months pregnant, she was relishing her meal while watching Netflix in her new home. Having just woken up, she needed to log into her laptop in an hour. Her employers were fairly easygoing and didn't pressure her to adhere to strict hours. She followed a flexible schedule and completed her tasks at her convenience. This situation was a silver lining of the pandemic; without the lockdown, she worried she would have to commute to work and exhaust herself during her pregnancy.

It was usually around 4 PM when she and Christopher finished their tasks. Even though they did not have many visitors due to the shutdown, they made an effort to take leisurely walks around the neighborhood, wearing their masks a few times during the week. Since they had recently moved into this neighborhood, Chris thought it necessary to go out and socialize with other neighbors while keeping social distancing guidelines in mind. However, they still restricted themselves from attending crowded social gatherings and parties.

Where an easy work-life balance and a relaxed routine were a perk of the pandemic, Ivanna's parents would also regularly visit her and ensure that she was okay. They would visit her on weekends, when Chris and Ivanna usually had no work.

It was the last week of her eighth month when her parents called, telling her that they were coming. Ivanna had woken up early that morning and cleaned up the house a little bit. It was just before noon when her parents arrived. She ordered food online, and they had lunch together before enjoying a cup of tea. The living room was flooded with soft light filtering through the blinds that spilled warmth across the furniture. Ivanna sat curled up on the couch, a blanket draped over her legs, one hand resting lightly on the swell of her belly. The news hummed quietly from the TV with another update on rising COVID-19 numbers, but she wasn't really listening. Chris was helping her mother in the kitchen while Ivanna and her dad rested in the living room.

Her mother poked her head out of the kitchen window, wiping her hands on a dish towel. "You want some more ginger tea, sweetheart? It's good for the nausea."

Ivanna smiled. "Thanks, Mama. That'd be nice."

"You know," her mother began as she turned back toward the kitchen, "when I was pregnant with you, there was a heatwave and I still had to walk to the market every morning. You girls have it easier now. Working from home, everything delivered..."

Ivanna chuckled, resting her head back. "Working from home has its perks. No one sees me snacking every ten minutes."

Her father, seated in his armchair, read the paper, looking up over the rim of his glasses. "We're just so glad you're safe. That's the only thing that matters." He folded the paper slowly, as if making a deliberate point. "This whole pandemic thing... It's scary. But at least you're not out there in those crowded offices."

Just then, the bell rang. Her husband stepped out of the kitchen and went to pick up the groceries, "Sanitized my hands twice before touching the doorknob," he announced with mock drama. "And the groceries are here. Left them outside to 'de-virus' first, as instructed."

"You're learning," Ivanna teased.

He leaned over to kiss her forehead, then paused and looked into her eyes. "You feeling okay? You woke up rather early today."

"Better. I slept a bit more last night."

He nodded, glancing at her belly with that familiar mix of awe and protectiveness. "I know people are worried about pregnancies during the pandemic," Chris said gently, sitting beside her. "But honestly? I'm not. You're working from home. We're careful. We wear masks. We clean everything. And you've got your family around you."

Her mother returned, handing her a steaming cup of tea. "Exactly. No need to let fear steal your joy. You're bringing a life into this world, that's a blessing, not a burden."

Ivanna took the cup, her fingers wrapping around the warmth.

"I am thankful to all of you," she whispered, her eyes misting. "I feel lucky. Really lucky."

One day after another, the last trimester passed. And before she could realize it, it was time for Ivanna to be admitted into labor. Chris and she were both first tested for COVID, and a screening test was conducted. After an hour, the results came back, and they proved to be negative. At that time, Ivanna's main concern was whether Chris would be permitted to join her. Fortunately, after receiving his negative COVID results, he was allowed to accompany her to the delivery room, although he had to wear a mask while Ivanna did not need to.

Compared to many stories she'd heard, her delivery was surprisingly smooth. Surely, the pain of delivering a baby was there, and Ivanna was tired. However, she had been ready for this moment. Her excitement eclipsed any exhaustion or pain.

The hospital room was quiet, dimly lit except for the soft glow from the monitor beside the bed. Ivanna shifted carefully in the bed, wincing just slightly as she settled into a more comfortable position. Chris sat beside her, one hand resting on the edge of the bassinet, the other still clutching the mask he had just taken off.

"Katie's so tiny," he whispered, looking down at their newborn daughter, bundled up in a pale pink blanket.

Ivanna smiled with a glow on her face that only new mothers had. "I keep thinking she's going to open her eyes and just… tell us who she is."

There was a knock on the door, and a nurse stepped in. Chris quickly pulled his mask back on.

"Just checking in," the nurse said with a warm smile. "Everything looks great. Let me know if you need anything."

When the door closed behind her, Ivanna sighed. "It's strange," she murmured. "I imagined this room full of people. My mom, my sister, maybe even some of my aunts. But now it's just… us."

Chris glanced at her. "Is that a bad thing?"

She hesitated. "No. Not bad. Just not what I pictured. I mean, it's peaceful. No chaos, no crowd, just space to breathe. That's been nice. But I also wanted Katie to be surrounded by love from the moment she got here. And now it's like...the world has to meet her through phone screens."

He reached for her hand and gave it a gentle squeeze. “She’ll be loved either way. And she’ll meet everyone eventually.”

“Eventually,” Ivanna repeated quietly, then looked at her daughter again. “I still worry, you know? Even with the vaccines. Even with masks. It’s like I’m always second-guessing whether it’s safe for Katie to be near people. I want to show her off. I want to walk down the street with the stroller and not flinch when someone leans in to say hello.”

“You will,” he said.

After a day under observation, they were allowed to take Katie home. Ivanna had not taken maternity leave from work. She had decided to continue working. However, she had taken a week off to regain her health, while Chris still had to return to work. As soon as they returned home, they sanitized themselves and the entire house before Chris locked himself in the study to work.

Ivanna took Katie into the bedroom and called her mother and siblings on Zoom. All of them greeted the new angel with big smiles and excitement. They wished to share that moment with Ivanna, and they longed to hold the baby. Her parents promised to visit her soon.

A week passed, and Ivanna began working again. She could easily manage childcare along with work and was extremely grateful for such an opportunity. One evening, after they had finished their tasks, Ivanna and Chris sat in their bedroom with Katie, marveling at her.

Ivanna stroked her baby’s hair, which was just beginning to grow in. “Working from home has helped a lot, you know. I can move things around, take breaks when I need to. It’s given me time to be with her in ways I might not have had otherwise. But I miss my family. I wish our daughter could meet them. I wish we could have a baby shower, and everyone would love her. Yet, I am also grateful that during this pandemic, she is safe and secure without many hands touching her.”

Chris leaned back on his pillow. “So... positive and negative?”

Ivanna gave a short laugh. “Exactly. Less people around means less germs, less stress. But it also means less warmth, less joy.”

There was a quiet moment between them, filled only by the occasional rustling of the wind through the open window.

"I guess what I'm saying," Ivanna said softly, "is that I don't regret anything. It wasn't what I expected, but it was still good. Everyone was kind at the hospital as well. I felt cared for. I feel safe with you. But there's nothing that can replace the family."

"You are right, sweetheart," Chris said, looking at their daughter sleeping peacefully. "But she's safe now, too. Focus on the bright side."

Ivanna reached down and ran a fingertip gently over her daughter's cheek. "I just hope the world becomes a little kinder soon. So, she can grow up surrounded by people. By real faces. Not just eyes behind masks."

She didn't say all of what she felt out loud, but it lingered in her thoughts: that she wanted her daughter to know a world that felt open again, where connections weren't filtered through worry.

For now, though, the three of them were together. And that, for Ivanna, was enough.

A few days later, after spending a week in quarantine, her parents and siblings came to visit her. They all ensured they were virus-free before meeting the newborn. Ivanna's excitement was through the roof. Everyone cooed at and gently held the baby, showering her with warm hugs. They also brought along a variety of gifts. Staying with Ivanna for a couple of days, they helped her with household chores to ease her burden. Before leaving, they all hugged and kissed her, promising to return soon. Their departure left a void in Ivanna's heart, yet she was grateful.

Her postpartum period unfolded as one of her fondest memories. She didn't have to leave work; she could be with Katie constantly, making it easier for her to handle everything and remain rested. Additionally, her family frequently visited her. Despite adhering to a set of guidelines and safety measures, she appreciated the benefits she received. All in all, it was a win-win situation.

13
Emily

Emily Murphy gave birth to her third child right in the middle of the pandemic. Life had been reshaped into something foreign and uncertain, but this child, this tiny life, was planned.

She and her partner had always dreamed of having three children. They had waited patiently through the anxious bloom of spring in 2020, watching the world tip on its axis, before deciding that summer felt safe enough, or at least safer, to try.

They conceived in October. Emily remembered the moment clearly, not in the clinical sense, but in the way her heart had thudded with cautious hope mixed with fear.

Pandemic Pregnancy. It felt as if the title had been plastered on her forehead, warning her each day that she had to be more careful than others. That others would need to take better care of her.

But the happy parents were ready. Or as ready as anyone could be when the air itself felt poisoned.

At that time, Emily was teaching at a high school and had a student teacher to help share the workload. Thanksgiving break was just around the corner. She had assumed they would continue teaching remotely after the break, as they had been. However, the school announced a return to in-person instruction. The announcement was casual, part of an email whose subject line only read "Post-Thanksgiving School Update."

Her heart dropped when she read the email. She tried to ready herself, to tell her body that everything was fine. But it wasn't, not for her.

"It's like... my body just isn't cooperating anymore," she whispered that evening to her husband, Andy, as they sat side by side on the couch. "I feel it in a physical way. The stress. It's like it lives inside me. I don't know what to do. I feel so stressed that I'm sure I won't even have a good time during the holidays."

Andy had reassured her and promised her that all would be well. But Emily could not help it. She had cried while carving the turkey, and wept while taking her shower before bed.

She tried to convince herself that she could handle it all, summoning the strength to return to the classroom. But each morning, the anxiety threatened to overwhelm her. As the day she was due back at school neared, her chest would tighten as she imagined the masks, the shifting protocols, the students who came from families that didn't, or couldn't, follow the rules. How much risk was too much?

Then she decided she had to try. Try to keep her baby safe.

She sought medical approval to teach from home. For a brief moment, she thought it might work. The doctor stated clearly that being indoors and near children would be a significant risk.

But the school's administration denied her request.

Her breath caught when she received the final answer. All hope vanished.

"Then I think I'm done," she told Andy. "I can't do it anymore. I will definitely get COVID if I start teaching in person!"

"I think that would be for the best. You don't have to worry about anything. I got it."

She smiled.

"You concentrate on taking care of the kids and of yourself. And of course, our little one. Everything else comes second."

Together, they made the decision. Emily would step away from the classroom. It wasn't easy. She felt like she was abandoning her students. Her heart was heavy.

"I feel guilty," she admitted, pressing her palm to her chest. "But I also know… I know I can't keep going like this." She had been having panic attacks regularly at this point, and she knew that would not be good for anyone. Her family needed her.

Slowly, clarity began to take root. After many panicked conversations with her husband, calls to her mother, and appointments with her doctor, she decided she no longer needed to justify it. Choosing her health and her baby's safety wasn't a weakness. It was the right decision.

Once she made it, she reflected on what her students were going through. Many of her students had reached out to her while school had been shifted online. Teenagers had been stripped of their social circles, their structure, and their sense of safety. There were more suicides. A noticeable rise in mental health struggles. Even the strongest ones seemed to be completely lost. Emily knew that she was not alone in her mental health struggles, but she also knew she was privileged. She had a home. She had financial stability. And most of all, she had a loving, supportive family.

After having experienced yet another panic attack, she stood at the kitchen sink, staring out the window as her children played in the backyard. They screamed and laughed without a care in the world. Emily always loved that they could still play outdoors, even though she wished she could take them to the zoo, parks, and museums.

Life during the pandemic had been a balancing act; it was an unrelenting, exhausting game of risk assessment. Her youngest child's genetic disorder added another layer to the already towering stack of concerns. Every sneeze, every errand, every decision seemed fraught with potential consequences. There was no room for error.

"It's like living in a constant state of fear," she thought. *"Like I'm trying to keep spinning plates in the air, and I can't afford to let a single one fall."*

Everyone kept telling her that she was doing a great job. She was managing her home and taking care of her kids, all while pregnant. But nothing felt enough. She was constantly worried, continually stressed, and always sad.

At some point, Emily had to let her guard down. She needed help, especially with childcare. She was stretched thin.

She remembered the decision clearly. The fear. The guilt. And the necessity.

"I couldn't do it alone anymore," she admitted to a friend over a distanced video call. "I let someone come help with the kids. I had to."

"Oh, your mom?" Cindy asked.

"No, a nanny."

"Must be expensive."

"It is."

"Well, that's okay. You're pregnant. You need it now."

"Yeah. I just wish I could do it all on my own."

They talked some more, but the conversation left Emily drained. Recently, Emily had not only been sad but also angry. She was afraid that anger could one day be directed at her kids. And that was the last thing she ever wanted. She knew that part of it was because she had no personal space. She always had to perform and be the best mom she could be. But at times, she fell short. She knew the nanny would not help with the personal space issue, but that was something that she decided could take a backseat for now.

The nanny did help greatly. It meant that there was one more person in the house to pick up the slack. But Emily did not feel any less alone.

She did not even get to have Andy by her side at prenatal appointments.

But this wasn't her first rodeo. It was her third pregnancy, and the familiarity of it brought an unexpected steadiness. She knew what to do and how to do it. She knew that part; she could handle it on her own.

Still, there was something raw about going through it solo. She split herself down the middle, logical on one side, emotional on the other. It was survival mode, plain and simple. She had to become a survivalist, and the fact that she had to maintain her dual personalities was threatening to overwhelm her.

Regardless, there was some unexpected peace. Emily had always been a homebody, someone who didn't crave social gatherings or houseguests. The enforced distance brought her a strange kind of relief. Her home was her and her family's sanctuary, and she vowed that no matter what, she would make it so that she loved being home. She decided to redecorate, ordering items for her home online. She spent days making sure it all looked perfect. She cleaned often and thoroughly, sometimes to distract from her racing thoughts and other times just because she loved her home.

"It's...quiet," she told Andy one evening as they shared a quiet meal after putting the kids to bed. "And kind of beautiful, isn't it?"

He looked up from his plate, smiling. “It’s us. Just us.”

That quiet became a cocoon. Without visitors popping in and out, without the pressure of outside expectations, the Murphy family had space to simply be. There were no grandparent drop-ins, no well-meaning but overwhelming offers of help that often created more stress than support. The solitude allowed them to draw closer, to become a stronger unit.

“This pregnancy...it feels different,” she told her sister on a phone call. “More exciting, somehow. Like we’re ready. Like this little one is joining something complete.”

She couldn’t explain it fully, but there was a quiet confidence growing in her, in Andy, in their children. The storm of the world raged outside, but inside their home, they had carved out a safe haven. And perhaps that, more than anything else, was what made this pregnancy feel so profound. Now more than ever, they felt like one unit, one family.

Even so, even with all of the good, there was still a whole lot of bad. Her mental health was at an all-time low. She tried to focus on the joy of new life, but Emily couldn't ignore the worry that came with being pregnant during a global pandemic. It was like wearing her "Mom Hat" and her "Survivor Hat" at the same time, only her head was not big enough; it fit the two, and she kept losing her balance.

Every day brought questions she had no real answers to.

What if I get sick? What if the baby does? What if I bring it home to the kids?

With each passing week of her pregnancy, she clung to one belief: the longer she could stay home with her children, the better. Being close to them gave her comfort.

When it was finally time to go to the hospital to give birth, her anxiety surprised her. She’d imagined it would be a moment of relief, but instead, she found herself counting the hours until she could leave again. The hospital itself was lovely, modern, clean, quiet, and the staff were gentle and attentive, wearing their masks like armor and treating her with care.

“It was really nice,” she told Andy. “But I couldn’t wait to get out of there. I just wanted to be home.”

Home, where her world felt safe and familiar.

The postpartum period, oddly enough, was the smoothest it had ever been for her. Summer softened the edges of everything, the light, the routine, even her mood.

Compared to her earlier postpartum experiences, this time felt more balanced. The "baby blues" that had lingered like a cloud after her previous deliveries seemed to lift faster this time. Whether Andy didn’t notice them or they truly weren't as intense, she wasn’t sure. Maybe it was both.

But sleep deprivation was still the thief it had always been. That was always the case with newborns. She was lucky if she had more than three hours of sleep a night.

There were moments Emily’s exhaustion tipped into what she jokingly, but not without truth, called "mama rage." She decided that she needed help for that and sought mental health help.

“I’d be standing there, holding a crying baby, and I’d just...snap,” she admitted to her therapist during a virtual session. “Not at anyone. Just inside. Boiling.”

Yet she steadied herself more quickly now. She felt more aware of her limits and better at protecting her peace. She supposed that was what happened with more experience. This was Baby Number Three, and she already knew the ropes. Now she could climb out of tough spots more easily.

One thing that had surprisingly helped her was online shopping. No chaotic store trips. No, dragging a newborn through fluorescent aisles. Just click, add to cart, confirm, and wait.

“I should’ve done this with the first two,” she muttered more than once as packages arrived at their door like magic.

What bothered her the most during her postpartum was her family. Her family didn’t seem to worry much, if at all, about the pandemic. They had that stubborn, old-school belief that bad things happen to other people, not to them.

Her father had been more upset about not being able to hold his new grandchild than about anything else going on in the world. It wore on her nerves.

Her in-laws, by contrast, understood. Andy's grandfather had been one of the early casualties of COVID. They knew what was at stake. His family approached the situation with respect and care. Masks always remained on, visits were spaced out, and every hug was replaced with a wave or a smile from six feet away. Emily appreciated their support, their understanding. It made things easier. She wished her own family could have acted in the same way.

Andy, especially, had been her rock. From the moment they saw the second pink line on the test, he was all in, confident, calm, and entirely thrilled. He had encouraged her to take the baby's entire first year off from work. He was adamant that the kids, especially the baby, needed their mom home and safe.

And because of that support, Emily felt herself ease into motherhood again, this time with less resistance and more joy. No lesson plans to prepare. No early morning rush. Just her, her children.

Looking back, she felt no regrets.

She had wanted her children to be close in age, and the bond between them was already forming - giggly, chaotic, and loving. The experience had been challenging, yes, but also beautiful. In its own strange way, the pandemic had stripped away the noise, revealing something quiet and whole beneath it.

14
Evelyn

Evelyn Vaughn stood at the kitchen counter, staring out the frosted window as the early morning light glistened on the steel windowsill. A small stick lay on the counter behind her, just barely visible beside the coffee mugs.

"It's blue," she said softly.

Her husband, Kevin, stepped into the kitchen holding his phone and a mug of tea. He paused mid-step. "What?"

She turned, her eyes wide but calm. "The test. It's blue."

He set the mug down and walked over, almost too slowly, as if afraid the moment might crack if he moved too fast. Then he saw it. The pale blue cross on the pregnancy test. For a second, he didn't say anything. Then, his lips broke into a big grin, and he wrapped her in a hug so tight she had to remind him, laughing, "Okay, don't squish the baby already."

"C'mon! It must only be a couple of cells right now." They laughed again.

They had planned for this. Every bit of it. A couple of years earlier, they'd left their apartment in California, said goodbye to palm trees and crowded highways, and moved east. They wanted to be closer to family, closer to the quiet. They'd found a small town upstate New York, bought a house with creaky floorboards and a wide porch, and planted roots.

They had transformed the house into a home, ready to start a new family life. And now, they were expecting.

Then the world shut down.

The pandemic rolled across the world like a slow-moving storm. Lockdowns, rising case numbers, and overwhelmed hospitals. Evelyn stopped going into the office. Kevin's job shifted to a fully remote setting. Grocery stores emptied, and plans dissolved into questions.

"Well," Kevin said one evening, staring at their shared calendar on the fridge, "I guess we're having a baby in a pandemic."

Evelyn smirked. "Perfect timing, right?"

But she wasn't bitter. They'd waited for this. They'd built everything around this goal. "We just didn't factor in global disaster," she muttered once, folding baby clothes on the couch. They had started doing a little online shopping for the baby, which was a convenient service.

Pregnancy during lockdown became a quiet affair. Days passed slowly. She filled them with classical music. Vivaldi in the mornings, Mozart in the evenings, and books she read aloud to the baby in her belly, half for the baby, half to keep herself anchored.

They thought of the pandemic in thirty-day chunks. Just get through this month. Then the next. "Thirty-day bites," Evelyn called them. It helped. So did the calm of the shifting seasons and the stillness that ruled the world. She felt blessed that she got to stay home and avoid spending her pregnancy commuting back and forth to work.

Her family, all close by now, checked in regularly. Many of them were in medicine, and their caution helped ease her worries. Although visits were rare, they made sure to strictly quarantine themselves before visiting her and wore masks to ensure the baby's safety as well.

Evelyn was private by nature. She didn't want anyone near the baby unless she felt it in her bones that it was right.

Time passed steadily, and soon January came. Snow piled up along the streets, and Evelyn went into labor during a quiet, sharp cold snap.

In the delivery room, she wore a mask. So did Kevin. So did everyone. But it didn't bother her. She had become quite comfortable with the mask since it had been almost a year since the lockdown began.

"If this helps protect the baby's first breath," she told a nurse, "Then I'm happy to wear ten of them."

When the baby finally came, wrapped tight in warm, soft blankets and blinking at the dim lights, Evelyn cried quietly. Kevin stood beside her, holding her hand. Outside, the wind pushed snow across the empty streets. Inside, it was warm.

They brought their daughter home with extra care and caution. That day, when Kevin's mother asked what they would name her, Evelyn said instantly, 'Clara.'"

For the next few months, they barely left the house. It was still winter, and no one expected them to do anything but stay home. Evelyn was grateful. It gave them space to be alone, just the three of them, learning from each other and exploring. She and Kevin took turns rocking Clara to sleep. Evelyn sang old folk songs, some her mother had sung to her, and Kevin read aloud from dog-eared paperbacks while the baby dozed soundly on his chest.

Groceries arrived at the front door. Evelyn always tipped high because she always felt guilty that while they were safe in their homes, these deliverymen risked their lives daily to provide service.

"Someone else has to walk through those aisles for me," she said once, watching a delivery van pull away. "I think about that a lot."

By spring, the vaccine brought hope. Buds appeared on the trees outside their house. They expanded their bubble, carefully. A walk with friends. A visit to the park. Clara met more faces, but only the ones Evelyn felt sure about.

Her family continued to call, always gentle, always understanding, and cautious as ever.

"They know we're living small right now," Evelyn told Kevin when he suggested that now they should be open to more gatherings. "They get it."

Kevin was steady and thoughtful. When Evelyn spiraled with fear and overwhelming thoughts, when the news felt too heavy, he didn't offer solutions. He just listened. Even when she was pregnant and would react unreasonably to some situations, he would give her time and validate her emotions.

He felt like he needed to be "the rock" for their family, and he was. He would offer her comforting words to help her feel at ease. "You're doing great," he would whisper softly at night, gently brushing hair from her forehead whenever she experienced discomfort while sleeping during her pregnancy. "We're okay."

Throughout the pregnancy and the postpartum period, they talked about everything. The risks, the exhaustion, the guilt, the joy.

"We built this life," Evelyn said one night, looking around the nursery where Clara was sleeping. "It took a few years. But we made it."

Kevin nodded. "Yeah. We made it."

And they had.

By the time Clara was four months old, the world felt warmer. Literally and figuratively. Spring had transformed into a hot summer. Vaccines were rolling out. Parks were open again. Sidewalks were dotted with strollers and coffee cups. There was a sense, if not of safety, then of hope.

One evening, Evelyn pushed the stroller beneath the shade of maple trees. Clara dozed under the soft canopy of the stroller; her tiny fists relaxed against her chest. Evelyn and Kevin walked slowly, breathing in the scent of sun-warmed grass and basking in the golden hour.

"It's different now," she told Kevin as they watched their daughter sleep, her toys rattling in a small compartment in the stroller.

He nodded, feet kicking a stone off the sidewalk. "Feels like things are getting better."

The time went by smoothly, and by the time Clara was three months old, Evelyn stood again in the upstairs bathroom, holding another pregnancy test.

It was positive.

She stared at it, then let out a single breath, half disbelief, half wonder.

When she told Kevin, he blinked. "Already?"

She laughed. "I mean...not already. It feels right. Doesn't it?"

He crossed the room, hugged her from behind, and rested a hand on her stomach, where life had just begun again.

"I don't know what normal is anymore," he said quietly, "but this feels like a good light."

Both of them went out of the bathroom and called their families to deliver the good news.

Everyone was surprised, to say the least.

Two babies, back-to-back. Less than a year apart. But for Evelyn and Kevin, it didn't feel rushed. It felt natural. It felt like the next step in a story they had started writing long ago.

That summer between her two pregnancies, they slowed down. Evelyn's workload had eased as she decided to resume work and achieve a work-life balance. The world was still cautious, still uncertain, but it had opened up just enough to allow for long afternoons in the yard, bare feet in the grass, and quiet dinners on the porch. Both of them still spent their sweet time with Clara.

Evelyn's second pregnancy was going smoothly, and soon, autumn arrived. Clara sat in her high chair beneath the shade of the maple tree, gumming slices of peach while Evelyn lay on a picnic blanket beside her, hand on her belly, eyes closed against the sun.

"I don't want to forget this part," she said to Kevin. "The in-between. It's peaceful."

He glanced up from where he was helping Clara with her peach slices. "You won't forget. You live too fully to forget. Moreover, these naughty babies won't let you forget any of it," he said as he pinched Clara's cheek.

As the months passed, Evelyn's workload became increasingly arduous.

She had taken a few months of remote work after Clara's birth, easing back in slowly, but once the second trimester hit, she found herself boarding planes, standing in boardrooms, and shaking hands. All of it was back again. The heels. Lipstick. Business cards tucked into sleek bags.

It was exhausting.

She sat in hotel rooms late at night, reading client briefs, pumping breast milk, and checking in on Clara over FaceTime. Sometimes she cried in the quiet. Sometimes she didn't even have time to do that.

But she remained determined and steady.

"I need to prove I can still be that person," she said to her sister on the phone one night. "I want to be a great mom, but I also want to show them I haven't disappeared. I really thought I could be a great working mother who could balance work and family both."

"Maybe you don't need to prove anything," her sister replied gently. "Maybe you just need to become more of who you are. You have this determination in you, and I know you can do it."

The second pregnancy wasn't any easier on her than the first.

There was no lockdown, no snowstorm silence. She was a mother now, already split in two, one part work, one part home.

But there was still joy. She walked often, took Clara on long stroller rides on the weekends, talking aloud to the baby growing inside her.

"This world's messy," she whispered to her unborn one afternoon, "but we'll take care of you just like we did before with your sister."

Amidst fleeting moments of calm and chaos, her second pregnancy came to a close, and she delivered her second baby on February 8, 2022.

Just like her first, the second hospital birth was uneventful, and for that, Evelyn was grateful. The first time, there was uncertainty. Protocols were changing weekly, and doctors were moving quickly behind masks. The second time, things were more stable. But still, her mind wasn't just on the newborn this time. It was on Clara too.

"Will she feel forgotten?" she whispered to Kevin, the day after their second child was born.

"Not for a second," he said. "We're expanding her world, not replacing it."

They named the baby Miles. Evelyn held him in the crook of her arm, the hospital room quiet, soft beeping somewhere behind her.

"We're four now," she whispered. "Look what we made."

In the months that followed, life became a balancing act.

Two children under two. Work was creeping back in. A pandemic still lingering at the edges of things. But Evelyn and Kevin stayed rooted. Careful. Focused.

They still sanitized everything and still limited visits. They made sure each choice considered the health and safety of the smallest members of their home.

Some days were so hard that they didn't even have time to talk. Some nights were so sleepless that they had to talk to each other to pass the waves of insomnia. But there was laughter in between, bubbly and messy and constant. There were early mornings with coffee on the porch and babies in their laps, birds singing in the background before they set off for work.

One evening, Clara ambled through the grass, giggling, while Evelyn held Miles and watched the sunset paint the sky in hues of gold and lavender. She took in the view before her eyes. Her daughter was happily running toward them, her son in her arms, staring at the birds flying above, and her husband, her rock, still standing strong by her side.

"Would I do it again?" she asked out loud, half to herself.

Kevin, beside her, smiled. "Would you?"

She thought for a long moment, then nodded. "Not the pandemic part, probably. But the rest? Absolutely."

They hadn't imagined this version of the story. They'd had a different script in mind. But they had adapted, changed course, and grown together.

There had been bumps, yes. But the road had led them here. And Evelyn wouldn't change a thing about it.

15
Tessa

Tessa Preston and her husband, Adrian, sat in silence under the bare oak tree. The bench was cold, and the February air was chilly. It was their comfort spot. Whenever life got tough and they needed to figure things out, they would sit on this bench and listen to each other and the sounds of nature.

Adrian had just lost his job, and with a growing fetus in Tessa's belly, everything in front of them seemed to blur. They were almost down for the count by the end of the first trimester when Adrian received the grim email from his employers.

Dear Employees,

It is regrettable to announce that, due to current circumstances, we must shut down our firm. You must all be aware of how we have been struggling financially for the past few months. Without holding you all back, we wish you all a bright and prosperous future ahead.

Warm regards,

CEO

The dread had still not left his mind as he sat with his wife to figure out what to do next. Adrian's hands were stuffed deep in his coat pockets. He was staring straight ahead, not quite at anything. Tessa glanced sideways at him. Her hand instinctively rested over her growing belly, barely a curve yet, but already a weight she carried day and night.

"I know we planned this," Tessa said, her voice more fragile than she intended. "But I still panicked when the test turned positive."

"I did too," Adrian admitted, eyes still staring ahead. "And then I lost the job, and… yeah."

Everything had unraveled so fast. The pandemic had swept through like a fog no one saw coming, shuttering offices, cancelling appointments, closing doors that had always seemed permanently open. Adrian's company had folded practically overnight. Just like that, the security they'd counted on was gone.

And now, there was this baby. A wanted baby. A longed-for baby. But Tessa couldn't shake the anxiety. She thought she had planned this baby too soon out of the fear that "her clock was ticking." She loved kids, that was no lie, and that was why she wanted to have another one before her age caught up with her.

"It's different this time," she murmured. "With the boys, we had routines. Appointments were shared. You got to hear the heartbeat too, remember? And this time, we'd be on a tight budget as well, since we'll only have my income to rely on."

Adrian nodded. "I thought the company would recover from the losses. I thought it would all be fine. But I promise you I will try to look for another job as soon as possible."

Tessa sighed. "It feels like I'm doing this one alone. Finances aside, I'll have to go to the doctor's office alone for visits as well."

He turned toward her then, finally. "You're not. It's neither of our faults. We can't fight the system, right? If it were allowed by the doctor's office, you know I would love to accompany you."

"I know," she said, and she did. In the deepest part of her, she knew Adrian was trying. He was the one making breakfast for the boys every morning now, the one patching the leaky faucet, the one scouring job boards late into the night. He was always doing his best to be the rock for his family. However, this pregnancy still felt quieter. More fragile.

Even at home, everyone tiptoed. Her mother called every day, voice laced with worry. One day, asking if she'd gotten the vaccine yet, the next day begging her to wait. Tessa had stopped answering calls sometimes, letting them go to voicemail.

Her father, usually so sure-footed, had confessed one evening, "I don't know what's safest anymore, Tess. The rules keep changing."

The boys, just six and four years old, didn't fully understand. "Is the baby coming in a mask?" her youngest had asked seriously at dinner.

Tessa had laughed so hard she cried. Or maybe she'd cried so hard she laughed.

"We're going to be okay," Adrian said now, his voice low and certain.

"Are we?"

He didn't answer immediately. "I think so. I hope so. We've done hard things before."

She looked at him. His eyes were tired. But still kind. Still full of love for her.

"I guess we'll find out," she said.

They stayed there a while longer. Letting the silence hold them. The wind tugged at Tessa's scarf, but she didn't fix it. Her hand stayed on her belly, cradling the small life growing inside her. That evening, in the middle of February, even amidst problems and chaos, they still had each other.

And somewhere deep beneath the layers of fear, something else stirred: resolve. She *could* do this. She *was* doing it. Maybe not with hospital rooms full of family or hand-holding at every appointment, but with strength she hadn't known she had.

Tessa Preston stood, her hand outstretched toward Adrian. "Let's go home."

He took her hand and stood beside her, and together they walked back to their home, to their boys who must have turned the house upside down by now.

The earth continued to revolve, the pandemic persisted, months passed, and Adrian had found a new job. Their family was doing well again when Tessa's third trimester came to an end. It was definitely different from the last two times because of the uncertainty and fear in the air caused by the virus and the rising death tolls.

Tessa was the most worried when she was giving birth to her third child. She was ready to take a bullet to her chest, but feared the tiny virus that might affect her new daughter. She would not be able to bear it.

Her hospital room felt more like a sealed chamber than a place where new life began. The windows looked out onto the grey city skyline, but the room inside was cramped, with just four sterile walls, an uncomfortable hospital bed, and a small bassinet where her newborn daughter now slept, swaddled tightly.

Visitors were prohibited. No flowers. No hugs from her sons. Only muted voices behind masks and the constant clatter of gurneys and carts rolling down the hallway.

Adrian sat across the room on a narrow vinyl chair. He'd barely left her side since they'd arrived, but every time someone knocked and entered, be it a nurse, a tech, or a doctor, he had to mask up, even when holding the baby. Tessa hated that part most. Watching her husband cradle their daughter with a layer of fabric between them. They could not even kiss her.

"You're getting used to her already," she whispered, watching Adrian adjust their daughter in his arms.

He smiled behind the mask. "She's perfect," he said. "And tiny."

"How about we name her Hope? What do you say?" Tessa asked as she watched Adrian lightly brushing the baby's cheeks.

"I think it's perfect," Adrian smiled and kissed Hope's tiny fingers.

Tessa did not need to explain the symbol or meaning behind that name. They both had been through the toil of the virus together. Their daughter was the silver lining amidst the darkest clouds, the light shining at the end of the tunnel, the first bright ray of sunshine after a dark night. She was the *hope* that no matter how hard times get, the ending is always beautiful. Beautiful like their daughter.

Tessa's eyes drifted toward the door. The past few minutes were still fresh in her memory. Hours earlier, she'd overheard a nurse whispering in the hallway, her voice tense: *"The woman in 208 just tested positive. We'll need to double up on precautions."*

Her room was 209. Room 208 was just next door.

Her chest tightened. She and that woman had the same nurse.

"They must've changed clothes between deliveries," she said out loud for the third time that day.

Adrian glanced at her. "Of course they did."

"But what if—what if she didn't disinfect something properly? Or if it was on her hands? Or her badge, or—" Tessa paused, closed her eyes, and exhaled hard. Her eyes opened slowly and went to her daughter's frail body. So small. So defenseless.

The nurse, kind-eyed and calm, had reassured her earlier. "We follow very strict protocols," she'd said, her voice muffled behind the double-layered mask and face shield. "Your baby is safe, Mrs. Preston."

But fear didn't care about protocol. It curled around Tessa like a fog, whispering worst-case scenarios. Hope's immune system was new. Adrian's job was still uncertain. The pandemic hadn't slowed. There were still so many unknowns.

And then, there was the question she kept circling back to, the one that seemed to divide every conversation these days: *Vaccinate or not?*

Her mother had called again that morning. "Tess, are you sure you're going to take it? While breastfeeding? Are you sure it's safe?"

The truth was, she wasn't. Not fully. She had read articles, spoken to doctors, and tried to weigh the risk. But the data was thin, and everyone seemed to have a different opinion. Even the nurses on labor and delivery avoided the topic when she asked.

"I just want to keep her safe," she whispered, holding her daughter and brushing a thumb across her soft cheek.

"I know," Adrian said. "Me too."

Her eyes met his over the top of his mask. They'd both aged during this pregnancy, more mentally than physically. The months of worry had etched fine lines around their eyes. The stress of not knowing what was right or wrong. The ache of isolation. The weight of choices they'd never had to make before.

"I miss the boys," Tessa said.

"Me too. They FaceTimed with your mom this morning. They were showing her how they made a 'Welcome Baby' sign for the front door."

She smiled at that, but her chest still ached. She wanted to hug them. Let them meet their sister. Let life feel normal again.

But nothing about this was normal.

They stayed another day in the hospital, confined to the same room, where Adrian slept on the stiff chair and Tessa barely slept at all. Each time a nurse entered, the mask went on. Each time a monitor beeped in the hallway, her heart skipped. Every decision, whether to breastfeed post-vaccine, whether to let grandparents visit later, whether to trust the rules or keep making their own, felt enormous.

By the time they were discharged, the weight of responsibility had settled like bricks in her chest. Yet as Adrian wheeled her out, Hope in arms, Tessa felt an epiphany dawn on her.

A kind of warm hug from the heavens.

She realized that she had carried a child through a pandemic. Given birth through fear. Faced uncertainty and still found a way to keep moving forward. She felt like an invincible woman, a mother.

At the hospital exit, the dry August air met them like an old friend. They sat in the car and kept the A/C off to keep Hope warm.

"We made it through the hard part," Adrian said softly.

Tessa looked down at her daughter's pink face, nestled against her chest. "One hard part," she corrected gently. "But we'll get through the rest, too."

Adrian knew she was referring to the upcoming days of the postpartum period. He would be working from home, but wouldn't be able to help her much since he had just started his new job and couldn't request paternity leave. It would also be challenging for her to manage their two sons.

Upon returning home, they were met with joyful cheers and "Welcome Baby" banners, which the boys had enthusiastically decorated. They marveled at the adorable banners. Tessa desperately wanted to hug them, but first, she needed to take a bath and rid herself of any trace of the virus.

The days after bringing Hope home, Tessa settled into a gentle routine, quieter than Tessa had ever known in the early days of motherhood. The virus was still disrupting the world, still raising the questions that no one could fully understand, but inside their home, a kind of peace had formed.

This time, there were no unexpected visits. No distant relatives asking to come hold the baby. No need to explain boundaries. This time, everyone already knew. That, to Tessa, was an unexpected blessing.

In her past postpartum experiences, she had felt like she was being pulled in every direction, hosting well-wishers, coordinating visits, letting others hold the baby before she was ready. But now, the silence was soothing. No one reached out to touch her belly in the aisles of the grocery store during her pregnancy. No one questioned her choice to stay home. For once, her space was hers.

"It's kind of strange," she told Adrian one night while feeding Hope in their dim living room, "but I love this peace. I love just being...us."

He smiled, cradling a mug of tea, his laptop open beside him. "We're in a bubble," he said.

"And I like it that way."

Adrian had started a new job just weeks before their daughter was born. It didn't offer paternity leave, and his schedule was busy, full of virtual meetings and unfamiliar names. But he worked from home, and in the little moments between calls, he was there. Helping her with lunch. Rocking Hope while answering emails. Sitting beside her on the couch, even if only for a minute. It wasn't perfect, but it was something. Tessa was grateful for that.

Their boys went back to daycare in the fall. It gave her breathing room, space to learn her daughter's cues, to nap when she could, to feel a little more like herself. She had resumed working after giving birth. And her job, too, allowed her to stay home. She could care for Hope, meet deadlines, and take breaks when her body needed rest.

The pandemic, for all its fear and unknowns, had made space where before there had been none.

Tessa often reflected on how different it all felt this time. With her first two children, there had been joy, yes, but also chaos. The pressure to entertain, to share, to include others in every milestone. This time, there was stillness. She could lie on the couch with her daughter on her chest and just *be*. No expectations, no obligations.

She remembered her mother saying, back when Hope was still in her belly, "It's a hard time, honey. But maybe it's also the right time."

She hadn't believed it then. But now, watching her daughter sleep, the house quiet around them, she did.

What had once terrified her—the timing, the uncertainty, the looming question of "What if?"—had turned into something rare. A time to slow down. To bond. To learn her baby's cues. To watch her boys become responsible brothers, their tiny fingers gently stroking their sister's hair.

Yes, there had been worry. So much of it. She still remembered how unsure everyone was at the hospital, how even the doctors admitted they didn't have all the answers. The vaccine questions. The safety protocols. The haunting unknowns of a virus still being studied. She had spent many nights awake, wondering if she was doing everything right. Wondering what "right" even meant anymore.

But through all of it, one truth had remained clear: she needed this baby. She needed *Hope.*

"I didn't feel complete before her," she admitted one afternoon during a quiet call with her sister. "I didn't know I was waiting for her, but I was."

She didn't regret the fear. Or the timing. Or the long, anxious nights. Because the joy outweighed it, the gratitude settled deep in her bones. She was happy. She was whole.

If she had to do it all over again, even in the middle of a pandemic, she would. Because the pandemic hadn't just changed the world, it had changed her home. It had brought them inward, closer. More aware of what truly mattered.

Hope stirred, stretching in her bassinet. A soft cry escaped her tiny lips.

Tessa crossed the room, picked her up, and held her close, inhaling the warm, newborn scent.

She smiled.

She was exactly where she needed to be.

16
Melissa

Melissa Bennett had always wished, hoped, and prayed for those two lines to appear on a pregnancy test. What she hadn't imagined was seeing it during a global pandemic.

She stood quietly in the bathroom, the stick trembling slightly in her hand. Her breath caught. She blinked.

"Doug?" she called softly.

From the hallway came her husband's footsteps, quick and light. He saw the test, then her face, and then his whole expression shifted.

"You're pregnant?" he whispered, staring at the test in disbelief. "But… how?"

She nodded, barely able to smile through the tears that suddenly spilled over. "I'm really pregnant."

They hugged, tighter than either of them expected. Because behind that joy was a history, a story of doctor appointments, lab results, hormone shots, and a conversation, months earlier about starting IVF. They had just begun the process when everything came to a screeching halt.

COVID-19.

The doctor's office closed. Appointments were postponed indefinitely. Hope was paused. But then, somehow, this.

"I don't know how," she whispered into Doug's shirt, as he held her, "but it happened. On its own. It happened."

"It's a miracle," he said.

And it was.

Despite the joy, their pregnancy was laced with anxiety. Melissa, ever cautious, took no chances. She wiped down every surface, sanitized packages at the front door, and never went anywhere without her mask. Even as the weeks passed and her belly grew, she maintained distance from everyone, even family.

"I have waited for this for so long," she whispered to herself as she opened the door on her way to work. "There is no way I'm risking it."

As a middle school teacher, her biggest concern became her students. So many kids were often sick. So many who could be potential carriers. All in one small classroom.

The day she made her decision\Melissa didn't even go to her classroom. She headed straight for the principal's office.

"I don't feel safe coming in," she told the principal.

She had rehearsed the conversation a dozen times in her head. To her relief, the principal was a mother herself, and she knew what Melissa was going through. She was understanding and approved her request to work from home immediately, effective from that very same day.

Though she was overjoyed to have this added layer of protection as well as job security, Melissa couldn't help but feel nervous. They had pursued IVF for a reason; she was getting older, and her pregnancy would have an at-risk status. Therefore, Melissa's first trimester passed in quiet secrecy.

A month later, when her boss, Amy, the school principal, asked why Melissa had requested that she keep her news a secret, she responded honestly and openly, grateful for all the support Amy was giving her.

"The early part of pregnancy is already scary," Melissa admitted. "You don't want to tell anyone too soon. Plus, I was doing IVF before I got pregnant. My baby is a miracle. I don't want to jinx it or disappoint my loved ones later."

"How would it be a disappointment, Melissa?" Amy said. "You are doing one of the hardest things a person could ever do. You should be proud of yourself, no matter what."

"That is true, but I need some time."

"I understand."

"How have you been faring so far?" Amy asked with genuine care in her voice.

Melissa laughed, adjusting her mic and wiping a speck of dust from her screen before she replied. "In a way, COVID makes it easier. No one expects to see me. I stay at home, do my work and enjoy my pregnancy."

She and Doug had turned down every invitation for dinner, every request to drop by, and every invitation to a party.

"Why don't you guys come out?" a friend texted Melissa when she had just started her second trimester.

"Honestly, it's just too cold. And COVID, you know?" she replied. COVID was the perfect excuse.

If they saw people, it was only outside, always masked, and always brief. Their home became a cocoon, a quiet place where their miracle could grow.

Melissa's pregnancy was incredibly enjoyable. She found herself humming while folding baby clothes, marveling at the strength of her body. Her skin glowed, her energy surprised her. She felt like a woman fully alive. But there was still a soft ache for the moments they missed.

"I wanted to show off my belly," she told Doug one night as they folded tiny onesies together. "I wanted people to touch it, to see it. To celebrate with us."

Doug nodded. "Especially with the family."

But there was also a sweetness in their solitude. Evenings spent cooking together, laughing on the couch, setting up the nursery bit by bit. They held onto each other more tightly because the world outside was so uncertain.

When Melissa finally shared the news with her family, her excitement overflowed. Their reaction only fueled her enthusiasm further. They were thrilled, shouting at the top of their lungs while on the call. Her brother hooted and fist-bumped the air. Her mother cried. Her older sister immediately launched into a rant about the need for more safety before rushing to the attic to retrieve one of Melissa's old cribs that they had kept in storage, awaiting this very moment.

But it was bittersweet. Her father was sick with COVID when she told them—too sick, in fact, to even react much at first. He was later hospitalized with severe pneumonia.

Through it all, what hurt most was how much Doug had to miss. He couldn't go to any appointments. He wasn't allowed in for ultrasounds. They FaceTimed through the anatomy scan. She held the phone steady as the sonographer pointed to their baby's spine, tiny fingers, and fluttering heartbeat.

"This is her," she whispered. "Can you see?"

"Yeah," Doug said, through tears. "She's perfect."

At 38 weeks, he was finally allowed to attend an in-person ultrasound. That was a moment that Melissa cherished.

Soon enough, it was time for the baby to be born. But after passing 41 weeks, the doctors grew worried. Yet Melissa herself was still in high spirits. She loved being pregnant and felt better than she ever had before.

The doctor's in consultation with Melissa and Doug decided that a cesarean section was necessary. A date was set, and when the time came, Melissa and Doug made their way to the hospital with packed bags and high hopes.

After the flurry of activity during check-in, while filling out the forms and being prepped, Melissa tried to stay positive, but a creeping anxiety threatened to consume her. Then, she was brought to her room. The delivery room was quiet, fluorescent lights casting a sterile glow over the floor. Melissa lay on the bed, breathing slowly, her hand gripping Doug's tightly, knowing that soon, they would be performing surgery on her. The nurse had just confirmed that her COVID test was negative.

"No mask for you, Mama," she said kindly, adjusting the fetal monitor. "But Dad, you'll need to keep yours on."

Doug nodded, his eyes full of concern above the light blue mask that had become second nature by now.

For Melissa, the delivery was nothing short of traumatizing.

It went smoothly, yes. The baby was healthy, yes. But Melissa felt broken.

Once she held her daughter Emma in her arms, all of the negative feelings took a backseat, and all she could feel was joy. Melissa and her husband were able to hold onto their gift, their miracle, their daughter.

Melissa laughed as she held her and said, "I think I would've kept Emma inside forever if I could."

Looking into her daughter's eyes, she reminisced about the glow she felt, the private bond with her baby daughter the world even knew. Remembering the quiet nights with Doug and the deep, overwhelming love that anchored them through a storm.

Melissa felt a flood of relief. Seeing Emma's face without her own mask in the way felt like a gift. Even with all the rules and restrictions, they got the experience they had long dreamed of—a birth that, despite its challenges, ended with their baby safe and in their arms.

"*We did it. She's really here.*" Melissa thought as she watched Doug cradle their daughter.

Those first hours in the hospital felt like a slow exhale. They soaked in every second, holding Emma, whispering her name, learning her tiny expressions. Time seemed to slow in that small room, where only the three of them existed.

But once they returned home, the stillness turned heavy.

Melissa sat in the nursery one morning, rocking gently as Emma finally drifted off to sleep. Her eyes were raw from crying again.

She didn't know why it happened every day. She only knew that it came like a wave, unexpected and relentless. Sometimes it hit while washing bottles. Other times it came when she heard laughter from someone outside, someone visiting a friend, someone who wasn't scared to have people over.

"This isn't what I imagined," she whispered to her daughter. "Not being able to go anywhere… not being able to share you."

She kept asking her parents and siblings to wear masks, even inside. She sanitized door handles. She avoided visits. Every person, no matter how close, was a potential threat.

The weight of that anxiety sat heavily on her chest, even when the house was quiet. Especially then.

In the past few weeks, Melissa had changed. She was constantly anxious, weepy—emotionally afraid.

Postpartum anxiety was what she had. But while it had gripped her by the throat, she had not known what it was. It was only later that her doctor confirmed her condition.

Doug saw it. And he responded in the way he always had, with gentle consistency.

When he returned to work, he rearranged his schedule so he could stop by the house once or twice a day, even for just 15 minutes. Melissa clung to those visits like a lifeline.

Her family, too, became her safety net.

They came often to help her, to take up chores and tasks that Melissa had no energy to do. To make sure that both mom and baby were safe and sound.

It had felt like they came to babysit her at times, not her daughter. Sometimes, it felt suffocating, but deep down, Melissa was always grateful. In hindsight, she realized that without them, things may not have turned out this well.

She was cared for. She was supported. She got better. She coped. Slowly. Steadily.

As the weeks passed, her parents began caring for the baby once a week, giving Melissa precious time to shower, breathe, nap, or just sit in silence. They also began planning for daycare.

They had found a facility all her friends raved about, but she hadn't been able to tour it in person.

"I spoke to the teachers over the phone," she said to Doug. "They sent a full video walkthrough. And it was... perfect. Really comforting."

The video showed cheerful rooms, labeled cubbies, and gentle music playing in the background. It was enough to make her feel like she was leaving her daughter somewhere safe.

Months later, Melissa sat on the same rocker where she'd once cried in silence. Emma, now bigger, cooed in her bassinet across the room.

She knew what she had missed—baby showers, shared dinners, family hugs. She knew what had been lost.

But she also knew what had been gained.

Outside, the world had changed. But inside, in their little home, a family had bloomed—carefully, quietly, and full of love.

17
Bethany

It was already 2021, and the coronavirus pandemic was no longer news to anyone in the world. It had been more than a year, and Bethany Paige was well aware of the consequences when she conceived her pregnancy in the summer of 2020. At that time, the virus was at its pinnacle, and Bethany's town was no exception. It was swarming with reported cases on a daily basis.

A few months earlier, she had flown twice a week for client pitches, sprinting through airports with carry-on in tow and AirPods jammed in her ears. But COVID had grounded the world overnight, and the agency converted to remote work in a single breathless weekend. Video calls replaced conference rooms; sweatshirts replaced pencil skirts. In the sudden stillness, Bethany and her husband, Fred, had found themselves wandering the same thought: *If we're home all the time... why not try?*

They had planned it once before the pandemic began, but at that time, they had delayed the plan because both of them were constantly moving due to work. They did not think they could manage being full-time working parents. When the pandemic began, Bethany was convinced that with no stress of work, the increasing number of reported cases and death toll, and with no medical improvement in sight, it was the best time to have a baby, as both of them were at home and had all the time in the world to spend together as a family.

She used the adverse situation to her advantage, hoping that when the baby arrived, everything would be better, and the healthcare professionals would come up with a cure. And they did. By the time her baby was born in March 2021, vaccines were already out, and the daily death tolls had eased.

When she got pregnant, both she and her husband were elated. She was enjoying the soda that she had ordered online when suddenly she felt the liquid in her stomach flip in her belly. She ran to the bathroom and vomited. That day, she took a pregnancy test, and as expected, the result came out positive. They had planned it, and she was happy to succeed. She ran to the bedroom where Fred was sleeping soundly. She woke him up with an excited shriek.

"We are pregnant!"

Before he could even open his eyes, she shoved the pregnancy test strip with two red lines in his face.

"What?"

"I said we are *pregnant*!"

He stood up and took the pregnancy test strip in his hands. For a couple of minutes, he just kept staring at the two parallel lines, then he looked at his wife. With a hand clasped to his mouth in astonishment, he just stared before he hugged Bethany so tight he could crush her. They shared a laugh, followed by tears, all while the chaos outside faded into the background.

The first few months passed in a blur. The nausea, when it came, felt like seawater sloshing under her ribs. But at home, she could slide onto the couch, bury her face in a cool pillow, and breathe through it. Fred, laptop balanced on the armchair, would lift an eyebrow—*another ginger ale?* —and wordlessly cracked open a can. On the worst mornings, she'd lie in the tiny bathroom, fan blasting to muffle her retches, grateful she wasn't on the A train pressed between strangers' backpacks.

Still, isolation pried under her skin. She wanted to see her mother's face in person when she broke the news, holding up the sonogram photo with a big smile on her face. She wanted to let her best friend, Harper, place a palm on her belly and feel the first fluttering kicks. Instead, she pointed her phone camera at the ultrasound printout while her mother dabbed tears on the other end of a video call, pixelated and delayed. Harper squealed through the speaker, but it echoed off Bethany's kitchen tiles, hollow.

One October afternoon, thunderclouds gathering over Manhattan's ghost-gray skyline, Bethany sank onto the living-room rug and folded herself into a gentle yoga stretch. A surge of emotion tightened her throat, half joy, half ache. When she had conceived, she was happy to be off work, but now it aroused a bittersweet feeling in her. She closed her eyes and pictured her office: the floor-to-ceiling windows, the hum of copy machines, the smell of fresh Sharpie ink during brainstorms. She imagined walking through those glass doors in seven-month glory, coworkers applauding, someone taping streamers to her desk.

Lightning flashed outside, spotlighting the half-assembled crib propped against the wall. Fred would finish it after his 5 p.m. client call, and they'd eat take-out Chow Mein on the floor beside it, debating whether the nursery should be sage or sunflower yellow. She touched the smooth wood rail, already seeing the future: a sleepy newborn in fleecy footies, the world outside uncertain, but this room steady, safe.

"Ready for the next meeting?" Fred called from the hallway.

"In a sec." She rose slowly, palms on her lower back, feeling both ancient and brand-new.

The meeting included a rare client camera-on moment. Bethany's screen filled with the CEO's mahogany-paneled study, trophies glinting behind him. Halfway through discussing campaign key performance indicators, a tiny foot jabbed beneath her ribs. A sharp, insistent kick from the baby. Her breath hitched. She muted the phone call, hand pressing down as if to soothe the baby and keep the secret a little longer. All these months, she had kept the news from her colleagues.

Suddenly, she couldn't wait anymore. When the CEO finished, she unmuted the call, cheeks flushed.

"One quick personal update," she said, voice trembling just slightly. "I'm expecting—due in March."

A beat of silence, and then her manager's square on the screen lit up. "Beth! Congratulations!" The chat erupted in heart emojis and virtual confetti GIFs. For a moment, the screen felt like a window thrown open; warm air rushed through.

After the call, she sat back, the room silent except for the noise of the rain pelting on the window. It wasn't the hallway applause she'd imagined, but it was joyous all the same. She snapped a photo of the chat thread, sent it to her mother, and laughed when the reply arrived: a string of crying-smile faces and fireworks.

That night, rain drummed down on the fire escape while Bethany and Fred tightened the last screw on the crib. They stood shoulder to shoulder, surveying their handiwork, the dim lamp casting a soft glow on unfinished walls of the nursery.

Bethany placed both hands on her belly. "He kicked during the meeting," she whispered.

Fred grinned.

She laughed, leaning into him. He was the only one with whom she could share her little joys. She missed her parents, her siblings, and her friends. No matter how peaceful it was with just two of them, it was the moments like these that she missed being around people and sharing her pregnancy experience with them.

Fred was very attentive to Bethany's emotional well-being during the nine months of pregnancy. However, it was during her obstetrical appointments that he was not allowed to accompany her. And in those moments, Bethany felt the most scared. She had imagined the two of them walking into the room together, nervous but excited, hearing the baby's heartbeat for the first time and maybe even laughing through their nerves. She had pictured him asking questions, holding her hand.

But instead, he would walk her to the office doors, kiss her forehead, and stand on the sidewalk waving as she went in alone. That image stayed with her—his face behind his mask, his eyes trying to be strong for her even though she knew he wanted to be there more than anything.

The first antenatal appointment was the toughest one for Bethany. Being alone in that exam room made her feel small and overwhelmed. She wasn't just scared of what the doctor might say, she was scared of doing this without him. She wiped at her eyes and tried to steady her breathing. The doctor was kind, but it still didn't feel the same. This was supposed to be a moment they shared. And instead, she was sitting in a paper gown, trying not to cry behind a mask.

Throughout the pregnancy, this pattern continued. Every appointment, every check-in, she went alone. Fred always walked her there, always waited outside, and always listened carefully when she came back out and filled him in on the updates. He never once complained, and she knew he understood why it had to be this way. But she also knew it hurt him, too.

Bethany often felt like something was missing, like the invisible thread that tied them together during this time was pulled too tight, stretched across the doctor's office doors and no-visitor policies. They were sharing a life-changing experience, but from different sides of the glass. And it was no different for Fred. He felt like he was losing the emotional connection with his son.

Until he was born, and Fred held him in his arms for the first time.

On March 18, 2021, after months of a rollercoaster, Bethany finally gave birth to Asher. She had been vaccinated and tested negative for COVID-19 before being taken to the labor floor. Asher came out pretty easily, too, and luckily, throughout Bethany's labor, Fred was allowed to be by her side.

It was a comparatively unseasonably warm day, and Bethany was already on edge. When the nurses confirmed that she wouldn't have to wear a mask, she was extremely relieved. The whole hospital staff who attended to her were very sweet and helpful. They calmed her down and made sure that her first pregnancy was a good memory.

Until he held the baby, Fred was very calm and collected, and helped Bethany. When the nurses brought the baby out after cleaning all the blood, and Fred held Asher for the first time, it was then that he broke down.

"I didn't know it was going to be like this. I am already in love with him. He can have my life, my soul, anything."

All the doubts that he had about losing emotional connection with his son went out the window. He kissed Asher and refused to put him down for even a second.

When they went back home, her parents also came to visit Bethany and the Asher. All of them got tested and spent two weeks in quarantine before finally arriving. They brought a bunch of presents and offered support during the postpartum period.

"No, Mom. I am on maternity leave anyway, and I also have Fred with me. Thank you so much for the offer, though. I might go for it later," she finished with a wink.

They stayed for a couple of days before going back home. Bethany and Fred received calls from different relatives who wanted to come and see the baby. Even though they were concerned for the safety of their son, they were still very happy to have family members visit Asher. Hence, as a precautionary measure, they developed a list of dos and don'ts, which they called the Baby COVID Rules.

For additional support, Bethany also joined a Mom's Group, an online group consisting of new mothers in her neighborhood. Since she could not meet her friends very often, and they often failed to understand the new Bethany, the mom that she had become, the neighborhood mommies became her newfound best friends. They understood her, validated her emotional struggles, and provided her with tried-and-tested solutions.

When Bethany's work resumed on-site, the mothers on the Mom's Group helped her by babysitting her son along with theirs. And when she could, she also returned the favor. However, Bethany felt a little guilty dumping her responsibilities onto someone else's shoulders.

So, she soon started to look for childcare, which wasn't hard for her since New York, being a bustling city with a majority of working moms, had a lot of good childcare facilities.

Asher was almost 6 months old when Bethany sat at the kitchen table, her laptop open to the daycare's registration portal, her finger hovering over the trackpad. Fred stood behind her, holding their sleepy son against his chest, gently swaying side to side. The apartment was quiet except for the soft hum of the dishwasher and the occasional creak from the old radiator.

The form was nearly complete. All that was left was the payment, which was a hefty deposit and, on top of that, non-refundable.

Bethany let out a long breath. "What if they shut down again?" she asked, not really expecting an answer. "We could lose all of it."

Fred rested his chin on her shoulder. "We might," he said softly. "But we also might not. And if they stay open…"

She nodded. *If they stay open*, their son would be surrounded by other children. He'd sit in a circle of little voices and little hands, hearing songs sung in different accents, learning games from kids with stories unlike his own. That mattered to her. Growing up in New York, she had always loved the way people came from everywhere, all mixed together. She wanted that for him, even now. Especially now.

Still, signing a contract that didn't protect them if COVID changed the rules again felt risky. Frustrating, even. But what choice did they have?

She tapped the trackpad and clicked "Submit." A message popped up: *Thank you for your deposit.*

Bethany closed the laptop and leaned back. "I just want Asher to be around kids who aren't exactly like us. I want him to make different friends," she said quietly. "That feels important."

Fred kissed the top of her head. "It is."

They both looked at their son, now fast asleep, his fingers curled loosely against his dad's shirt. Bethany smiled, a mix of nerves and hope fluttering in her chest. A question popped into her brain.

Would she do it again?

She thought about how she had always wanted to grow her family, have mini-Freds and mini-Beths running around the house, and the answer was clear as ice.

A million times over.

18
Olivia

The city outside was still and quiet, as though the whole world was holding its breath, just as Olivia was. But in her heart, there was only warmth, excitement, and a little tangle of nerves.

Her husband, Noah, sat cross-legged on the living room floor, his laptop balanced on his knees. He looked up and caught her gaze, offering her a tired but genuine smile.

"Are you sure about this?" he asked her months earlier when she first floated the idea.

Olivia had smiled, brushing a strand of hair behind her ear. "Yes. I really am. We're ready, Noah. I know it."

The truth was, they had both wanted this for a while—a family. It was Olivia who nudged them over the edge, who gently convinced him that now, despite the virus, it was the right time. He was working from home. She had been laid off in March.

They got pregnant fairly quickly after that.

When her job finally called her back in July, she solidified her decision, her vision.

"I'm not going back," she told Noah, her hand resting protectively over the small life growing inside her. "I can't take the risk. This… this baby matters more."

He hadn't argued. He had only nodded, wrapping his arms around her shoulders. Choosing to leave her job was the first major sacrifice Olivia made for her child. It was a decision she stood by in the coming months and years.

The couple never considered COVID a deterrent, but in the months that followed, the pandemic profoundly shaped every moment of Olivia's pregnancy. She became an early riser, setting her alarm for dawn so she could be one of the first through the sliding doors of the grocery store. Masked, gloved, and sometimes even wearing a plastic face shield, she would glide silently through nearly empty aisles, the faint buzz of fluorescent lights overhead, the only sound in the store.

She felt safer that way—safer for herself, safer for her baby. Each decision, every small action, was another sacrifice. And yet, in the solitude, there was also gratitude. She knew how lucky she was to stay home, to control her exposure, to create a small safe bubble around the life inside her.

Still, not every part of it was easy.

One chilly afternoon, she had been crying silently, thinking about the parts of her pandemic pregnancy that she wished were different. "I just wish you could come with me," she murmured, glancing toward Noah.

"I know," he said gently, setting aside his laptop. He looked tired, more from worry than from work. "I wish I could, too. I hate that I'm missing everything."

They both knew there was no choice. The doctor's office allowed no partners, no visitors. Ultrasound appointments came and went, the soft whoosh of their baby's heartbeat playing through sterile rooms where Olivia sat alone. Noah waited outside in the parking lot, sometimes for hours, always ready to drive her home.

"He's a trooper," Olivia later told a friend with a small, bittersweet laugh. "He drove me to at least half of my appointments. He never complained. But I could see it in his eyes; he felt left out. He's been so anxious about this whole thing. I feel that if he were able to come with me to my appointments, it might allay some of his anxiety."

Her heart ached for the little things they lost: the joy of hearing the heartbeat together, seeing the tiny feet on the ultrasound, sharing quiet tears over the first flutter of movement. Noah's nervous energy sometimes filled their home, but his excitement never faded. Olivia knew he longed for reassurance, something tangible, something real, but until the very end, that would not be possible.

The other losses weighed on Olivia too. She dreamed of wearing pretty maternity dresses and stepping out into the world, her belly on proud display, accepting smiles and congratulations from strangers. She imagined the baby shower she'd always wanted—the games, the laughter, the shared joy of friends and family gathered in one room.

Instead, her "babymoon" was nothing like the pictures she'd saved on her phone in better days, like the Pinterest board she had carefully curated. She and Noah checked into a quiet hotel, ordered pizza, ate junk food in bed, and binge-watched old mystery movies. There were no walks along the beach, no romantic dinners. Just them, the baby, and the world outside still on pause.

She thought at times that maybe this isolation was good. The world outside, the crowds, even her own family, were too anxiety-inducing at times. When Olivia thought back to how her family had reacted to the news of her pregnancy, she felt a pit in her stomach.

"Sweetheart, you're going to be a *hot mess,*" Helen, her mother-in-law, had stated. "You'll be begging for help. Just wait."

Her brothers, Mark and Jason, had reacted terribly. The pregnancy had opened the floodgates to arguments, particularly over whether or not she should take the COVID-19 vaccine while pregnant.

"You *need* to take it," Mark had insisted over the phone one evening, his voice tight with worry.

"I can't!" Olivia protested, pressing her palm to her forehead. "I'm not eligible yet."

Jason had chimed in too, sending her endless links—studies, articles, opinions—until her phone buzzed every few minutes with new "advice." One message in particular made her laugh bitterly through her frustration: an article about how pregnant Labrador Retrievers had received the vaccine without complications.

"I'm not a damn dog!" Olivia had snapped.

The constant pressure, the bombardment of opinions and information, sent her spiraling. One night, heart pounding, breath hitching in her throat as she held her phone in her hand while trying to reply in her family group chat, she realized she was having a full-blown panic attack. Noah had found her curled on the bathroom floor, shaking, and had sat with her quietly until her breathing steadied.

"It's going to be okay," he murmured, brushing damp hair from her forehead. "We've got this."

Olivia realized then that she needed no one else's support. All she required was her husband, and he was the best she could ask for.

When labor finally came, it was both unexpected and beautiful.

The hospital felt like a strange, sanitized cocoon, the air filled with soft beeps and the rustle of gowns and gloves. To Olivia's relief, the nurses treated her like royalty, checking on her constantly, offering warm encouragement and gentle smiles. She felt like a queen.

Noah, on the other hand, looked as though he might faint at any moment. He hated hospitals, hated the sight of blood, hated seeing Olivia in pain. When the nurse asked if he wanted to cut the cord, his face turned ten shades paler.

"I'm good," he mumbled, swallowing hard. He walked around the delivery room with his head down, deliberately staring at his feet so he wouldn't have to see anything too graphic.

Olivia managed a laugh. "Big, tough guy," she teased weakly, her hand gripping his. She told him she was nauseous.

The delivery itself went well, and soon their son Wyatt was in her arms, feeding at her breast. For a while, the world outside faded into nothing.

They hadn't even made it home from the hospital for more than thirty seconds before Helen's car pulled into the driveway, her face alight with joy as she rushed to help with their son. "I just couldn't wait another minute!" she beamed.

To Helen's surprise, and to Olivia's own, things were nothing like Helen had predicted them to be. Olivia was, in fact, not a hot mess. Motherhood came naturally to her. She felt comfortable, grounded, and surprisingly at peace as a new mom.

Soon enough, Olivia decided to forgive Helen and put what she had said behind her. After all, Helen, to her credit, was ecstatic to be a grandmother.

But the real test came later.

Five weeks postpartum, Olivia was startled awake in the middle of the night by sharp, burning pain that radiated through her upper abdomen and into her back. She had felt this same pain during her second trimester, but back then, she had attributed it to the pregnancy. Now, she knew she had to get checked out by a doctor. The agony grew so intense she could barely breathe. Nausea swept over her, and she vomited until her body trembled. Noah rushed her to the emergency room.

The sterile white of the emergency room blurred around her as she lay curled on the narrow bed. Morphine dulled the edge of the pain, and the CT scan confirmed what she had feared: gallstones—cholelithiasis.

"Drink lots of fluids, stick to low-fat foods," the ER doctor advised gently. "Let's try to manage it conservatively for now."

But a week later, the pain returned. Worse than before. Another trip to the ER confirmed the diagnosis of cholecystitis. There were no surgeons immediately available, and Olivia found herself being transferred to another hospital, waiting for the weekend to pass, her body aching, her mind consumed with one thought: she needed to get back to her baby.

By Monday morning, she'd had enough.

Sitting upright despite the pain, she fixed her eyes on the attending physician. "Look," she said, her voice hoarse but firm, "I know you've got all the degrees and the experience. But I'm six weeks postpartum. I haven't breastfed my baby in two and a half days. I haven't pumped. I'm engorged. I'm exhausted. I need to have this surgery *now.*"

The doctor hesitated, then nodded, clearly taken aback by her resolve. A nurse was sent to Labor and Delivery to find her a breast pump, and within hours, Olivia was finally wheeled into surgery.

When she woke, groggy but relieved, the pain that had haunted her for weeks was gone.

The experience, the fear, the helplessness, and the physical separation from her newborn had changed the way she looked at her postpartum period. The sweetness of those early weeks was now tinged red.

Still, as she cradled her baby again and her heart softened. The storm had passed. And in the end, despite everything, her arms were full. Her son was safe. And that was enough.

When people asked her, sometimes with curious eyes, sometimes with pity, what it had been like to be pregnant during a global pandemic, her answer never wavered.

"It was…good," she would say. "Because in the end, you end up with your baby. That's what matters."

And it was true. Every sleepless night, every masked appointment, every canceled plan, all of it had led here. It was why she could feel the warmth of tiny hands curling around her finger, smell the sweet scent of Wyatt's breath. All of it had given her a life that felt more precious than anything she could have imagined.

To make things even sweeter, Noah's company offered him sixteen full weeks of paternity leave, and when he finally returned to work, it was from the comfort of home.

There were so many things to enjoy: family walks beneath pale winter skies, lunch breaks with the baby gurgling between them, and watching their son nap.

Because of COVID, Olivia made the decision that felt most natural to her: she wouldn't return to work that first year. She wanted to be home. She wanted to see every yawn, every roll, every gummy smile.

"I couldn't have missed this," she told Noah one evening as they sat together on the living room floor, Wyatt kicking happily on a soft blanket between them. "I've wanted this for so long. I needed to be here."

Though the anxiety had often felt overwhelming, she held onto the quiet triumph that she had done it.

"I did such a good job keeping Wyatt safe," she said to herself.

Motherhood had changed her in ways she never expected. It had slowed her down, cracked her heart open, and taught her the sweetness of relishing the present.

The days were not always easy. She had faced pain, both physical and emotional, that had pushed her to her limits. But the small, perfect weight of her son in her arms made it all worth it.

19
Lena

It was around eight in the morning when Lena strolled her cart through the aisles of the grocery store. She had a list of items that she needed to buy in one hand and her phone in the other. The world outside was vibrant and pleasant because of the bliss of spring.

The store had just opened, and the staff were still arriving for their shifts. There were only a couple of customers besides Lena. She took her time examining the items and added them to her cart, reading each ingredient. It was the only time she came to the grocery store.

Wearing a mask, she spoke to her husband on the phone, her voice muffled. “I bought everything on the list. Is there anything else we need that I might be forgetting?”

“What about the multi-purpose cleaner and vinegar solution? I think I forgot to write that.”

Lena looked at the list and then back at her cart, which was full of grocery items. She did not see any cleaning supplies. A frantic worry overcame her. She knew how much of a germophobe she was. In a hurry, she bought more cleaning supplies than were needed and headed for the checkout.

A short woman in her mid-forties stood at the checkout counter with her mask dropped down to her chin.

“I think you should pull your mask up to your nose. The virus hasn’t gone yet.” Lena did not want to sound rude. She just could not control her urge to warn her. Being a clean freak, she was always reminding her family and friends to maintain good hygiene.

The cashier looked at her with a frown, yet without any disagreement, she pulled her mask up. Her eyes judged all the cleaning supplies Lena had in her cart, and as she scanned every item, her judgmental look intensified.

Lena realized that she might have upset the lady. She stood there, adjusting the strap of her cloth mask as the cashier scanned a second bottle of disinfectant spray with a soft beep. The judgment radiating from the woman's eyes didn't faze her as much as it might have six months ago. She was used to it by now.

"I know it might seem like a lot," Lena said suddenly, her voice soft through the mask but laced with nervous energy. "I've always been a bit neurotic about germs, even before the pandemic. But ever since I found out I was pregnant again...I've been even more over the top with COVID precautions."

The cashier looked up, her brow easing slightly. She looked at the guilt dwelling on Lena's face.

Lena pressed on, almost as if confessing made her feel lighter. "I only come to the grocery store around this time. That's when the shelves are freshly stocked, and the crowds are thin. COVID has made me overly cautious. I always wear at least one mask, sometimes two if the news has been particularly alarming. And I try to make it quick, like I'm on a timer. I need to leave before more people crowd it."

She gave a short, breathy laugh, almost embarrassed at herself. "It's just… I want to be sure I don't get sick. I want to protect the baby. It's one thing to be anxious for myself, but when there's a life growing inside you, that anxiety takes on a whole new dimension."

The cashier nodded slowly, still scanning. There was something softer in her demeanor now, less judgment and more understanding.

"My older kids still go to school," Lena continued, shifting her weight and checking her phone as it buzzed with another message from her husband. "But their schools are not that populated. Masks are mandatory, and everyone's serious about social distancing. Their schools have done a great job, honestly. Better than I expected. I feel safe sending them."

As she placed a pack of wipes into the last shopping bag, the cashier finally spoke. "That makes sense," she said, her voice quieter, maybe even sympathetic. "It's been a hard couple of years. We all have our ways of coping."

Lena nodded. "Mine just involves a lot of Lysol and Clorox."

They both chuckled softly. They had not become friends in that moment, but understood each other, a tiny moment of human connection amidst the invisible boundaries the world had drawn.

As she paid and gathered her bags into the cart, Lena felt the familiar ache in her lower back. It was mild, but persistent. Her doctor had said it was normal, especially with her being in her second trimester. Still, every twinge sent her spiraling for a moment.

Pushing the cart toward the automatic doors, she stepped into the spring morning. The air smelled like wet pavement and blooming jasmine. She paused, letting the warmth touch her forehead. A breeze caught the hem of her coat, and for a moment, she forgot the masks, the wipes, the endless sanitation.

She went back home, and the daily routine followed. Her husband, Jacob, who had been granted work-from-home arrangements by his employers, had already tidied up the house. In her previous pregnancies, as well as this time, he made sure to be with her through every step. If she did groceries, he cleaned the house. If she cooked, he did the dishes. If he picked up the kids from school, she made lunch. And the same went the other way round. They worked like two wheels of a cycle, riding the ups and downs of life together.

As her due date approached and her belly grew, so did her worries about the baby's health. Her other children were planned and were not born in such a unsettling period as COVID. Even before COVID, she had always been finicky about hygiene and cleanliness. However, with COVID as the cherry on top, she had grown more perturbed and made sure to follow all the CDC policies.

Whether it was grocery runs in the morning, or evening strolls around the neighborhood, she met people who would rather touch her belly or, even worse, bend down to hear the movements. These interactions made Lena rather angry than upset.

Can they not see this big belly? They should be staying six feet away from me without even having to ask. I don't know why people can't follow basic social-distancing rules.

She had made her rules clear to her family as well. Although with all the restrictions and shutdowns, her family did not meet her very often, still they respected and appreciated her for prioritizing her health and the baby's.

During all her antepartum visits, she wore a mask and sanitized her hands frequently. Jacob was not allowed to attend the appointments with her, but he was pretty laid back about it. He and his daughters Sarah and Hannah celebrated and cherished the ultrasound pictures that Lena would bring back after the visits. Her son was a big blessing for all of them, and even though Jacob was a little disappointed at not being able to be there for her appointments, he still made sure to be elated about their perfect little blessing.

The last trimester passed in the rhythm of cleaning protocols, taking care of her older children, and doctor visits. Soon, it was June, and she was admitted to the hospital in labor.

The labor itself had come in waves. It was quick, powerful, and consuming. After approximately four hours and the final push, the doctor delivered her baby boy Gabriel. The doctor herself was covered in a hazmat-like suit and held Gabriel with extreme gentleness. The boy's body was fresh and red with blood dripping from it, and the placental remains were still attached.

"Can I hold him?" Lena asked, her voice trembling. "I mean… do I need to sanitize? Should I wash again? Is he okay?"

"He's perfect," the nurse said, placing the baby carefully on her chest. "Skin-to-skin is safe, and it's good for both of you. You're safe here."

As Gabriel settled onto her, his tiny fists curled against her gown, a deep wave of emotion crashed over her. Love, fear, joy, and that relentless anxiety braided together into something fierce and maternal.

She kissed the top of Gabriel's head, her voice barely a whisper. "Welcome to the world, little one. I'm going to do everything I can to protect you… even from the things I can't control."

The monitors beeped steadily. The staff continued to move around her, quiet and precise, cloaked in their protective gear. But in that moment, Lena heard only her son's breath and felt the warmth of his body rising and falling against her.

She didn't know what the next hour would bring, or the next day, or the next wave of news from outside. But for now, in this sterilized cocoon of hospital light and filtered air, *she had him*. And that was enough.

After she was done and cleaned, the nurses told her to rest while they took the newborn son to the nursery. Lying there, her mind wasn't wholly in the room. It drifted toward one thought over and over again: *Where is my son right now? And who is he being exposed to?*

The nurses had reassured her. The protocols were strict. Masks were required. Sanitization procedures were followed like sacred rites. But Lena had learned, over the last year and a half, that protocol didn't always mean compliance. What if someone lowered their mask to speak? What if a tech brushed against a contaminated surface and then adjusted her IV? What if, what if, what if?

She turned her head slightly, eyes scanning the figures moving in and out of her room—nearly all dressed in full PPE: gowns, gloves, goggles, masks, sometimes even full-face shields. They looked like astronauts navigating an alien terrain, and somehow, that comforted her.

"It's interesting," she whispered to Jacob, standing at her side, with a mask on his face and gloves on his hands, "when your baby is inside you, you're frightened… but once they're outside, it's worse. You realize how little control you really have. You can't shield them from everything."

He gave her hand a gentle squeeze, his gloved fingers cool against Lena's skin. "That feeling might never go away, I guess," he said with a soft smile behind his mask. "It just shifts."

Lena nodded, eyes welling. She was tired and exhausted, really, but more than anything, she was wired with the kind of adrenaline only mothers feel. It was not like she was feeling this for the first time, and her body was fighting through the pain, but her mind was still cataloging every breath in the room, every hand that touched her or an instrument, every corner that might harbor a stray germ.

Once visitors were allowed, Sarah and Hannah rushed in, masked and holding their aunt's hands. All three of them came in and hugged Lena excitedly.

"You guys just came in from the outside. Sanitize yourselves first," she said, lightly pushing them away. With a little laugh, they obeyed and sat on the couch.

"The nurses said they will bring Gabriel back from the nursery in an hour or so," Jacob informed.

"Okay, then. We'll be waiting here for him with you guys," Lena's sister said.

It had been just a few days since she came home from the hospital, and everything still felt surreal. The house smelled faintly of lavender detergent and hand sanitizer. There were disinfectant wipes by the front door, an air purifier humming in the corner, and hand soap stocked in triplicate in every bathroom. Yet, somehow, despite all the protocols, the anxiety, and the exhaustion, Lena felt a deep and anchoring sense of peace.

"Who cleaned the house?" Lena asked with relief as she walked out of the room, waking up from a long nap.

"Of course, I did. Who else?" A voice came. It was her older sister who was sitting with Sarah, Lena's older daughter, on the couch.

She looked over at her daughter, gently flipping the pages of a picture book, her mask still looped around one ear from when she had come home from school. It made Lena smile. "You can take that off, sweetheart," she said softly.

Her daughter did, carefully placing the mask in her school bag. "I just didn't want to bother Gabriel," she whispered.

Lena's heart swelled. "You're not bothering him. He loves hearing your voice. You can go and see him."

Sarah stood up and went to lie with her brother on the bed.

Lena leaned her head back against the couch and sighed—not from fatigue, but contentment. "I know not every family has experienced this pandemic the same way," she said quietly, almost as if she were talking to the room itself, but her elder sister listened quietly. "Everyone's had their own story, their own struggles. But I'm so grateful that our family responded the way we did."

She adjusted the blanket around her feet and continued, her voice warm and steady. "The pandemic was terrible—of course it was. It was scary. Uncertain. But… it was also not *that* terrible. It gave us something, too. Time. Stillness. Togetherness."

From the kitchen, her husband emerged, holding three mugs of tea. He handed one to Lena with a knowing smile and one to his sister-in-law. "She is getting philosophical again," he said to her.

Lena smiled up at him. "I can't help it. I just keep thinking about how close we've all become. You stayed home. I stayed home. The kids were more aware, more involved. They learned how to help, how to care, how to protect. They knew why we wore masks. They knew what social distancing meant—and not just at school. They carried that mindfulness home with them. They understood that we were doing it for our son, our baby." She looked down at the hot mug, cradled securely in her palms.

"It's been like glue," she said. "This strange, unexpected glue that kept us all connected when the world was falling apart."

"You are right," her elder sister said.

Jacob sat beside her on the floor. "We have all come close as a family. It is a little sad that our whole family cannot be here, but still, we have to cherish what we have."

Lena nodded, tears quietly building in her eyes, some from sadness, some from the fullness of gratitude. "Being pregnant at any time is a blessing. But to be pregnant during all this...and to still feel this loved, this supported, this protected...I can't take it for granted."

She looked out the window, where the trees swayed gently in the early summer breeze. The world was still uncertain, but inside this home—her home—there was certainty. There was safety. There was growth and love.

Everything was perfect at that moment.

20
Lacie

Lacie Bernard had known she was running out of time to have more children. At thirty-six, with each passing month, her longing to have another child grew more insistent. However, she faced an obstacle that made her reconsider her plan – COVID.

Working as an ICU nurse during the storm of the early pandemic showed her just how fragile life could be. Back then, life was utter chaos. The outbreak had begun in February, and the fallout had not yet settled. The hospital corridors were filled with the sounds of ventilators, alarms, and the quiet sobs of loved ones receiving impossible news.

By September 2020, though, things had shifted—at least it felt that way.

"I think it's finally calming down," she had whispered to her husband, Aaron, one night as they sat on the back porch. She had just gotten home from a twelve-hour shift at the hospital. She could feel the ache in her back and the dull throb behind her eyes, which was slightly helped by the cup of green tea in her hands. The air was crisp, and the world was temporarily still. "They're working on vaccines. I think...I think it's time. The vaccines will be here by 2021, and since both of us work in healthcare, we will probably have easy access to them."

Aaron was an EMT who had seen just as much devastation as she had. His eyes were tired, but soft. "Are you sure?" he asked gently. "I mean, we can wait—"

Lacie shook her head. "I don't want to wait anymore," she murmured. "My uterus wants a baby," she added with a nervous laugh, but her heart ached. She wanted life, she wanted hope, she wanted something beautiful to come out of the ashes of the year they had just survived.

They began trying that month.

By the time the vaccine became available in early 2021, Lacie hesitated. She stood in the small waiting room of her doctor's office and felt her stomach twist. There was little data available on the side effects of the vaccine, especially for pregnant women, and she was already pregnant. She could hear her own heartbeat in her ears, and her head spun with raging thoughts.

"What if—" she began, but she stopped herself. She thought of the women she had watched deteriorate on ventilators. The helplessness. The fear. She exhaled slowly, rolled up her sleeve, and took the shot.

A week later, she found herself standing over a young woman in the ICU, pregnant and critically ill with COVID, her life hanging by a thread. The woman was pale, frail, her belly just barely rounded with new life. She was on life support. It was a scene Lacie prayed she would never have to see again. Because of her job, she had already encountered too many heartbreaking images.

Her hands trembled slightly as she adjusted the tubing. "You can't unsee this," she thought grimly. Any doubt she had about the vaccine was completely erased. She would protect her baby. She would protect herself. Whatever it took.

Back home, things had to change. Lacie and Aaron sat their family down (on a video call, of course): her parents, her brother, their kids. The rules were clearly laid out.

"No one visits if they're sick," Lacie said firmly. "Vaccinated or not. And everyone who comes into this house has to be vaccinated."

"A bit of a different vibe to your pregnancy announcement," her teenage niece said as she chuckled.

Her mother's face crumpled slightly. "But—Lace, we just saw your brother's new baby...There were no issues there."

"That's their family, Mom," Lacie replied. She knew that she had to remain resolute. "Aaron and I have decided on these rules after much thought. This is what we feel we need to do to protect our baby, your grandchild."

"But I want to be a part of my grandbaby's life!" her mom protested.

"And you will. Of course you will. It'll just happen with a few rules in mind."

The rest of the family stayed quiet, but they nodded.

Lacie's heart ached. "Since you have just been to Mark's place, you will have to wait for a while before you can see us. I think you need to quarantine for about a month," she said softly. "We can't risk it."

"Okay." Her mom looked upset, but she still managed a smile.

"What about Bella and Rachel Lace? Are they being safe too?" her father asked.

"Yes, Dad. Aaron and I have had a separate talk with them. They are fully on board."

"That's great, hon. We will be too. I promise."

It hurt—God, it hurt—to keep distance from the people she loved, but the stakes were too high. Her family had always been social, always gathering, laughing, hugging close. Now? They hunkered down. It was just Lacie, Aaron, and their two girls, cocooned in their little house.

She worked only three days a week, which meant she was home more, helping with online school, sitting cross-legged on the living room floor with Bella and Rachel, drawing, reading. Even though she loved the extra time with her kids, she could not fully shake off the feelings of anxiousness. She was constantly worried about what would happen if one of them got infected. She was not just trying to protect her fetus; she also needed to protect the girls. The fact that she and Aaron both worked in healthcare made things even scarier.

Her last two pregnancies were not this difficult, especially mentally. Some part of her wished that this one could be the same. But she knew that was not possible; COVID was not something she could control, nor was it something that she could devise a foolproof plan against.

Every time she came home from the hospital, she and Aaron would enter the house through the basement, their quarantine zone. They had to make sure the door to it was always unlocked. Even though it did increase the risk of break-ins, she decided that was less of a concern than COVID.

Once they got in, they had a system. Shoes off. Scrubs stripped. Straight to the shower. Work clothes tossed straight into the washing machine. The girls knew not to come down, even though sometimes they'd stand at the top of the stairs, little faces peering down with wide eyes.

The routines kept them safe, but Lacie also built an invisible wall around her heart. She lay awake some nights, hand resting protectively over her unborn child, wondering: Was it enough?

Then came the accident.

It was a stupid, ordinary moment. Lacie had been cutting something in the kitchen when suddenly there was blood. So much blood. Lacie stared down at her hand as her Emily spilled.

"Aaron!" she gasped, and within minutes, he had called for an ambulance.

She remembered the flashing lights, the concerned faces behind masks, the sting of panic as she was loaded onto the stretcher. The ER was a blur. Blue scrubs, gentle voices, hands working quickly to stop the bleeding.

Even in that chaos, every single person followed COVID protocols. She saw it in their eyes—the determination, the care, the exhaustion. These were her people, her healthcare family. They cared as much as she did. They were as cautious as she was. She was safe. Her baby was safe.

When they brought her home, hand bandaged, nerves frayed, Aaron held her close on the couch. She let herself cry, soft, exhausted sobs that shook her thin shoulders.

"I'm okay," she whispered more to herself than to him. "We're okay."

And somehow, through it all, the fear, the stillness, the ache of separation, the quiet joy of family, Lacie carried on. One heartbeat at a time.

On the day her water broke, the labor suite was quiet except for the rhythmic beeping of the monitors and the muffled voices of nurses behind their masks. Lacie gripped the sides of the bed, her knuckles white, her breath shallow beneath the suffocating mask stretched across her face.

"I can't… I can't breathe in this!" she yelled.

Aaron sat by her side, masked too, his hand firm around hers. His eyes, the only part of his face she could truly see, were filled with worry. "You're doing amazing," he whispered, squeezing her hand. "Just breathe, Lace. Just breathe."

But breathing was the hardest part.

"Get this thing off me!" she shouted.

"Once your rapid test comes back negative, we will take it off Lacie." The nurse was calm and poised. Just what Lacie needed, even though she was probably being rude with all the yelling.

All she could think about was how unnatural it felt, laboring behind layers of fabric, behind fear, behind rules she knew were necessary but still resented in that moment.

When the results finally came in—negative—she wept. Not from the physical pain but from the overwhelming relief of being able to pull the mask down and draw in air without restriction. She could finally meet her baby face-to-face, skin to skin, as she had with her daughters.

The rest of her experience was as wonderful as her previous deliveries.

And when her son was placed in her arms, everything else faded into the background. Ethan was perfect. He was here. And her heart, despite the bruises of the past year, felt whole.

The first days after leaving the hospital, though, were unlike anything she had experienced with her other children. The exhaustion was bone-deep, the kind that settled into her very soul. In the past, her babies had been passed from one loving arm to another, grandparents, siblings, friends, each showering them with kisses and warmth.

Not this time.

This time, the house was still. There were no visitors. No gatherings. No celebratory chaos. Just her, Aaron, the girls, and the fragile new life they had brought into the world. She looked down at Ethan one evening, her fingers gently feeling the softness of his hair, and felt both gratitude and sadness.

"Ethan's missing what his sisters had," she whispered to Aaron, her voice thick. "No one to hold him, no one to love him the way they were loved…"

Aaron slid an arm around her shoulders. "You're kidding. Am I the only one whose phone is ringing 24/7? Your mom has FaceTimed Ethan five times already. And that's just today."

Lacie laughed.

"Everyone loves him to death. They love him so much that they are doing all they can to keep him safe. And besides, Ethan has us," he said softly. "And one day he'll know how hard we fought to keep him safe."

Lacie nodded, tears slipping silently down her cheeks. It was true. This wasn't the postpartum experience she had known before. It was more isolating, more fragile, but the blessing of her son outweighed the losses. She wouldn't have changed a thing. She was proud of the choices they'd made, especially the choice to get vaccinated. It wasn't just for her; it was for Ethan too. Her son was safer than her daughters currently were.

But the anxiety never fully left her. It gnawed at her, coiled tightly around her nerves. She remembered the way her blood pressure had spiked during one prenatal visit, how her heart had raced with the stress of work and the weight of every terrifying possibility. It seemed as if that feeling had never quite left.

She wanted to be calm. She wanted peace. But sometimes, all she could do was worry.

Bella and Rachel adored their baby brother. Every morning, they'd rush to his side, eager to touch his tiny fingers, to lean in close and kiss his soft cheeks. Lacie found herself pulling them back gently, her voice apologetic but firm.

"Not his face, sweetheart," she'd say softly. "Let's keep him safe, okay?"

It broke her heart to say it. It felt unnatural to teach her children to withhold affection, to ask them not to kiss the brother they loved so fiercely. She could see the confusion in their eyes, the little flicker of hurt. But they adjusted. They always did.

One change she hadn't expected, but came to appreciate, was how much they stayed home. Before, life had been a blur of activity: birthday parties, playdates, errands, social events. Now? Now there was time. Time to sit on the floor and build towers. Time to curl up together under blankets and read books. Time to simply be.

Lacie breastfed Ethan longer than she had the girls, her heart set on giving him every ounce of protection she could. She didn't mind the long hours or the sleepless nights. Every moment she held him close felt like bliss.

When she returned to work, it was only two days a week. Aaron, whose schedule had blessedly shifted, stayed home with their son. They didn't need daycare, and for that, Lacie was deeply grateful. They made it work. Their little family adjusted, reshaped by the pandemic, but still whole.

Her own family, her parents, her siblings, had been scared for her. They had worried endlessly about her working in the hospital, about being pregnant while surrounded by risk. Lacie had shared their fear, but she had carried on because that's what she knew how to do: care, protect, survive.

COVID had stripped so much away. It had demanded vigilance, sacrifice, and constant caution. But in its own strange way, it had also given them something, a pause. A breath. And of course, at the end of it all, she had gotten the biggest gift of all, a healthy baby boy named Ethan.

21
Maya

The city was still in semi-lockdown, the kind of eerie quiet that blanketed the world during the second year of the pandemic. In a small townhouse tucked away in a leafy New Jersey suburb, sunlight filtered in through gauzy curtains. Maya Whitfield sat cross-legged on the couch, enjoying the morning sun, a steaming mug of ginger tea cradled in her hands.

Her husband, Jordan, walked in from the kitchen with a plate of toast and peanut butter.

"You okay?" he asked, crouching beside her as he set the plate down. "You didn't sleep again, did you?"

"I did," Maya replied, then sighed. "Sort of… I don't know, it's been weird. Everything aches and feels so heavy, and it just feels wrong. The mask makes it worse. Every day, I wake up nauseous. Then I have to deal with going outside and wearing that damned mask. I smell my breath and want to puke even more."

Jordan gave her a reassuring, sympathetic smile.

This pregnancy wasn't an accident or a surprise. It was a deliberate, carefully calculated decision. Maya had been diagnosed with a chronic autoimmune disease in her early twenties. The disease shaped every major decision in her adult life; it was always something she had to work around or work with. Before even trying to conceive, she had spent two years stabilizing her condition, with the help of doctors, of course. She worked closely with her neurologist, weaning off medications, tracking blood panels, and undergoing tests until she got the green light. Pregnancy had been a deliberate path paved in spreadsheets, appointments, and sleepless nights filled with hope and anxiety.

Jordan had always been supportive. He already had two children from a previous marriage and was familiar with the terrain of parenthood. But this was different; this was Maya's first, their first together, and it was happening during a global pandemic.

"You sure we're doing the right thing?" Maya had asked him months earlier, when the pregnancy test turned positive. The pandemic did not help things either.

Jordan had taken her hand. "We planned this. We're ready. We'll take every precaution. And we'll face it together."

It helped that he'd already received the COVID-19 vaccine through his work with the transportation authority. Maya had felt a wave of relief when he received it. It meant that not only was he better protected, but it made her feel just a bit safer, too. Still, the thought of being pregnant during COVID sometimes made her stomach drop.

Her parents reacted with unrestrained joy. They were thrilled, of course, but they were aware of the risks. So, they promised to be the best grandparents they could, but from a distance, until a time came when they could all gather freely. Maya's younger brother, Jake, was less composed.

"I just—Maya, I don't know if this is safe. You're already dealing with your illness. What if COVID hits you worse? What if something happens to the baby?"

She had tried to reassure him. "I've consulted every doctor I have, Jake. Every one of them signed off on this. I'm okay."

"You *seem* okay," he had replied. "But this virus is unpredictable. You're taking too many chances."

She didn't blame him for worrying. In truth, she worried about it every single day.

But she kept going. She pushed ahead.

Prenatal appointments were nothing like either of them had expected; they were a strange, lonely routine. The doctor's office didn't allow Jordan to attend, and FaceTiming was prohibited. Maya would sit alone in the waiting room, masked, trying not to breathe too deeply, trying to ignore the scent of her own breath, keeping her mouth stuffed with mints. Some days she wore a double mask, even when it made her lightheaded.

Jordan waited outside every time, parked with a podcast on or sipping coffee from the café down the street.

"How'd it go?" he'd ask as soon as she climbed back into the car.

Maya would smile weakly. "Heartbeats strong. She's doing fine." Something of that sort. She would always keep it short. There was no way to fully describe the emotions she felt in there upon seeing the little life growing within her. Neither the positive nor the negative could be captured in words.

“She?” he’d asked on the day when they finally hit 19 weeks.

Maya had nodded. “They confirmed it today. We’re having a daughter.”

That night, Jordan brought home a small pink onesie that said “Princess” on the front. Maya cried happy tears when she saw it.

So much of it felt perfect, and yet, she could not let herself relax.

The hardest question, the one she asked herself over and over again, was about the vaccine. As a woman with an autoimmune condition, she knew what it meant to be cautious. Vaccines were rolling out, but the data on pregnancy was murky at best. Every doctor had a different opinion. Every article contradicted the last. She knew other people who had her disorder who did receive the vaccine, and she watched how they fared, but of course, none of them were pregnant.

Ultimately, it was a support group that helped her make the decision. Other women, some with her condition, some without, shared their stories online. One woman, also immunocompromised, wrote: *“I chose the shot so I could be here to raise my child.”*

Maya reread that line ten times.

She received her first dose in April.

“I’m proud of you,” Jordan said, brushing a curl from her face when they were on the way back home.

“I just want her to be okay,” Maya whispered.

“She will be. Because you’re a rockstar,” he smiled.

As her due date approached, Maya counted kicks and drank raspberry leaf tea. She kept her distance from nearly everyone, FaceTiming her mother instead of visiting, waving at neighbors from the porch instead of stopping to chat. She missed her friends. She missed her family. She missed the version of pregnancy she had dreamed about—the baby shower, people feeling her belly, the hand-holding at appointments. Nothing about this was anything like what she had imagined.

And yet, she considered this the most beautiful part of her life so far.

Maya often sat in the nursery, hand on her belly, speaking softly to the life within her.

"We made you with so much love," she'd say. "So much care. You were not an accident. You are a dream we built, brick by brick. You're a miracle."

The baby kicked in reply, and Maya smiled.

The world outside was uncertain, but inside that room, inside that womb, her baby was safe.

Because of her autoimmune condition, Maya was under the close care of Maternal-Fetal Medicine specialists. What she expected during a time when hospitals were continually full, and healthcare professionals were constantly overburdened, was dismissiveness or vague reassurances. However, what she did receive surprised her and helped ease some of the concerns she had about her condition. She received vigilant, thoughtful care. Her providers understood the complexity of her body. Every medication, every symptom, every dip in energy was documented and discussed. They didn't treat her like a statistic. They treated her like a person, like a woman, like Maya.

"They take you seriously," Jordan told her one evening, after one of her longer visits.

"I know," she said excitedly, "I feel...safe. It's not just me they're watching. It's her."

One doctor, a silver-haired MFM physician named Dr. Kline, looked her in the eye after a long consultation and said, "Your autoimmune disease is the major concern here. COVID? It's just the icing on the cake."

It was blunt. But it was honest. And for Maya, it meant that people saw the full picture, not just the pandemic headlines, but the deeper, chronic realities she'd lived with for years.

The doctors cared for her diligently. Still, her fear didn't disappear entirely. She made two emergency visits to the hospital during her third trimester. The first visit to the ER was especially upsetting. As she was being wheeled alone through the sterile corridors, with nurses in full personal protective equipment protecting their faces, panic was all she felt.

"I need Jordan," she had said through tears. However, due to COVID-19 restrictions, he wasn't allowed in.

That night, she cried into a hospital pillow until exhaustion took her.

The second emergency, in Labor & Delivery, was better. She was allowed one support person. Jordan never left her side.

"I can breathe here with him," she thought to herself. She hadn't told Jordan just how scared she had been during her last hospital visit. She hadn't wanted him to worry. He had enough on his plate and was frustrated because of all the rules.

Their daughter came a few weeks later. Healthy. Happy. Perfect.

It was just Maya, Jordan, their daughter, and the team of doctors and nurses.

They decided to name their little girl Liat, which was Hebrew for "I have been given."

For the next three months, Maya and Liat were inseparable, and though caring for a newborn was tiring and difficult, Maya could not have been happier.

Returning to work three months after giving birth was a bittersweet experience. Maya hated to be away from Liat, but she knew it had to be done.

The pandemic hadn't lifted, and in-person daycare visits weren't allowed. Choosing a daycare over a Zoom call felt surreal.

"Just a video tour?" she asked Jordan, scrolling through websites. "No walkthrough? No, seeing how they hold the babies?"

"I know," he said, frowning at the screen. "We'll trust our instincts. We've made it this far."

Still, Maya felt like something was stolen; a little rite of passage she didn't get to have. But it was a small loss in the grand scheme of everything they had overcome.

They had done it. They'd taken a leap of faith when the world was spinning with fear. They'd navigated a minefield of medical appointments, loneliness, policy changes, emergency visits, and tough choices. But they had done it together. And more than that, they would do it again.

22
Sierra

Sierra Lynn Goldman and her husband, Ronan Goldman, had planned to travel to Japan when the news of a deadly pandemic shook the world. They had both worked hard and saved the money for this trip, but when the world went under a lockdown in March of 2020, both of them had no idea what to do.

They could have continued with their jobs, kept their savings secure in a bank account, and waited for the pandemic to end. Yet, when summer came and the summer vibe got the best of them, they decided to invest the saved money in something similarly healing and transformational. They decided to have a baby.

"This damned virus isn't going anywhere soon. Better have a baby while I have leisure time," was what Sierra thought when she made her decision.

Amidst the lockdown, the global economy was declining rapidly. People were losing jobs, stores were shutting down, and the market was severely affected. Quitting the job at such a time was a diabolical thought. Yet, Sierra decided that as soon as she conceived, she would quit her job for a year. Of course, Ronan tried to talk her out of the decision, trying to stop her from taking an irrational step. He thought the decision to get pregnant at such a time was desperate, nonsensical, and stupid.

"I don't think that this will result in any loss, Ronny," Sierra persuaded, "We already have a lot of savings in the bank. We are doing well financially. I think we will be able to manage just fine, if not better, if we have a baby in the picture."

"But… Okay. Let's see. We can go to our primary care physician tomorrow and listen to his advice. I don't want to take any risks during this already trying time," Ronan replied.

"Our baby would be no *imposition*. I promise," Sierra said.

The next day, they visited Dr. Foster, their primary care physician. They consulted him regarding their decision to get pregnant and if the ongoing pandemic would cause any hiccup.

"It is completely fine to get pregnant. It would be even better because if Mrs. Goldman decides to stay home, then there would be less to no chance of contracting the virus. In my opinion, the world is stagnant right now; it's at peace. What better time to plan a baby than now? And the healthcare professionals are working on different vaccines. I am fairly certain that by the time you deliver, you, along with the rest of the world, will be vaccinated. You just need to be extra careful with following the precautionary guidelines. Here is a booklet issued by our hospital that can guide you well," Dr. Foster finished as he took out a glossy booklet from his drawer and handed it to Sierra.

Sierra and Ronan were pretty relaxed after the conversation with Dr. Foster. Sierra thought about other problems, like finding a good daycare center after the baby's birth, and how to arrange gatherings so the family could meet the baby. But these were the things she would think about later. She hoped that the future would be better. They planned and calculated everything, described and jotted down their roles as parents. They completely agreed on one thing: that they would do it all on their own. Whatever responsibilities the future holds, they would not ask for help from anyone.

As planned, near the end of the first pandemic year, Sierra got pregnant. The period began as an overwhelming rush of vomit and nausea. Even the thought of sleep was a far-fetched dream. She would spend the nights tossing and turning, resting on the pillow, and then throwing it at Ronan, feeling breathless and crying as she had lost her will to live. One night, she woke up from severe itching on her belly. It was the end of her second trimester. The belly was red with thin skin peeling off. She immediately decided to see her obstetrician. Ronan was not allowed to join her in any of the antenatal appointments, and it added to her unwelcome anxiety. The obstetrician examined her rashes and concluded that they were just pruritic urticarial papules and plaques of pregnancy (PUPPP). She said that it is very common and equally harmless for both the mother and the baby.

After the second trimester, both the rashes and nausea stopped. Sierra had come to peace with her pregnancy and started enjoying it. By the time 2021 started, new vaccines for the COVID-19 virus were out, and both Sierra and Ronan had gotten vaccinated. They were no longer disturbed by the ongoing pandemic and enjoyed the last three months of the pregnancy. The cherry on top was that Ronan was also allowed to join her at the antenatal appointments after getting vaccinated.

She also felt deeply fortunate that the vaccine had become available during her pregnancy. It gave her a sense of agency. With every dose, she felt like she was protecting not only herself but also the fragile little life growing inside her. It brought comfort on the long nights when her thoughts spiraled and fear pressed against her chest like a stone. The vaccine didn't just offer immunity, it gave her space to breathe, to plan, to hope.

Sierra had planned to have a natural delivery. She, however, went into premature labor, and the doctors ultimately had to perform a cesarean section on her.

After a blur of activity a beautiful baby boy was delivered. The nurses, covered in their white hazmat suits, ran here and there. One carrying the baby, the other carrying the towels and instruments. All of them had masks on and made sure to minimize human contact with the baby as much as they could.

For Sierra and Ronan, their son was all they had ever dreamed of. Ryker was both a mixture of every blessing they had ever asked for, and an angel from heaven that they could never even have ever fathomed.

"Isn't Ryker more beautiful than Japan?" Sierra joked.

Ronan laughed and replied with utter awe, "More beautiful than anything in this world."

Even though they had planned to have him, they could never have been prepared for him.

Or for the new rush of problems…

It had only been six days into Sierra's postpartum when she awoke suddenly in the middle of the night, her heart pounding as if she had sprinted a mile in her sleep. A crushing weight clamped down on her chest, and each breath was a desperate, shallow gasp. Panic gripped her like a fist. She reached for Ronan, trembling. The anxiety twisted her insides before she could even speak. He sat up immediately, his face contorted with fear.

“I can’t breathe,” she whispered, clutching at her chest.

Within minutes, they were on the phone with a provider. The verdict was immediate: go to the emergency room. But Sierra hesitated. The thought of entering an ER during the pandemic, with cases of COVID still rampant, sent a fresh wave of fear over her. Ryker was just six days old. She was breastfeeding. How could she take him there? How could she leave him?

But there was no other option. She and Ronan bundled up their son, his impossibly small face peeking from the blanket. When they arrived at the hospital, the security guard glanced at the infant and shook his head firmly.

“No babies inside,” he said sternly.

That moment, standing outside the glass doors of the ER, sick, scared, and alone, felt like a cruel joke. Ronan offered to wait in the car with Ryker. Sierra walked in by herself, her breath still erratic, her mind spiraling into worst-case scenarios. She waited for hours. Time didn’t just slow; it melted into an agonizing stillness, interrupted only by cold fluorescent lights and the sound of footsteps echoing down the hallway.

Eventually, she made the decision to leave. She had not yet seen a doctor. She had waited too long, and something in her gut told her she would be fine. Perhaps it was the intense desire to be reunited with her baby. Maybe it was exhaustion winning out over fear. She signed herself out, walked out of the hospital, and climbed back into the car.

Ronan looked at her, eyebrows raised. “Are you okay?”

“I think...I think I just need sleep,” she said, leaning her head back.

In the weeks that followed, she would think about that night more than once. It hadn’t just been physical. The shortness of breath, the racing heart, they were as much about anxiety as anything else. The pandemic had heightened everything: her fears, her vulnerability, her protective instincts. The sleep deprivation twisted it all into something darker.

There was another night, one she remembers vividly, when she woke up trembling, teeth chattering uncontrollably. She pulled the covers tighter, but couldn’t stop the chills. Her forehead burned with heat. Her temperature hit 102°F. She tried to get up, but her legs felt like rubber.

"Go to bed. Please, sleep. I will take care of Ryker," Ronan urged, gently pushing her back onto the mattress.

She woke up five hours later, drenched in sweat but alive, calm, steady. It had passed.

The delivery itself, in retrospect, didn't seem like it had been drastically impacted by COVID. But there were jarring pieces of it that reminded her she had given birth in a global health crisis. She wasn't allowed to hold her son for hours. The doctors and nurses hovered like ghosts, masked and gloved. She wore a mask too, after she had delivered, even during those first surreal moments with her newborn son. She still remembers the way his tiny lips searched for her, and how all she could do was breathe shallowly, her heart aching to feel him closer, skin to skin.

But despite everything, Sierra felt lucky. She delivered in the summer, when the world was beginning to open up again. Everyone around her had been vaccinated. There was sunshine, and there was some sense of safety. She invited her family to the ceremonial circumcision. Her parents came, and so did Ronan's parents. There were masks and sanitizer bottles on every surface, but there were also smiles beneath the masks, warm eyes above them.

Her mother stayed afterward. She had quarantined, tested, and waited patiently before arriving. By the time she walked into their home, Sierra and Ronan had begun to fall into the fragile, beautiful routine of diaper changes, bottle sterilizing, soft lullabies, and sleepless nights. Having her mother there was a gift, even though she had once promised herself she wouldn't need anyone's help.

Then came the visit from her mother-in-law. She had barely stepped inside before she scooped the baby into her arms. Sierra stiffened, her stomach clenching. It wasn't that she didn't trust her; it was the timing, the risk, the invisible virus still hovering in the air.

The next day, as she feared, Ryker spiked a fever.

Panic surged again, raw and heavy. They rushed him to the hospital. Tests were done. Observation overnight. Sierra sat by the tiny bassinet, hands clasped together, whispering prayers.

Fortunately, it turned out to be nothing serious. The fever passed. But the imprint of that night stayed with her.

Motherhood was not how she had imagined it. It was both more terrifying and more beautiful than any vision she had once scribbled in her journal or whispered into Ronan's ear. And in the backdrop of a global pandemic, every moment felt amplified and more sacred.

However, throughout it all, her family held a crucial role. They had been thrilled. Genuinely overjoyed. In the midst of a world going haywire, the thought of new life had felt like a miracle. Her pregnancy, she realized, had been a rare light in a season so darkened by illness, fear, and loss. It became, as she often thought of it, "a beacon of joy." A small, steady flame burning against the backdrop of a chaotic time.

Her family had embraced the news with open arms. They were delighted with the thought that they were going on with a new life. Even as fear of the virus lurked in the background, there had also been celebration, hope, and the gentle reassurance that something beautiful was unfolding.

If someone had asked her whether she would get pregnant during a pandemic again, her answer would have been clear. She was thrilled that she did it. She knew that the pandemic was not going anywhere and that she had made the right decision for them.

The pandemic, of course, brought isolation. There was no denying that. The days could feel lonely, stretched out, and muted. But there had also been something wholesome about the slowness of that time. Sierra had returned to work after the first month of postpartum, and with both she and Ronan working from home, they had been given an unexpected gift: uninterrupted time together. No commutes, no packed schedules. Just the three of them, learning how to be a family and grow together.

There was a warmth to those memories of early mornings, watching their son's eyes flutter open, afternoon naps on the couch, Ronan reading baby books aloud while Sierra breastfed in silence. Those months stitched together the fabric of their family in a way no parenting book could've prepared them for.

If she could go back, would she wish that her delivery hadn't happened during a global health crisis? Of course. It wasn't ideal. She would have loved to hold her baby without a mask, to have visitors come freely, to not feel the constant tension of risk and exposure. But she wouldn't change anything. Not really.

They had managed to parent side by side, sharing every decision, every challenge, and every joy. And in doing so, they had built something that felt uniquely theirs. A closeness. A home.

She knew, if given the chance to do it all over again, she'd approach it with a different mindset. A little less anxiety. A little more grace. But that knowledge only came because she had lived it. She had made it through. She had learned that she could, in fact, do it.

Pregnancy during a pandemic, the rocky postpartum recovery, the sleepless nights clouded by uncertainty, all of it had pushed her to her limits. But it had also shaped her. It had shown her what she was capable of. What she and Ronan were capable of, together.

Sierra knew this with a quiet certainty: they had done it their way. And it had been exactly right.

They were happy. Truly happy. And that, she realized, was everything.

23
Louisa

Louisa Mitchell hadn't planned on having another baby, not now, not with the world still spinning in the throes of a pandemic. But life, in its usual defiant way, didn't consult her calendar or her sense of timing.

The moment the news sank in, Louisa's mind turned to her health. She had an autoimmune disorder, and her doctors had already warned her, *getting COVID was not an option*. With case numbers still climbing and new variants emerging, Louisa and Shareef knew they had to take every possible precaution.

That week, they pulled their toddler, Miles, out of daycare.

"He's going to miss it," Louisa said, watching him play with his blocks.

Shareef, her husband, shook his head. "Not as much as we'd miss you if something went wrong."

Louisa knew he was right. Not a day went by when she didn't feel nervous about possibly contracting the virus. They decided to go all out in preparation for this pregnancy and make the necessary changes to their lifestyle. They switched to grocery deliveries, double-masking, and social distancing—even outdoors. Friends became faces on a screen. Louisa felt like she was living inside a snow globe, sealed, fragile, and far from everyone else.

They were fortunate because they both could work from home. They were especially lucky to be able to hire a nanny to care for Miles while they worked. Choosing her was a difficult process. They needed someone they trusted, someone who would keep their child safe, and someone who was just as meticulous about COVID precautions as they were. But once they selected her, a friendly woman named Jenise, things were as close to perfect as they could have been given the circumstances. The next few weeks went very smoothly, with Louisa receiving all the support and love she needed from both her husband and her son.

But then, at eight weeks, it happened.

The pain started as a dull ache in her right side. She tried to ignore it, but by evening, it had sharpened to a knife.

"I don't want to go to the emergency room," she said through clenched teeth. "There's COVID everywhere."

Shareef looked at her, his face pale. "You *have* to go, Louisa. We can't mess around with this. The baby…and I know you never overreact when it comes to something like this."

Louisa grunted as she clutched at her stomach. "Fine. Let's go."

They drove to a smaller hospital on the outskirts of the city. Louisa walked in alone, masked and anxious, while Shareef stayed in the car with Miles. Policy didn't allow visitors, not even husbands. She felt like she was entering a war zone. The small tents, busy staff, and crowd made her feel really on edge.

They evaluated her quickly. Something was definitely wrong, but they couldn't handle it there. She was transferred alone to the main hospital downtown. She called Shareef and told him to go back home, promising to keep him updated as much as possible.

Once she entered the hospital, the fear truly set in. No family. No comfort. Just a cold hallway and throngs of sick people waiting for help. She did not even get a room because all of the wards were full; instead, she was told that her doctor would examine her right there in the hallway.

A doctor finally approached her after she had waited for hours.

They suspected that her pain might be coming from her appendix or gallbladder and sent her for testing.

"We may need to operate," he said gently. "It's likely appendicitis. But...you should know, given how early you are in the pregnancy, there's a risk of miscarriage."

Louisa's throat tightened. She was taken to another hallway so they could do an ultrasound.

"Can't you check? See if the baby's okay?" Louisa asked the technician and the doctor.

"We're only scanning your appendix and gallbladder for now. Right now, we're focused on diagnosing the source of your pain. An obstetrical resident will check on the pregnancy as soon as they can. We just don't want to delay the surgery."

"Okay." Louisa felt the smallness of her voice, but she knew that the hospital was too overburdened already.

The doctors concluded that she needed surgery to remove her appendix. It was urgent. Had to be done that same day.

After they gave her the news, Louisa felt her senses dulling. What felt like a few hours later, she picked up her phone to call Shareef, and that's when she realized her phone had died.

She scoured the place looking for a charger when a nurse noticed that she was on the verge of panicking.

"Hey, hon—what do you need?" the nurse asked her.

"Yeah, I need to tell my husband that I'm going to have surgery. But my phone is dead."

"Come with me, dear. I'll get you a charger." The nurse guided her to a break room.

After putting the phone on charge, she thanked the nurse with all her heart.

"You can call your husband," the nurse said warmly. "Let him know."

Louisa did, and from that minute on, neither she nor Shareef could fully control their fear.

At 9:00 AM the next morning, they operated.

They said that the baby was healthy and that Louisa would make a full recovery.

She was relieved, but all she could think about was getting out of there, out of that petri dish.

By 12:30 PM, she was discharged. Too soon, too weak, but the hospital was overwhelmed. Shareef arrived to pick her up, only to find blood soaking through her shirt.

"Louisa, Jesus, your stitches!" he cried, alarmed.

Back inside she went. The staff rushed her to the recovery room, sealing the incision with more glue. Finally, she was allowed to go home.

The weeks that followed were filled with obstetrical appointments, high-risk maternal-fetal medicine, and her rheumatologist. Louisa juggled it all. She missed the comfort of having Shareef by her side during those long visits.

"It's like walking a tightrope alone," she told her sister on the phone. "Every scan, every test, I'm terrified something bad will show up, and I'll be alone when it does."

But everything stayed on track. The baby girl growing inside her was strong. She was grateful that she had so many involved providers; they gave her excellent care, and she felt like the luckiest mom in the world.

Both Louisa and Shareef decided to get vaccinated, and since both were scientists, there were no questions about whether it was a good idea or not. A few months later, they were actually relieved that she had been vaccinated, as the evidence showed that the antibodies passed to the fetus.

She and Shareef set up a cozy office, tag-teamed parenting, and avoided every risk they could. Louisa called it "living in a bubble," and Shareef made sure it stayed sealed. As a virologist, he was adamant about safety. He insisted she double-mask when they went out, even to medical appointments.

At night, they curled up on the couch and watched TV while the baby kicked gently beneath her ribs.

"Are we really doing this?" she whispered one evening. "Having a baby in the middle of all this?"

Shareef kissed her temple. "We already are."

The delivery was smooth. Louisa cried when she heard her daughter's first cries. They named her Ivy Grace, a name that felt like hope after so many months of fear.

What came next surprised Louisa most: *no postpartum depression*. With Miles, it had hit her like a wave she hadn't expected. This time, she knew the currents. She felt prepared, centered. Empowered.

After her delivery, the COVID numbers began to increase once again, and they returned to their hibernation, but both being scientists, they understood and accepted the protocols without hesitation. Louisa already knew what it took to be a mother and how to juggle all that life threw her way. She felt her confidence growing with each day as she watched Ivy Grace grow.

"I think I'm stronger now," she admitted to her therapist. "We've already survived so much."

Louisa felt calm. Ivy was healthy. Their family was whole.

"I miss the celebrations," she said to Shareef one quiet afternoon. "No baby shower. No visitors. No one came to hold her."

Shareef nodded. "I know. It's been lonely sometimes."

"But... I'd still do it again," she said.

He looked at her, surprised. "Even during a pandemic?"

Louisa smiled, watching Ivy sleep in her bassinet, sucking her little thumb. "Without a doubt. Look at her. She completes us."

24
Keisha

Keisha and Malik had been trying to have a baby for so long that her husband no longer waited patiently outside the bathroom for her to take the store-bought test. Instead, he was now busy in the kitchen, preparing a nice meal of steaks, green beans, and a family dipping sauce recipe.

The first snow had dusted the rooftops of Brooklyn when Keisha Baron saw the two pink lines. She was curled up on the couch in their tiny apartment, blanket around her shoulders, the test clutched in shaking hands.

"Malik!" she called out, eyes wide.

He emerged from the kitchen, wiping his hands on a dish towel. "What? Are you okay?"

She didn't speak. Just held up the test.

He stood still, processing. Then he dropped the towel. Keisha's face broke into a smile that could light up any room. Eyes filled with joyful tears, she nodded and stretched out her hands towards Malik, who was already crossing the room. He swept her into his arms.

"Keisha...we're having a baby?" His voice cracked mid-sentence.

Tears were slipping down her cheeks. "We planned this, I know, but...It's real now."

And at that moment, everything felt perfect.

They spent the next few weeks laying the foundations for their dream to become a reality: browsing cribs online, arguing playfully over names, and looking for ideas for baby bump photoshoots. There was talk of a spring baby shower, maternity shoots in Central Park, and long walks with the stroller down leafy brownstone-lined streets.

Keisha's first trimester was as perfect as could be. Aside from the typical morning sickness, she felt completely confident about this, with no doubts, second thoughts, or anxiety.

But by early March, New York City's usual lively rhythm had been silenced. Something invisible had begun to spread.

"I think we should cancel dinner with your cousins," Keisha said one evening, her bump just beginning to become noticeable. "The virus...It's not looking good."

Malik looked up from his phone, where news alerts screamed about rising infection rates. "Yeah. You're right. I'll send them a text."

Then it all began. Busy streets emptied. Sidewalk cafés were silent. And Keisha's dream of the perfect pregnancy was shattered.

Keisha spent all of April 2020 indoors. The couch became her office, her bed, her bunker. This couch was where she took her virtual prenatal appointments with Dr. Lancer, her solo practitioner, who thankfully allowed Malik to accompany her when she did have to make her visits in person. But for Maternal Fetal Medicine (MFM) appointments, which were already nerve-wracking enough, she had to venture out of her safe zone, and she had to go alone. Always alone.

One afternoon in late June, after a long subway ride with masked strangers, Keisha sat stiffly in the MFM exam room. She sat on the bed, eyes wide, nibbling the edges of her fingernails. They had already been raw and bleeding, but she barely noticed the sharp pricks of pain.

The ultrasound technician barely made eye contact. "We'll do the ultrasound first."

Keisha watched the screen, heart pounding, as the wand glided over her stomach. The tech's brow furrowed.

"I'll go get the doctor," she said too quickly. Pulling off her gloves, she rushed out of the room, disappearing before Keisha even had a chance to open her mouth to question her.

A few minutes later, a physician Keisha had never met walked in, mask tight against his face.

He put on a new set of gloves and picked up the wand, examining it himself. At this point, Keisha was too scared even to ask him what was wrong.

"The baby's growth is lagging, and today's readings worry me," he said. "You need to go to the hospital now. We may need to induce you."

Keisha's ears rang. "What? Alone?"

"I'm sorry. Protocols. But we will take good care of you."

She texted Malik from the Uber: Going to the hospital. It's early. I'm scared.

Five minutes later, Malik saw the message and immediately called her. He stayed with her on the phone, consoling his crying, terrified wife as she reached the hospital.

"Hey, listen. I am already on my way there. I'll be right there with you. I'll find out if I can get in to be with you."

As Keisha pulled up at the hospital entrance, she said goodbye to Malik. The call had calmed her frayed nerves a bit, but she felt as if her heart was pounding in her throat.

Inside the hospital, there was pandemonium. Every inch of the place seemed to be occupied. Keisha was glad she had chosen to double-mask this morning.

In triage, Keisha lay on a narrow bed separated by only thin fabric from other laboring women. She had hoped for a separate room, but those were reserved for the COVID-positive patients. She heard a woman coughing in the next stall. Were they tested? Were they positive? Panic ensnared her, threatening to overwhelm.

When she was finally moved to a delivery room, the relief of solitude was immediate, though the mask remained. Here, her husband was allowed to be with her. As soon as he got the green light, he rushed to her. When the contractions started, Keisha gripped Malik's hand, both of them trembling with fear and adrenaline.

Their son arrived just past midnight. She wept as he was placed on her chest.

"He's perfect," Malik whispered.

They named him Micah.

Their postpartum room was not private; she shared it with another mother. She knew that everyone admitted to the hospital had been tested for COVID-19, including her, so the other mother would not be a carrier. However, her Significant Other was in the room too, untested. He kept taking off his mask when no one was looking, and even though Keisha had already asked him not to, he dismissed her, calling her stupid.

To make things worse, the room did not have a shower. There was only a communal shower in the hallway, which all the patients in the wing were expected to use. So, she decided to go without one and wait until she got home.

Her anxiety at this point was through the roof, bordering on frantic. Her husband, in contrast, was calmer, at least outwardly. She knew that inside, he was nervous too, because no one truly knew the best way to deal with situations like these, given the pandemic.

She longed to escape the hospital where danger seemed to be lurking in every corner. That wish, at least, she was granted. She was asked to leave as soon as she had been determined to be stable, since they needed the space.

Back home, exhaustion set in like concrete.

Over the next few days, the couple tried to establish a routine. Malik took night shifts, paced the hallway with a colicky baby, and made meals that went cold before Keisha was even able to touch them.

"I feel like I'm doing this all wrong," she said one night after Micah was finally asleep on her chest.

"You're doing everything right," Malik assured her.

But she missed her mother. Her parents couldn't visit as they weren't vaccinated yet. She longed for her mom's hands guiding hers, showing her how to bathe Micah, soothe his cries, and rock him to sleep. She was fiercely protective of her little boy.

One day, she asked their pediatrician, "Is it safe to take him for a walk outside?"

The doctor blinked. "Yes, just avoid crowded areas."

Even fresh air came with a warning label.

At pediatric visits, only one parent could attend. Without a car, Keisha packed diaper bags, wipes, bottles, and masks, pushing the stroller through the streets alone. Every journey felt like an expedition. But she was thankful for this. She did not trust ride-sharing services anymore, not with her baby in tow. Walking seemed like the best option, and since they lived in the city, they had been able to choose a pediatrician who practiced nearby.

They had already decided that they wanted to move. Now their plans were set in motion. They knew they couldn't raise Micah in a box with sirens outside the window.

The move to Westchester was bittersweet. They left behind the city that had raised them and welcomed them as a couple. Moving as new parents with a newborn was almost as difficult as being pregnant during a pandemic. But Keisha knew that this had to be done. Just six months after giving birth, she soldiered through it, knowing that once it was over, she would never look back. After moving, they gained space, grass, and most importantly, proximity to family.

"I can breathe here," Keisha said as she watched Micah play on a blanket in their new backyard.

Her parents could finally visit. There were still precautions, still hand sanitizer and masks, but at least Micah had grandparents now. Malik's parents were still unable to meet the baby because they worked in healthcare and had to take extra precautions.

Though the early months had been traumatic, Keisha began to find a rhythm. Motherhood no longer felt like a trial by fire. She started to trust her instincts. She was also grateful that she was not expected to host guests because of the pandemic. She knew that if it weren't for the fact that they were in lockdown, her home would constantly be overrun with people clamoring to meet the new baby.

"I think I understand myself more," she told Malik one night over tea. "I never wanted to be this isolated. But I had to rise to the moment."

He smiled. "You didn't just rise. You soared."

Even when Micah turned one, the world still had not returned to normal, but it had adjusted. Vaccines were rolling out. Schools were reopening. Life was reshaping itself.

When Keisha stared at a new pregnancy test one summer morning, she felt something unfamiliar.

Calm.

Micah was toddling now, clapping and calling her "Mama." And inside her, a second life had begun.

A few months later, she stood barefoot in the backyard of her suburban home, morning sun warming her face. Micah was chasing butterflies through patches of daffodils, his giggles filling the air.

She rested her hand on her slightly swollen belly and exhaled. "You're already growing fast," she murmured to the child inside her. "I can feel you."

When Malik came out holding two mugs of coffee, she smiled.

"You've got the glow again," he teased, kissing her forehead. "That or Micah's rubbed his oily hands on your face again."

"Probably both," she laughed.

This pregnancy was different. It was also affected by the pandemic, but no longer ruled by it. There were vaccines now. Testing. Mask mandates. People knew what COVID was, and though it hadn't vanished, it no longer felt like a monster under the bed. It was just part of the landscape.

She had changed too. Keisha was far more confident and less afraid. She knew she had what it took to be a mother, a good mother at that. She was stronger now.

Still, Keisha remained smart and cautious. The world demanded it.

Because she was considered high-risk, Keisha was referred to Maternal Fetal Medicine for her care.

On a hot August afternoon, she sat in the waiting room, masked, surrounded by other women with swollen bellies and nervous eyes. This had become routine now, and she no longer felt uneasy about being alone, but she was on edge because she knew that during any one of these visits, she could be given bad news.

A nurse stood at the door asking each patient, "Any COVID symptoms today? Fever? Loss of taste?"

Keisha kept her gaze low. She didn't like this. The air was heavy. There were too many people in the room. Her pulse ticked faster.

She texted Malik: They're still not letting partners in. Feels like last time.

His reply came instantly: Breathe. You got this. I'm right outside.

Getting back home felt like stepping into paradise. This time, Keisha wasn't in a cramped apartment, but she was still alone in many ways. She had a toddler to care for, a baby on the way, and Malik now working full-time from a home office that doubled as Micah's playroom and her own nap space.

She often stood at the stove, stirring oatmeal while balancing Micah on one hip and counting fetal kicks with the other.

"You okay?" Malik would ask during breaks, finding her standing too long in one spot, zoning out.

"I'm fine. Just tired."

And she was tired. But not just physically. Emotionally, too.

What made it different, though, manageable, was support. Her parents visited weekly. Malik's parents, both finally vaccinated, had flown in and met Micah for the first time when he was nine months old. Keisha had cried watching them hold him. Now, they came as often as they could.

The second trimester brought with it the familiar nausea and fatigue. But this time, Keisha didn't have to wake up at 6 a.m. to commute. She didn't have to plaster on a smile for coworkers or pretend she wasn't exhausted.

"I get to rest," she said to her mom one morning as they sat together in her living room. "During my first pregnancy, I had to be everything to everyone all the time. Now I can slow down. Tackle one thing at a time."

Her mother nodded thoughtfully. "Sometimes hardship teaches us what really matters."

Micah sat before them on the floor, playing with his toys. He was half asleep.

"Thanks for babysitting again," Keisha told her mother. "It's so nice not having to put him in daycare. I have no idea what could be going on in those places or if the caretakers are taking COVID precautions. Having you supporting me in this is...I can't thank you enough."

"Oh, please, it's no bother. You know I love spending time with him. Can't wait to do the same with this little one." She placed a hand on her daughter's belly.

They spent the rest of the evening talking, and Keisha said goodbye to her mother with her heart feeling full.

That night, Keisha journaled before bed. She wrote about how her first pregnancy had forged her into something unshakable, how she had learned to trust her instincts, even when no one else was there to guide her, how the loneliness had also brought clarity.

"I thought I had to figure motherhood out alone," she wrote. "But in doing so, I found myself."

She laughed. "I should get this framed and look at it each time I feel unsure of myself," she whispered to herself.

At 38 weeks pregnant, Keisha once again sat in a doctor's office. But this time, things were calmer. She had a car now. She had her mother waiting at home with Micah. She had knowledge. Tools. Backup.

She didn't feel helpless.

Her doctor, a kind woman with silver curls and a gentle voice, tapped her chart.

"Everything's looking good, Keisha. Baby's growing right on track."

"Thank God," she murmured.

She looked down at her belly.

"Almost there, baby girl," she whispered.

Her second baby came right on time, exactly on the due date. Once her labor began, Malik drove her through winding roads to the same hospital where Micah had been born, but now, protocols had changed. Masks were still required, but partners were allowed to stay. Testing was quick. Triage felt safer.

When Keisha was wheeled into a private delivery room, she smiled at the nurse.

"I didn't get this last time," she said, looking around.

The nurse smiled back knowingly. "Things are a lot better now. The past two years have been hectic for sure, but now the world is beginning to recover."

Her labor went smoothly. Their daughter, Nyla, came into the world just before noon. Keisha held her against her chest and whispered, "Welcome home."

Unlike last time, when they got back home, there were visitors—masked, careful, but present. Her parents brought food. Friends sent flowers. Micah toddled around saying "baby" and offering Nyla his stuffed dinosaur.

She breastfed in the sunlight. She slept when the baby slept. She held Nyla and sang lullabies that she hadn't known she remembered.

Malik sat beside her one night while she rocked Nyla, who had hiccups.

"You're different this time," he said.

She looked up. "What do you mean?"

"Calmer. Stronger. Like you already know how to do it all."

Keisha smiled. "Because I've done it once before."

"I was surprised you wanted another pandemic baby. That's what they have started calling them these days, you know. There's a whole hashtag for it and everything."

Keisha laughed. "The new generations deal with heavy stuff in such interesting ways." She paused for a second, reflecting. "When I realized that COVID was going to be longer than we predicted, longer than scientists even predicted, I knew I could not put my life on hold. I wanted this. I wanted her. I didn't want to change my life plan just because of the virus.

"Sometimes…I think that only those who have been pregnant during the pandemic could truly understand what it has been like. For Micah, we came in totally unprepared. COVID wasn't even a thing back then. We all expected it to be over within a few months and then within a year. For Nyla, at least we had some idea of what we were doing. Not fully, but we had an idea. And it's been so beautiful, I wouldn't change a thing about it."

Malik stroked her hair. "Yes. You have got to be present with them both. You're with them almost 24/7. I get to be here more often too."

Keisha chuckled, “Thank God for work from home. I didn’t have to do commutes. That might have been my tipping point.”

Malik was laughing too now. “We saved a fortune because of your mom too. No day care.”

“Both our families’ support has been game-changing. And you.” She cupped his face with her hands. “You are the best husband I could have ever asked for.” She kissed his cheek.

“It's all you, babe,” he said. “You're so self-confident now. It's been amazing to watch you grow so much stronger.”

“Comes with being a mother,” she replied.

She sank back into the couch, feeling a wave of tranquility wash over her. Everything was just right. Calm. Peaceful. Secure. It was a moment of pure perfection.

25
Kassidy

The summer of 2020 wreaked havoc worldwide. And it wasn't any different for Kassidy Lane and her family. With the news channels listing death tolls and rising number of COVID cases, pregnancy was the last thing Kassidy wanted.

Like ninety percent of the world, Kassidy was homebound with her precocious son Leo and working remotely. She and her husband, Patrick, had discussed taking advantage of such a time to plan a baby when the world was on pause; there was nothing much to do except stay home and see the earth go about its orbit.

When they had discussed the possibility of a baby, they had also immediately refuted it. The mental instability and disrupted routine that COVID brought made them give it a second thought. They decided to wait it out a little and plan once the virus situation was over.

But it was already too late.

After a couple of days of constant nausea and an obstetrical visit, Kassidy found out that she was already about five weeks pregnant. Even as they dismissed the idea of a second baby, the little mischief was already eavesdropping from her belly, probably smirking.

Beneath the shadow of a global pandemic, this pregnancy left her with a multitude of uncertain questions. Her first concern was not her new baby; it was her son, whose daycare might close without warning. It was on Patrick, who still had to leave the house every morning for work, exposed in a way she couldn't control. It was on the baby inside her, and what little anyone knew about how COVID might affect a pregnancy. She had searched for answers, surfing through websites, medical journals, and parenting blogs, hoping to find something reassuring. But all she found were question marks. There were no definitive studies or real statistics. Just a growing weight of anxiety.

And yet, life carried on.

By the end of summer 2020, restrictions began to loosen. People were moving around more freely. Stores opened. Parks began to fill again. For some, it was a sigh of relief. For Kassidy, it was a slow panic unfurling. She had spent the early months of her pregnancy sheltering herself and her family like a fragile secret. And now, the idea of being exposed to strangers, of walking into a store or touching a gas pump, felt reckless. Her instincts screamed at her to pull back, to stay hidden. And so they did.

As the second trimester began, they locked themselves down again, voluntarily this time. She banned any visitors and stopped sharing meals or taking her son to playdates. Her world narrowed to the walls of their home, and even those felt like they were closing in some days. Her mother, who had been her rock during the first pregnancy, now dropped off groceries and baby supplies at the door. She'd stand back on the porch and wave through the glass, eyes misty, smile tight behind her mask.

"I wish I could hug you," she would say.

Kassidy nodded, her eyes always tearing up. "Me too."

There were no baby showers and no brunches with friends. No laughing over tiny onesies or guessing the baby's weight. Everything that had once made pregnancy feel magical had been stripped away, leaving only the physical experience: the nausea, the cravings, the exhaustion, and the worry. She felt invisible in her own life, the mundane routine getting the best of her moods.

She didn't complain out loud. But she felt the absence of celebration. Her first pregnancy had been marked by joy, but this one? By quiet. She often thought about the difference and recognized how both pregnancies were only a couple of years apart in time, but miles apart in feel. Both pregnancies defined "love" differently for her. That sometimes, the greatest acts of love were invisible ones. Isolating herself was love. Staying away from her own mother was a sign of love. Refusing to go out, even when it made her feel lonely or restless, was love.

She was building a safe cocoon not just around her unborn child, but around her entire family.

And in that stillness, something began to shift.

There were small rituals that anchored her. Leo's laughter in the early mornings. The flutter of baby kicks during long work Zoom meetings. The way Patrick would come home, immediately wash his hands, and hug her and Leo before anything else.

They were isolated, yes. But they were together. Kassidy took the isolation as a blessing in disguise. She started working on herself and her closest relationships. She gave the house more attention to turn it into a home. She utilized her time to do mundane chores in an enjoyable way, savoring every move and minute. In the quiet, their family grew closer.

That sense of unity became her comfort. Even in the absence of family gatherings or medical certainty, there was something powerful about the way they showed up for each other. Her husband might not have been home during the day, but he made sure the evenings were sacred. He took over bedtime with their son. He cooked simple meals. He rubbed her back without her asking.

Every night, before going to bed, Kassidy would place both hands on her belly and whisper the same thing: *We're okay. You're okay. You're safe.*

She missed her mother's touch. She missed the way her friends would have fawned over her baby bump, the photos they would've taken, the gifts they would've wrapped in pastel tissue paper. But she also found strength in the solitude. She had never felt more protective, more attuned, more determined.

Through summer and winter, spring finally came. On April 13, 2021, Kassidy finally gave birth to her second born.

The day she went into labor was chaotic, not because of the contractions or timing, but because of everything else.

Right before labor, Kassidy was tested for COVID, and to her shock, she tested positive. The hospital staff shifted her to the COVID ward, where the delivery room wasn't a room at all. It felt more like a glorified storage closet: cramped, with barely enough space for the medical bed and a tray of supplies. She labored alone. The lighting was harsh. The air, too sterile. The walls, too close. It wasn't the kind of space where you welcomed new life with open arms, it was the kind of place where you held your breath and hoped nothing went wrong.

Her nurses, distracted or simply overburdened, didn't respond promptly when she voiced discomfort. When she called for help, it took longer than expected. Questions went unanswered. The sense of security that Kassidy so badly needed never arrived.

But oddly enough, when the baby was born, her worries melted. He was tiny, warm, and wailing against her chest. The world suddenly softened. In that moment, the rest of the room faded into background noise.

And then came the unexpected gift.

Because of COVID restrictions, no one was allowed to visit. And Kassidy was happy with no flowers, no balloons, and no stream of relatives filing in and out. Just her, her newborn son, and the quiet hum of a hospital wing locked in isolation.

It was, surprisingly, everything she didn't know she needed.

There was no advice from experienced mothers. No hovering. No comparisons to how someone else had done things. She could stare at her baby uninterrupted. She could nurse without an audience. She could learn the shape of his face in silence. That time was hers alone. She called it sacred. And in some ways, she described it later as the only part of her COVID pregnancy that felt wholly, blissfully peaceful.

At night, she swaddled him with calm and quiet under the fluorescent lights. There was no pressure to entertain. No need to smile for pictures or pass him around. It was just mother and child, breathing the same air, the exact thing she could not have with her first born. She would later tell friends, "That part… that part was beautiful. No one could touch our bubble."

But outside of that quiet pocket of time, things felt fragmented. Where she was at peace, she missed the true excitement.

Unlike her first pregnancy, there was no celebration or hugs from her friends and family, not even from her husband. Even during the pregnancy, there were no prenatal visits with her husband beside her. She would meet the obstetrician alone, bring the ultrasound images home in an envelope, and then slide them across the table. Her voice was the only bridge connecting Patrick to the pregnancy. He would nod, try to picture what she described, but it wasn't the same.

And now, because she tested positive for COVID, her husband could not accompany her during labor. The nurses brought him in, masked face and muffled voice. Yet, his eyes said it all. She could see that even after all the detachment and indifference throughout pregnancy, he could not suppress the emotions now. The baby was no longer just a picture. It was real and breathing.

They brought him home and named him Carlos Christopher Lane.

One night, weeks after their son was born, they sat on the living room couch, both of them exhausted. Leo was asleep. Carlos finally dozed off after a long evening of cluster feeding. Patrick turned to her and said, quietly, "I didn't feel like I was part of it this time. Not really."

She knew what he meant. He had missed the heartbeat appointments. The kicks during scans. The nervous hand-squeezing in the waiting rooms. All the touchpoints that had made their first pregnancy feel real and shared were absent this time. He had received updates, not experiences.

"I tried to keep you in the loop," Kassidy said, gently. "I told you everything the doctor said."

"I know," he replied. "But hearing about it isn't the same as being there."

That admission stayed with her. Because it was true for her, too, even as she had carried the baby, felt every movement and change, she too had felt alone in the journey.

But now, their family was very much present and complete. It had grown, both in blessings and responsibilities.

There was no village around her like before. No popping over to a friend's house for tea. No bringing the baby out for brunches or lazy afternoons at the park. Everything was risk-assessed, calculated, and filtered through the ever-present question: *Is it safe?*

She didn't feel as free and secure as she had the first time.

She hesitated to take the baby anywhere. Even grocery runs gave her anxiety. Every public surface, every uncovered cough in the air, felt like a threat. They had skipped family holidays. No birthday dinners. No random mornings at her parents' place. Her parents, especially, had been cautious, understandably so, but it only deepened the sense of distance.

Still, she was grateful for what they did give.

Once vaccines became available, her mother, mother-in-law, and sister-in-law began to visit again, one night each week, rotating like a gentle support system. Her best friend would come over when she could, offering company and folding laundry without being asked. These women didn't just visit. They showed up. Their presence didn't erase the isolation of the early months, but it helped cushion it.

Her mother would arrive with casseroles and fresh fruit, placing them on the counter. Her sister-in-law, herself a COVID delivery survivor, would recount her own story with a weary laugh.

"Felt like I was in solitary," she'd said once, folding tiny clothes beside Kassidy. "I don't remember seeing anyone for hours. Just this constant beeping and fluorescent lighting. It was awful."

Kassidy had nodded, silently grateful that at least she hadn't been separated from her baby. They had stayed together, even if it meant standing in a closet-sized delivery room.

But the lack of family connection still weighed on her.

Pregnancy had always seemed like a communal experience to Kassidy the first time around, where people reached for your belly, shared stories, and passed down swaddling tricks like heirlooms. But this time, it was something private and solitary.

It wasn't that people didn't care. It was just that they couldn't come close even if they traded everything for a single moment together.

And even now, months into postpartum, that distance still lingered. Leo had adjusted well, showing flashes of protectiveness toward Carlos. But Kassidy sometimes caught herself watching the baby nap, wondering what kind of world he'd grow up in. *Would caution always define their choices?* Whether celebrations would return. Whether "normal" was still ahead or already behind them.

In moments like those, she'd breathe in deeply and remind herself: they were safe. They were healthy. And though the journey had been lonely, it had also made her resilient.

She didn't feel the same as she had after her first pregnancy. She felt older, maybe. Quieter. A little more tired, but a lot surer of herself.

And would she do it again? Be pregnant in COVID? Survive the isolation again?

A hundred times, "Yes."

Even through the harsh storm, she had her husband and two beautiful boys, whom she would choose over anything any day.

26
Kamille

Kamille Voss and Bryce had been wanting children for years, measuring the right time against their savings, careers, and readiness. Kamille was a nurse at St. Michael's Hospital, and had imagined a joyful pregnancy shared with family, friends, and colleagues, the kind of experience where everyone's hands seemed to reach out to touch her swelling belly and ask the same excited question: *"When are you due?"*

But as the pale blue line appeared on the pregnancy test, the news on the television in the other room was speaking a new word into the world: *COVID*. They had no idea what it meant, not really. Only later would she think to herself, *if I had known there was going to be a pandemic, maybe we would have waited.*

"Twins," the sonographer had told her at her first ultrasound, her voice muffled behind a surgical mask.

Kamille had laughed in disbelief. "Two?" she said, looking over at Bryce, who grinned like the happiest man alive.

Two babies, two little heartbeats. The joy was undeniable.

But under it all, there was fear. Fear of what would become of the world in the next few months.

As it turned out, this was the last antenatal appointment in which she would have her husband there with her, able to hold her hand, look into her eyes, and share in her joy right when the news was being broken. His absence during the next few appointments was one of the hardest parts of her pregnancy.

Once protocols began being implemented and COVID began spreading more rapidly, things shifted. Though she was a nurse, Kamille was spared caring for COVID patients. "They're keeping me away from the ward," she told Bryce one evening over tea. "Too risky with the twins."

"Good," he replied. "That's one less thing to worry about."

In some ways, COVID became a shield for her. The relentless nausea and fatigue kept her mostly homebound anyway, but the pandemic gave her an unarguable excuse. No visitors. No crowded grocery stores. No one leaning too close.

Still, it was just a bit more than she was comfortable with, a bit too lonely.

All medical appointments were taken alone, were stripped of comfort. The doctor's were unable to give any sort of reassurance. They had to stick to the bare minimum: examine, diagnose, treat. They were too short-staffed and overwhelmed for anything else. When she was told she needed to have genetic testing, the news came during a short visit. Cold. Quick. Then, even scheduling genetic testing became a puzzle, since doctor's offices were avoiding in-person visits.

After finally being told she needed amniocentesis to check for genetic disorders, birth defects, and other conditions in her fetuses, she expected at least to be allowed to bring Bryce with her. But no. Again. Alone.

The amniocentesis was the worst. She remembered walking into the dimly lit procedure room alone, clutching the strap of her bag. Kamille lay there, heart pounding, staring at the ceiling tiles as the needle slid into her belly. She had no one to hold her hand, no one to whisper that it would be all right.

Later, she drove home in silence, wincing from the ache in her abdomen, fighting back tears.

Through it all, she stayed strong, but Kamille could not shake the feeling that she might be doing something wrong. *What if I get sick? What if they get sick?* She wore her mask faithfully, even inside the house when others visited briefly. She told Bryce, "I'm not taking any chances, not with them."

Fortunately, the news was good. The twins had no genetic disorders.

When the twins finally came, the hospital's fluorescent corridors felt like a foreign land. One daughter, Lila, was whisked away to the NICU, her tiny body underweight and needing constant monitoring. The other, Sophie, stayed with Kamille.

Visiting Lila was complicated. COVID's exposure rules meant she couldn't stay with the her for long, especially with Sophie needing her too. Kamille felt torn in the middle. She knew Sophie was just an infant who needed her mom 24/7. Even though she was healthy, Kamille knew that even a few hours away would stress her baby. But then there was Lila, who was hooked up to beeping, loud machines. Being cared for by the NICU nurses and medicine, sure, but still, completely isolated and away from her mother, the woman who could give her comfort as she gained strength.

Staff shortages made it worse, almost unbearable; for two days, no one spoke to them about Lila's condition.

Then, at 2 a.m., the phone rang. "Mrs. Voss," a tired voice said. "You'll need to buy a new car seat for your daughter. She's too light for the one you brought."

Kamille sat up in bed, blinking in confusion. "Couldn't you have told me in person? During the day?" she asked, but the person on the line was already moving on to the next instruction.

When it was time to bring Lila home, only one parent could go into the NICU. Kamille stayed behind, cradling Sophie, while Bryce walked out hours later with Lila wrapped in a blanket strapped into her car seat. She would always remember the hollow ache of that moment, feeling as if she had abandoned one of her twins at birth, feeling guilt for not being able to stay by her side as she fought to live those few precious moments of her life in a healthy way.

She blamed the hospital and the rules for not considering her individual experience. But she knew that this was the best way to keep her entire family safe.

After that, it didn't get much better. Her postpartum care felt like an afterthought. No lactation consultant spoke to her. Education was minimal. The staff shortage seemed to excuse everything, but Kamille didn't accept it. "COVID or not," she told Bryce one night, "our care was unacceptable. It wasn't good enough for them, or for us."

Bryce had been happy through it all. He didn't seem fazed by the pandemic. "We got lucky," he told her. "Lila and Sophie are healthy. That's all that matters."

Kamille would always remember the fear that had lived in her chest for nine months, the quiet hours spent counting kicks, the lonely office visits, the way her mask became part of her body, the wait for Lila to come home. But what he said was true. Her babies were with her; they were perfect, they were healthy.

With her daughters' laughter bouncing off the walls, it was hard to imagine anything else, to imagine them coming into the world any other way.

27
Kinsley

It was the year 2021. It had been a year since the pandemic, and COVID had become a routine, something people handled as the rest of the mundane tasks of life. They worked, played, lived, and did everything while wearing masks. Almost all of the world had been vaccinated at this point, and people had gotten used to the reality, to the death toll, to the constant number of COVID-positive cases being reported in hospitals.

In that same year, Kinsley Monroe and her husband, Jeremiah, decided to try to have a baby. It was more of a hit or miss. Since Kinsley was in her forties, neither she nor Jeremiah expected that she would be able to conceive. As a precaution, both of them got vaccinated and wore masks every time they went outside. There wasn't much they could do anyway.

One smart move they made was to track rising COVID-19 case rates and continually move between the states with the lowest reported case rates. Moreover, both of them were lucky enough to be able to work from home. That way, they were more relaxed and could actually think through the situation rationally and with practicality.

It was in April of 2021 when they found out about their pregnancy. Spring was at its pinnacle at that time, with flowers blooming here and there. On weekdays, they avoided leaving the house unless absolutely necessary; however, on the weekend, for a change of scenery and to enjoy the weather, they geared up, wore their masks and went to the nearest park in town or to meet their family.

Jeremiah was over the moon ever since he found out about the pregnancy. He, especially, carried the joy of their news like a light inside him. He was thrilled to think of becoming a father, to imagine the small hands that would one day reach out to him, the little footsteps that would echo in their home. At the same time, there was a shadow of worry that followed him. Although he was overjoyed, he couldn't help but think of the unknown risks. The way COVID still hung in the air like an uninvited guest. No one truly knew what pregnancy during a pandemic meant for the health of mother and child.

Still, he clung to the fact that they were home together. That they had turned their little house into a cocoon, a shelter where the chaos of the outside world could not penetrate. They wore their masks faithfully, washed their hands until their skin was raw, and kept their distance even from those they loved. It wasn't easy, but it gave them peace. Jeremiah told himself again and again that they were protecting their growing family the best way they could.

He would shop for the groceries, clean around the house, help Kinsley with nausea and morning sickness, and do everything that he could to make this time easier for her. Since Kinsley was older, it would get physically tiring for her sometimes, and that was when Jeremiah made sure to be there for her. He would make soothing ginger tea for her (her favorite) and give her foot massages.

The first two trimesters were a routine mix of work, household chores, obstetrical appointments, and family getaways on weekends, all while wearing masks. As the seasons changed, the year rolled into December, and soon it would be January 2022, the time for them to deliver the baby. Another year with its own challenges and bounties.

When it came time to make a decision about where she would deliver, Kinsley felt a strange sense of relief when Florida seemed the most practical choice.

"Florida?" Jeremiah asked as they sat on the couch, Kinsley's head resting on his shoulder. The light blue glow of the muted television flickered across the room.

"Yes," she replied, rubbing her belly absentmindedly. "It makes sense. We can be outside more, and you've seen the numbers—COVID rates are so much better there compared to here in Connecticut."

Jeremiah tilted his head, considering her words. "And you feel like we can control things better?"

"I do," she said firmly. "I don't want to feel trapped inside hospital walls up here, with staff stretched thin and so many restrictions. Florida gives us… some breathing room. Some control. We can bring our child back here after delivery when the condition gets better. So, it's a win-win."

Jeremiah nodded slowly. He had grown used to trusting her instincts during the pregnancy, and though he worried, he could see that she sounded certain when she spoke of Florida. "Then Florida it is," he said, giving her hand a squeeze.

When the time finally came, the hospital in Florida felt like a different world compared to what she had feared. Sunshine streamed through the windows in the days leading up to labor, and the air outside carried warmth and salt from the ocean. Both she and Jeremiah felt reassured that their decision had been the right one.

But not everything went as smoothly as she had hoped. After delivery, her body ached in ways she had not anticipated. She asked for additional pain management, but she felt that her requests went unheeded.

"Excuse me," Kinsley said after several hours of pain, her voice tired but steady. "I need something more for the pain. It's… It's been harder than I thought it would be."

A nurse adjusted her mask, glanced at the chart, and offered a vague smile. "We'll check on that for you, okay?" Then she slipped out of the room, leaving Kinsley staring after her.

Jeremiah sat by her side, his brow furrowed. "That's the third time you've asked. I don't know what's the matter with them," he muttered, frustration creeping into his tone.

"I don't understand," Kinsley whispered. "I don't know if they're ignoring me, or if there just isn't enough staff to follow through. Everyone looks so… overworked." She paused, trying to swallow the lump in her throat. "Is it because of a staffing shortage? Or are they just not listening to me?"

Jeremiah leaned closer, brushing a strand of hair from her damp forehead. "Either way, it isn't right. You deserve to be heard." His voice softened as he looked at her, his eyes holding both worry and love. "I'll keep asking for you. You focus on getting some rest."

Despite Jeremiah's words, Kinsley couldn't shake the unease. The joy of holding her newborn was real, fierce, and overwhelming, but when the baby slept and the room was still, her mind reverted to the aches in her body. It felt like every joint had been twisted and broken. And she wondered if this was the reality of postpartum care in the shadow of a pandemic, where even the most essential requests were sometimes lost in the shuffle of a strained system. Or was it the normal postpartum pain? *Being a mother, delivering a whole human out of you was not an easy thing,* she thought.

The weeks after bringing their son home unfolded in ways Kinsley had not expected. She had braced herself for sleepless nights, for endless crying, and the fog of exhaustion that so many of her friends had warned her about. But her son was an angel, he made the experience so beautiful for her. Jaden was such an easy baby, content with their pattern of feeding and sleeping.

Jeremiah often joked, "He must have gotten your temperament, not mine." And Kinsley would laugh, shaking her head as she adjusted Jaden in her arms. "No, he's his own little person. He just… came to us peaceful."

Although she didn't have any other help except her husband, Kinsley didn't mind. In fact, she relished the challenge. She had always taken pride in herself as independent, someone who thrived on learning by doing. Parenthood, she decided, was no different. "I like the opportunity to figure this out with just us," she told Jeremiah one evening as they sat in the nursery, rocking their newborn between them. "No noise, no outsiders telling us what we should or shouldn't do. Just us, learning together. If it hadn't been for the pandemic and social distancing, then we wouldn't be doing it the same way as now."

Jeremiah smiled, brushing his hand over their son's soft hair. "I think we're doing okay," he whispered.

And they were. Since Jaden had adjusted to the sleep routine pretty well, the nights were quieter and calmer, punctuated not by panic but by soft cries that were quickly soothed. She learned the cadence of her baby's hunger, the subtle shifts in his face that told her what he needed. Jeremiah took turns with Kinsley, carrying their son through the house in the early mornings, whispering lullabies into the dawn while she rested.

Furthermore, visitors were few and carefully managed. Each one had taken a COVID test before coming, and all of them were comfortable masking as needed. The house filled with muffled voices, laughter from behind the masks, and the coos of relatives meeting the newest member of the family. Kinsley never felt worried. If anything, she felt reassured by the commitment her loved ones showed. "It's not the same as before," her sister admitted, eyes smiling over the edge of her mask. "But it's enough. Even though he can't feel our touch, he knows we're here."

Kinsley nodded. She was grateful enough.

In the weeks that followed, Kinsley often found herself reflecting on the timing of it all. Pregnancy in the middle of a pandemic had sounded daunting when she first imagined it, filled with unknown risks and fears of what could go wrong. And yet, as she looked back, her dominant feeling was gratitude.

When her friends asked her what she thought about being pregnant during a pandemic, she was honest. "I am really happy that nothing bad happened," she said simply, the words carrying a weight only she and Jeremiah could fully understand. The fear had been real, the risks ever-present, but somehow, they had made it through untouched.

She remembered the prayers whispered at night, the quiet bargains she made with God when uncertainty clouded her thoughts. "Please," she had murmured over her belly, "just keep him safe. Keep us safe." And when the third trimester arrived, she made the decision that gave her peace of mind: she got the COVID booster. She got it to protect her child before he was even born.

Jeremiah had been supportive from the beginning, reading every article, scanning every medical update about the booster shot, and holding her hand tightly when she scheduled the shot. "We're doing this for both of you," he told her, voice firm. And afterward, when the soreness faded and their baby continued to thrive, she knew she had made the right choice. "It was the best decision," she told anyone who asked.

In quiet moments, Kinsley reflected on how privileged their circumstances had been. Both she and Jeremiah worked from home even after delivery, laptops open at the dining table while their newborn slept in a bassinet nearby. They still moved between states, always choosing places with lower COVID rates, always keeping their circle small and controlled. "We are lucky," she admitted. "So many families don't have that choice."

Privilege wasn't a word she used lightly, but she understood its weight now more than ever. They had been able to carve out a life of safety and comfort while chaos raged elsewhere. For that, she felt a deep responsibility to never take her situation for granted.

One afternoon, as she watched Jeremiah pacing the living room with their son nestled against his chest, she felt a wave of emotion she could barely describe. "He's our best decision," she whispered, tears pricking her eyes.

Jeremiah turned, his expression soft, his gaze lingering on her as he rocked their child. "The best," he echoed. "Nothing else comes close."

The days blurred into weeks, and soon Kinsley no longer measured time in the old ways. Instead, she thought in terms of feedings, naps, and milestones. The first time her son grasped her finger with surprising strength, she laughed aloud, marveling at the tiny miracle of it. The first time he smiled in his sleep, Jeremiah rushed to grab the camera, his own grin wide and uncontained.

Despite the postpartum exhaustion that crept in at times, Kinsley's heart was full. She didn't crave outside help or elaborate routines. Instead, she cherished the small yet great bliss around her; the serene mornings, the calm evenings, the sense that their world was whole within the walls of their home.

When friends asked her later how it felt, how she managed pregnancy and new motherhood during such an uncertain time, she always returned to the same truth. "We were delighted," she said. "Delighted to have such a wonderful pregnancy, and now, our wonderful son."

Her words were simple, but they held layers of meaning. Delighted encompassed relief, joy, resilience, and awe. It meant surviving the fears of a global pandemic, carving out a safe space in the middle of a pandemic, and emerging not just unscathed but also grateful.

Months later, when Jaden learned to crawl and hold things on his own, when she looked back on those first fragile weeks, Kinsley remembered the sunlight in Florida streaming through their windows, the sound of Jeremiah's voice as he sang lullabies to Jaden, the reassuring presence of family who showed up masked and careful, but still present. She remembered her excruciating postpartum pain, too—but even that memory softened in the glow of everything that came after.

She smiled, seeing Jaden trying to make sense of things around him, recognizing foods and smells, crawling and trying to stand up, tightly grasping the table legs.

What remained clearest was the feeling of being exactly where she was meant to be: with Jeremiah, with her son, in a moment of history where uncertainty was the air itself, but love had been enough to sustain them.

As she rocked to sleep in the nursery one evening, humming softly, she whispered the words she had carried all along.

"We're so lucky," she said. "So, so lucky."

Jeremiah, standing in the doorway, smiled. "No," he corrected gently, "we're blessed."

And in the soft, warm glow of their little home, Kinsley knew he was right.

28
Chloé

Chloé Fisher was one of the many people around the world who took COVID as lightning in a bottle. With the world under lockdown, both she and her husband Adam were working remotely, which Chloé saw as a golden opportunity to conceive a baby. They did not have to go out; no one could visit them. They were at home and had ample time to focus on the baby. From Chloé's perspective, it was a once-in-a-lifetime chance.

Around the same time, a few other friends of hers were also either pregnant or had just become new moms. It was as if they had all caught baby fever.

Even though the dangers still lurked out there, Chloé and her friends were very excited about being moms around the same time. Even back when Chloé had not yet conceived, she and her friends had planned everything from baby showers to gender reveal parties together. They decided the themes, matching outfits, and one of them even created a whole mood board from Pinterest, manifesting all of their wishes.

All of it happened over Zoom calls. And even the day that Chloé found out about her pregnancy, and after she shared the wonderful news with Adam, they held a Zoom conference call. All of them were sitting in different corners of their homes, in their comfy PJs – that was the best thing about the COVID year, wearing PJs all the time and not having to dress up.

"I'm pregnant!" Chloé's voice burst through the screen.

All of them had been waiting desperately for this news, and as soon as it was out, they all high-fived and cheered. Their happy faces and big smiles were spread on Chloé's laptop screen when her long-held tears started to flow.

"Oh, please. You can't cry at such a moment. Now, all six of us are going to be big Mamas. This is a happy day!" Gabriella said. Her own daughter was in her arms, peacefully sleeping.

"I know. These are happy tears. I am so happy for all of us."

The conversation carried on for hours, and the plans about coordinating baby clothes and baby showers were repeated all over again with even more enthusiasm.

But things did not go as they had hoped. The COVID-19 pandemic worsened in the summer of 2021. Chloé's heart shattered along with her dreams. Still, she was grateful for the safety and security she felt.

Since the start of the first trimester, both she and Adam were on cloud nine. Even through the waves of nausea and exhaustion from morning sickness, they did not once regret the decision. They were happy, to say the least. Working from home, it was easy for them to deal with the first trimester. They did not have to go out and commute to work daily, interacting with people.

Initial obstetrical visits were done online via telehealth, and even though they were not very helpful, Chloé was still grateful she did not have to go out. However, it was her second month of the first trimester when she was went to the doctor's office to receive the COVID-19 vaccine. That was when a wave of fear surfaced in her veins.

What if I get COVID? What if the vaccines aren't actually helpful? What if the vaccines have some side effects on my baby?

The questions swirled inside her head, and even voicing them out loud to Adam was futile, as he was as clueless as she was.

Nonetheless, Chloé got vaccinated. Throughout that month, she waited for any adverse side effects, but nothing came. Her anxiety lessened and she accepted that she was overthinking it all because of her significant anxiety issues. No matter how hard she tried to tone it down and not overthink everything, the unknowingness of COVID made it impossible. Her anxiety often made her plunge into a cycle of overthinking.

Her only support throughout the whole pregnancy season was Adam and her fellow mommy friends. Two of them had already given birth, so they calmed her down by telling her their experiences. They told her that pregnancy makes one supersensitive and highly emotional, so it was normal that she was feeling a certain way. Adam, by her side, also helped her with such episodes. The on time he needed to leave the house for work he feared that Chloé would go into labor without him, or she would contract COVID, or maybe he would not be able to see his baby being born.

With numerous ups and downs and a rollercoaster of emotions, nine months eventually ended. Adam was there with her when Chloé went into labor. However, her brain was swirling with other worries.

What if I have to wear a mask during delivery? Would the nurses wear masks? What if I get COVID after delivery? Before delivery? What if my baby gets COVID?

The nurses, clad in white personal protective equipment and masked, pushed her wheelchair to the operating room. Adam was also allowed, after going through a screening test, which turned out to be negative. He set the room up with all of Chloé's essentials, and then it was time for the cesarean section.

The surgeon entered the surgical suite with a broad smile on her face. After warm greetings, she put on her gloves and mask. Soon, Chloé was anesthetized. After two hours, she found herself staring at her newborn in awe.

Their daughter was everything they had ever dreamt of. She was the image of heaven itself. And they named her Eden. Eden Colleen Fisher. Their heaven.

The world changed for Chloé after the delivery.

Her first challenge was with lactation and the shortage of formula. Her browser had a dozen tabs open: articles about breastfeeding positions, lactation consultants offering online classes, and forums where exhausted mothers posted in the dead of night.

She had taken so many of those online courses that she could recite the basics in her sleep. She knew the tricks, the way to hold her daughter, the way to encourage Eden to latch. And she was proud of herself for it. In a world cut off by lockdowns, she had used the internet to prepare herself. Yet, oftentimes, she would have problems lactating, and she would need formula to keep her baby from starving.

And the formula shortage was the cherry on top of everything COVID had already brought. Shelves at local stores were bare, photos of desperate parents filled social media feeds, and Chloé felt trapped. "I didn't even get a choice," she whispered to Adam one night, her voice heavy with exhaustion. "I wanted breastfeeding to be something I chose for Eden, not something forced on us because there's no formula left."

Adam reached for her hand. "You're doing an amazing job," he said, but Chloé could see the same flicker of worry in his eyes that she felt in her own heart.

Their families had been worried from the very beginning. Every phone call with her mother began the same way: *Are you sure this is safe? Are you sure it's okay to be pregnant during all of this?* The worry was constant, circling around them like background noise. Chloé could not deny that they worry had worsened after her cesarean section. The operation had been necessary, unavoidable, but the added stress of doctor visits and the looming threat of increased COVID numbers made it nearly unbearable for her.

With the passage of time, Chloé was consumed by emotions that she could not easily name. On one hand, she was ecstatic to finally hold her daughter, to feel her tiny fingers curl tightly around her own. On the other hand, her chest often felt heavy with an invisible weight. The anxiety she had battled for years seemed sharper, louder, more relentless now. COVID had worsened it during pregnancy, and in the loneliness of the postpartum period, it grew even more unsettling.

She began to notice how her mind never rested. If Eden coughed or sneezed, her thoughts spun into webs of "what ifs." What if it was COVID? What if she got sick from Adam? What if something happened while she was sleeping? At night, when the house was still and Eden finally dozed off, Chloé would lie awake, her heart racing, listening for the sound of her baby's breathing.

It was Adam who gently suggested therapy again. Because everything was remote, it felt doable. Chloé increased her sessions from once a week to two times, sometimes needing the extra space to pour her thoughts out, to have someone tell her that her fears did not make her a bad mother. Therapy became her lifeline. On the days she felt most fragile, those calls reminded her that she was not alone, that her anxieties were not her fault.

Still, the isolation gnawed at her. The pandemic meant her family and her very dear friends could not visit freely, and Eden's first smiles and coos were shared through pixelated screens. Chloé often felt robbed of the postpartum community she had imagined. She had always wanted her mother by her side, her friends dropping in with meals, and her cousins randomly stopping by to see the baby just because they missed her. Instead, there was silence. She and Adam did their best, but Chloé's worries became louder without the presence of others to soften them.

She admitted to herself that she was an anxious parent, maybe even more so because of COVID. The thought of daycare haunted her. Every news article about outbreaks in schools or daycare centers made her stomach twist. The idea of leaving Eden in the care of others, where she might be exposed to something beyond Chloé's control, seemed unbearable.

For now, Chloé clung to her routine of therapy sessions, daily walks with Eden in the stroller, and long conversations with her mommy friends online. These things gave her clarity and hope. She wanted to believe that with time, her fears would ease, and she could breathe more freely as a mother and be a good, healthy one to her little girl.

Their little girl – as Adam would often correct her – was beautiful, perfect in their eyes, but she was also a baby with a bad case of colic. Night after night, Eden cried with a force that made Chloé's heart jump out of her chest. Her tiny body would scrunch up, her face turning red, and the wails seemed endless. Chloé tried rocking her, feeding her, singing softly, anything to bring comfort, but nothing seemed to work.

The isolation of the pandemic only made those painful nights unbearable. If it had been a different time, her mother might have stayed with them, or a friend could have stopped by to lend a hand, to give her a break, even just for an hour. But because of COVID, visitors were scarce, and Chloé felt the burden of parenting rested solely on her and Adam. She had wanted that in theory, just the two of them figuring things out together. Yet in practice, with the colic and the anxiety layered on top of a pandemic, she often felt more alone than she ever imagined possible.

Adam tried to reassure her, to share the weight of the newborn stage, but Chloé admitted to herself that she sometimes felt like she was failing. Each little cry from Eden made her nerves fray a little more. She loved her daughter beyond words, but her postpartum period was undeniably difficult. The constant crying, the lack of sleep, and the never-ending cycle of feedings blurred the days and nights into a haze.

And yet, when her therapist asked her if she would do it again if given the chance, Chloé smiled. "I would do it again because of the results," she said, her voice both tired and filled with wonder. Eden was worth all the tears, the fear, the exhaustion. Even in the hardest moments, she never regretted their decision to bring a child into the world during COVID.

But she also learned lessons. One of them was practical, born out of experience. "Next time," she laughed to her therapist, "I'm going to stock up on formula before getting pregnant again. I'm not doing that scramble all over again." It was a small but important piece of wisdom, a marker of how pregnancy and postpartum had changed her, how they had made her not just anxious, but resourceful, too.

Reflecting on the whole experience, Chloé often described it as an experiment in creativity. The pandemic had forced her and Adam to adapt in ways they never thought possible. They held virtual baby showers, made playlists for Eden's arrival instead of hosting parties, and learned how to lean on telehealth appointments when in-person ones weren't an option. "We figured out how creative we could be," she said. "We ultimately made lemonade out of lemons."

The metaphor fit perfectly. COVID had taken so much from the world—lives, freedoms, gatherings—but for Chloé, it had also given her a chance to discover resilience she never knew she had. The anxiety was real, yes, and the postpartum struggle was raw, but the end result was a daughter who filled their home with light.

Chloé's final thoughts about pregnancy during COVID always circled back to gratitude. The hardships had sharpened her vision, helping her notice things she might have overlooked otherwise. She learned to be thankful for the quiet mornings when Eden would finally fall asleep on her chest, for the steady presence of Adam who whispered encouragement when she doubted herself, for the support of friends who showed up on Zoom even when they couldn't step inside her home.

"Looking back," she said, "I feel so grateful for everything. Both the good and the bad."

Chloé often thought about how much COVID had changed her story of pregnancy and motherhood. It wasn't the dreamy picture she once painted in her head, but it was real, full of unexpected lessons and moments that would shape her forever. She learned that motherhood was not about perfection but presence, not about everything going right but about being there, even when things went wrong.

29
Natalie

Natalie Ramirez still remembered the silence. It clung to their house like a second skin.

The world outside had shut down, and inside, she and her husband, Daniel, were preparing, bracing for the arrival of their first child.

The pregnancy had been planned, and she had conceived a few months before COVID-19 had started spreading. Back then, they were excited, certain, joyful. Now, all they felt was fear. The world was no longer safe. How could they make sure that their newborn would be safe?

The news was always filled with reports of overburdened, understaffed hospitals. How were they supposed to get good antenatal care? How were they supposed to cope when it came time to deliver?

For now, all they could do was wear their masks, avoid going outside, and use sanitizer regularly.

Daniel had been the worrier of the two. He confessed one night, "I just… I don't know what this virus means for the baby. No one does. What if there are long-term effects we can't see yet?"

Natalie, though equally afraid, placed a hand on his and whispered, "We'll be careful. We'll do everything we can."

When July came along, baby Krissy was born. Natalie went into labor, fearful yet strong, ready to tackle anything that came her way. She had tolerated the abysmal antenatal care after all. She knew that whatever happened today, she would get through it as long as her baby was healthy. And healthy she was—healthy and perfect." Healthy and perfect.

She remembered pressing the call button in the middle of the night, desperate for help as Krissy screamed and struggled to latch. The button lit up, but no one came. Staffing was short. Nurses rushed between rooms like ghosts, stretched too thin.

Alone, with breasts aching and her baby crying, Natalie had tried and tried. A wave of helpless guilt washed over her, making her feel like she was already failing her daughter. When nothing worked, exhaustion broke her resolve. Formula became the answer.

The struggles she faced in the hospital were nothing compared to the isolation.

Natalie's parents had waited their whole lives to be grandparents, but when the baby finally arrived, they could only stand at the doorway, masked and cautious, peering at the bundle in Natalie's arms. They didn't dare step inside. There were no family dinners, no women of her family gathered around to show her how to soothe or swaddle. Instead, there was Natalie, Daniel, and their daughter in a quiet house that felt too big.

Their families tried to be supportive, but COVID hung over every conversation. At the baptism, every photograph showed a sea of masked faces, only the baby's cheeks bare to the world. At holidays, phone calls replaced embraces. And in between, there were hard discussions about vaccines, masking, and who could be trusted inside their fragile bubble.

Daniel said once, after pacing the length of their kitchen, "This isn't how I imagined it. Becoming a father should've been different."

"I know," Natalie admitted, her throat tight. "But it's what we've got."

The one positive, the thing that kept him going, was the fact that he could spend all his time with Krissy. Daniel's job allowed him to work from home, and he often sat with the baby asleep on his chest between meetings. He told Natalie one evening, smiling softly, "I'm getting to see her grow. I wouldn't have had this before."

Natalie's employer was understanding and granted her a long maternity leave. It was a relief she hadn't expected, and together, she and Daniel began to stitch a rhythm into their days—cooking, cleaning, parenting, protecting. Alone, but together.

Over the next year, things began to calm down. Vaccines were rolled out, and everyone now knew about the virus and what it could do. Regulations and isolation were still in place, but now, due to more research, they were more effective. By the time Krissy was a year and a half, Daniel and Natalie decided they wanted another baby. They decided they no longer wanted to wait. They decided that even though the world had been turned upside down, they had the strength, as a family, as a unit, to take on anything and everything the pandemic threw their way.

In September 2022, when they saw the face of their healthy baby boy, James, they knew. They knew that the gift of their children was worth everything that they had endured.

30
Tanya

The ending months of 2019 hit her like a truck. Tanya Thompson was already three months into pregnancy when the news of a virus breaking out in the world burst from news channels worldwide. COVID-19 had spread rapidly across the world, and the number of positive cases was increasing day by day.

When March began, the world was shutting down. All businesses and stores were vacated and locked within 24 hours. When planning the baby, she and her fiancé, Steven, had no idea about the rollercoaster ride they would be taking.

At first, Tanya tried to brush it off. She told herself that the pandemic would pass in a few weeks, that life would return to normal before her belly really began to show. But the reality set in quickly. The days were filled with breaking news, government updates, and grim statistics flashing across the television screen. Every number felt like a warning, every cough in public like a threat.

At first, Steven was not at all scared of the virus. But once he understood that the situation was grave, he became supportive and helped Tanya in every way he could to maintain hygiene and safety in the house.

She and Steven developed routines they never imagined would be necessary. A bottle of Lysol lived permanently near the door, and anything that crossed the threshold, whether it be mail, groceries, or packages, was wiped down meticulously before being placed in its proper spot.

"I'll do it," Steven insisted one evening as she reached for the grocery bags. His latex-gloved hands held the disinfectant wipes like weapons.

"Steven, I can help—" she began.

"No, Tanya. You're pregnant. You're not risking anything." His voice was firm, but behind it, she could hear the fear.

So, she stepped back and watched him spray, wipe, and arrange their groceries where they belonged, as if their life depended on it. Maybe it did.

In April her employer, unsure of when things would open up again, decided to let her go. At first, it felt like relief. She enjoyed the time getting to rest and focus on her pregnancy. But soon it became suffocating. The walls of their home seemed to press inward. Days blurred together. The calendar on the fridge held canceled plans: prenatal yoga classes, visits with friends, the baby shower she had dreamed of.

Steven didn't have the luxury of staying home. As an EMT, he suited up every morning and walked straight into the unknown. Tanya tried to smile as he left each day, but the knot in her stomach tightened with every shift.

"Promise me you'll be careful," she whispered one morning, her hands resting on her growing belly.

"I always am," he said, pressing a kiss to her forehead. His uniform smelled faintly of disinfectant, and the smell lingered long after he left.

The hardest blows came one by one, like dominoes falling. Her baby shower, which was all planned, paid for, and dreamed about, was canceled. Friends sent their gifts in boxes, left at the doorstep without hugs or laughter. Tanya unwrapped tiny clothes and blankets alone in the nursery. All the while, she cried as tears wetted the wrapping papers in her hand.

Steven tried to cheer her. "We'll have a party later, after all this is over," he promised. But Tanya knew it wouldn't be the same. Pregnancy was fleeting. She wanted to share it now with her sisters, friends, and mother. Instead, her only company was loneliness, vaccines, and multivitamin supplements.

Even doctors' visits were lonely affairs. "I'm sorry Tanya, but he can't come in with you," the receptionist would say with a practiced tone. Steven would sit in the car, scrolling on his phone, while Tanya faced the sterile doctor's office alone. She longed for him to be there with her, to hear their baby's heartbeat for the first time, and to share every little moment together. Instead, she clutched her mask, eyes watering, whispering, "She's really in there, Steven," when she returned to the car.

But joy and grief collided in cruel ways. Her grandfather fell severely ill due to COVID and was admitted to the hospital. She wanted desperately to see him, to sit by his bed, to thank him for the years of wisdom he had shared with her. But the risk was too high. She stayed home, staring at her phone, waiting for updates. When he passed, she mourned from afar. No final goodbye. Just silence and the pain of loss.

Their wedding plans, too, crumbled under the weight of restrictions. The grand celebration they had imagined shrank to a modest ceremony, stripped of most of its guests. Tanya tried to smile through it, but the photographs told another story. Her eyes, hidden behind a mask, reflected the grief of a bride whose family could not be there with her on her big day, whose laughter was muffled by fabric on the day she was supposed to smile the most.

Tanya's isolation only grew as the days passed. Both Tanya's and Steven's sisters worked in high-risk environments, and visits became impossible. Holidays passed with empty chairs and phone calls instead of family gatherings. Tanya would sit on the couch, her hands tracing the outline of her belly, whispering to her unborn daughter, "You're not alone. Mama's here. Mama's here."

When the day of delivery arrived, Steven was finally allowed to stay with her in the hospital, a small consolation amid the restrictions. Yet even then, the rules were suffocating. He could not leave the room for food or air. They were confined within four white walls waiting for the fragile miracle of new life.

Holding their daughter Maeve for the first time, Tanya felt joy so fierce it nearly broke her. "She's perfect," she whispered, tears streaming down her cheeks. For a moment, the entire world did not exist except for the weight of Maeve in her arms and the warmth of Steven's hand on her shoulder.

The delivery itself had been great. After months of fear and loneliness, the hospital staff felt like a blessing. Nurses moved with gentle hands, checking on her and the baby with kindness that was contrary to the cold, white walls of the hospital room. Doctors reassured her with calm voices, answering questions she barely knew how to articulate. Steven was at her side the entire time, masked but present, and that was enough.

"I couldn't have asked for a better team," Tanya told Steven as she cradled their daughter on the second night. The room was quiet except for the constant buzzing of machines and the muted chatter of the floor outside.

"They're incredible," Steven agreed, rubbing her shoulder. "Even with all these restrictions, I feel like we're being cared for."

The absence of visitors was something that once would have broken her heart, but surprisingly, it turned into a gift. Within the silent hospital walls, there were no interruptions, no expectations. Just the three of them: Tanya, Steven, and Maeve, discovering what it meant to be a family.

But once they returned home, the reality loomed again. Friends and family only sent well-wishes through video calls. No one could hold the baby; no one could share in the soft wonder of newborn life. Nights felt endless, days felt heavy, and Tanya's loneliness grew into something darker. Postpartum depression.

She found herself staring out the window at empty streets, wondering what kind of world she had brought her daughter into. Sometimes she would cry without knowing why. Other times, she would sit in silence, numb. The loneliness, the missed milestones, the constant fear, it all wrapped around her like a shroud.

"I think I'm not okay," she finally admitted to Steven one night, her voice barely audible over Maeve's soft breathing.

He turned to her, his eyes full of worry. "We'll get through this," he said, pulling her close. "You're not alone. We'll find help."

Naming it postpartum depression was both terrifying and relieving. Tanya realized it wasn't just her. It was the pandemic, the silence, the missing people and voices that should have surrounded her.

Still, amid the shadows, there was light. Her daughter was a healthy baby. And she was growing well day by day. Every giggle from her daughter, every new milestone, reminded her why she endured. "For you," she whispered as she rocked Maeve to sleep. "I'd go through it all again for you."

Tanya's pregnancy during COVID had been nothing like she dreamed it would be. It was marked by fear, by loss, by deafening loneliness. However, it was also marked by resilience and a fierce love from a mother and father determined to protect their child. And as she kissed her daughter's forehead, she knew that even in the darkest season, life had found a way to bloom.

For weeks, they lived in a bubble. Family members called and FaceTimed. Screens lit up with faces eager to see the newest addition, and Tanya smiled, holding Maeve close to the camera. But when the calls ended, she felt a lingering ache in her heart.

"It's not the same," she confessed one night, scrolling through a string of missed calls. "She can't feel them through a screen. She can't know how loved she is just from voices and faces on a phone."

Steven kissed her forehead. "We'll get there. They'll meet her when it's safe."

It wasn't until their daughter was three months old that the families finally met Maeve in person. Tanya remembered the day vividly. It was an early winter afternoon when they arranged an outdoor visit in her grandparents' backyard.

Her grandmother's eyes welled with tears behind her mask. "She's beautiful," she whispered, her voice cracking. "Oh, I wish I could hold her."

Tanya's heart clenched. She wanted nothing more than to place her daughter into her grandmother's arms, to let her feel the warmth of the baby's skin, the softness of her breath. But instead, she held the baby tight, rocking gently as the family admired from a distance.

"She'll know you," Tanya promised, her own voice trembling. "She'll feel your love, even like this."

It was a bittersweet reunion. Love was there, thick in the air, but it couldn't be touched, couldn't be shared in the ways it had always been before. Tanya went home that night, grateful her daughter had finally met her grandparents, but the sadness followed her. She had imagined these moments differently, with a crowd of family, friends, and laughter, arms passing the baby from one to the next. Instead, it was quiet, restrained, and heavy with what was missing.

As the months stretched on, Tanya's reflections grew sharper. People asked her often, half-joking, half-curious: "Would you do it again? Would you have another baby during a pandemic?"

Her answer was immediate. "No," she said, shaking her head. "Not like this. Never like this again."

She was grateful, of course, for her healthy daughter, for a pregnancy and delivery that had gone smoothly despite the circumstances. But she could not imagine willingly stepping into that kind of isolation again. It weighed her down more than she had imagined.

"Knowing what I went through," she told a friend over the phone, "I wouldn't choose it. Not for myself, not for my family. I wouldn't want anyone to experience pregnancy like that."

It wasn't until her next pregnancy, after the pandemic had eased, when restrictions were gone and the world was breathing a little freer, that Tanya realized how different it could be. This time, she attended appointments with Steven by her side, his hand in hers as they listened to the heartbeat together. Friends visited, bringing food and laughter, filling her home with the warmth she had longed for before. She had a baby shower, surrounded by women she loved, opening gifts amid smiles and hugs.

"It's night and day," she said softly one evening, rocking her newborn son while Steven played with their daughter nearby. "This is what pregnancy is supposed to feel like. Shared. Celebrated. Not hidden away."

When she compared the two experiences, the truth became undeniable: the pandemic had taken so much from her first pregnancy. It had amplified every fear, every ounce of anxiety, until she felt like she was drowning. It had contributed to the postpartum depression she struggled with. The isolation and stress wrapped around her like chains.

"I thought it was just me," Tanya admitted during a counseling session, "but now I know. It wasn't just me. It was the pandemic. It stole things, not only from me, but from everyone in this world, the things we'll never get back."

And yet, as she held her daughter, healthy, vibrant, full of life, Tanya felt a deep gratitude. Out of all the uncertainty, she had gained her greatest gift. The experience had scarred her, yes, but it had also sharpened her perspective.

"Would I change it if I could?" she asked herself one quiet night while journaling. She paused, pen hovering over the paper. "I don't know. Because without it, I wouldn't have her. But if I could choose, if I could rewrite the circumstances, I would never choose pregnancy during a pandemic again."

Her reflection was not bitter but honest. When people asked her about her first pregnancy, she smiled at the memory of holding Maeve for the first time. But when they asked about the pandemic, her face grew somber.

"It changed everything," she would say. "It made something joyful into something traumatic. It shapes who I am today."

Yet Tanya also carried resilience. She had faced the darkest of seasons, walked through fear and loneliness, and still came out with a love deeper than she could describe. In the end, she knew the pandemic had not defined her daughter's life; it had only shaped the beginning of her own journey as a mother.

And with that knowledge, Tanya closed her journal, looked across the room at her children playing, and whispered, "Never again. But always, always worth it."

31
Kim

The first time Kim Williams saw the plus sign appear, she cried. Not from shock, but from relief, from utter, absolute joy. After years of endometriosis, thyroid struggles, and endless rounds of medical appointments, she had learned to temper her hope. Yet here it was, undeniable and glowing: she was pregnant.

She clutched the test to her chest and whispered Dimitri's name. When he found her in the bathroom, tears streaming down her cheeks, he froze.

"Is it—?" he asked.

Kim could only nod. He wrapped his arms around her, both of them laughing and crying. They had planned this pregnancy carefully, consulting doctors, adjusting medications, making lifestyle changes, and mapping out every possibility. And now, at last, it was real.

What they didn't plan for was a pandemic.

By her last trimester, COVID-19 swept across the United States. Kim packed up her office desk and retreated to the spare bedroom, where the glow of her laptop replaced the buzz of colleagues. She was glad to be able to work from home because it protected her precious baby from the virus, but the setup was less than ideal. Kim was an extrovert who drew energy from interacting with other people. She joked that the beige walls knew her better than her friends did now.

In every aspect of her life, she was forced to undertake a solitary mission. "No loved ones allowed, only patients may enter," the receptionist told her flatly over the phone as she tried to book an antenatal care appointment in March of 2020. Dimitri wasn't allowed to attend, wasn't allowed even to FaceTime. Still, Kim bore through the appointments like a champ, managing all of the stress and pain on her own. Her appointments had to be more frequent than most, considering her medical history, and she had become accustomed to fighting for her medical rights on her own since she had an illness that few doctors knew how to treat correctly.

One of these appointments was her most cherished and, at the same time, her saddest.

She lay on the exam room bed, the cold gel on her stomach giving her goosebumps as the doctor watched the screen.

"Twins," the doctor said. Though a mask covered her face, Kim could tell she was smiling widely.

Kim's heart soared. This was better than anything she had dreamed for this pregnancy. Her family would be complete. She decided that Dimitri needed to hear this in person, so as she made her way back to her car, all she did was send him a short text informing him that the appointment went well. But as she drove home, the joy was tinged with sorrow.

She peeled off her coat and rubbed her belly once she reached home. Dimitri walked by, eating a sandwich. "Hey, babe. How was it?"

Kim was out of breath but smiling.

"What? Is something wrong?"

"No, no. Everything is perfect. So so perfect!"

Dimitri was smiling too now. "A girl, huh? That's what you always wanted." He took another bite.

"Even better, Dimitri! Two girls! We are having twins!"

Dimitri froze mid-bite, his sandwich forgotten as his eyes widened. "Twins?" he repeated, the word catching in his throat. When Kim nodded, laughter spilled out of him, full and unrestrained. He dropped the sandwich onto the counter and scooped her into his arms, spinning her carefully despite her protests.

Tears stung her eyes as she clung to him, both of them laughing, both overwhelmed. In that moment, the fear, the masks, the empty waiting rooms, all of it disappeared. All that mattered was the miracle of two tiny heartbeats, already changing their world forever.

Later that night, they lay in bed together, Kim resting against his chest. They discussed how they would handle twins in the months to come and how COVID-19 would impact their plans. How would they have to adjust their lives to make sure their babies were safe?

Dimitri was anxious because he wanted to be there for them as much as he could.

"I wasn't there today with you. I didn't hear it. I didn't see them." He reached for her hand and kissed it, but his shoulders sagged. "I want to feel like this is ours, Kim. Not just yours."

She tried to be strong, but tears burned her eyes. "I felt alone in that room. Like I was carrying this by myself. I needed you to be there too. This was such an amazing moment. I wish we were able to experience it together."

"I know. Well, what is done is done. There was nothing we could have changed. But once they are born, I promise, I will never leave their sides."

Kim laughed, happy that her husband was as excited as she was.

Her parents worried too. During late-night video calls, Maria, Kim's mother, paced the living room behind the screen, wringing her hands. "This pregnancy is high-risk enough," she said. "Now with the virus…hospitals are overwhelmed, doctors are exhausted. It scares me. You can't take chances."

David, her father, leaned forward. "We'll come to help out once the twins are born. We can work remotely. You shouldn't go through this without help."

"Better yet, we will come now. I'm sure you need help around the house. It's the last few weeks; you could pop any time now." Her mother chuckled.

When they finally arrived, suitcases clattering against the porch, Kim's chest loosened. Their visit stretched from two weeks to months. They helped with meals, rubbed her back when the twins pressed painfully against her ribs, and promised they'd stay as long as she needed.

Dimitri became the guardian of their little fortress. He stacked groceries in neat rows, wiped down every package with disinfectant, and turned away well-meaning neighbors at the door.

"No one in, no one out," he muttered, lining up cans on the pantry shelf. "I won't risk you, or them."

Kim admired his vigilance, but loneliness crept in like a draft. Baby showers were canceled. No friends came to place their palms on her belly, to marvel at the life stirring within her. The house was quiet when it should have been full of laughter.

When August finally came, Kim was ready to see her baby girls. She remembered the hospital walls closing in, the mask strapped across her face, each contraction leaving her breathless. Dimitri wasn't there—no hand to clutch, no voice to steady her. Nurses whispered encouragement, but their words blurred in the storm of pain. When the twins finally arrived, she felt triumphant yet strangely hollow.

It wasn't until postpartum, when the mask was finally removed, that she wept openly. She pressed her daughters to her chest, inhaling them deeply, skin to skin.

Later, back home, she sat on the couch with Dimitri as the babies cooed beside them. "I wish you'd been there," she murmured.

"I do too," he admitted, tracing a finger along their tiny hands. "But we're here now. And I'll protect you. I'll protect them."

Childcare options vanished once her parents had to return home, and her maternity leave came to an end. Daycare tours were impossible. Eventually, they found a woman who ran a home-based program, her backyard wide and bright with sunlight. It wasn't what they'd imagined, but it was safe, and the girls thrived.

Some days, Kim would watch them from the porch—two small figures chasing bubbles Dimitri blew into the warm Southern air. Their laughter rang out across the yard, a sound bright enough to dissolve the shadows of isolation.

And yet, the ache remained. No grandparents' kisses. No aunts and uncles passing the babies from arm to arm. No communal celebration of their birth. The pandemic had stolen their village.

But as the girls tumbled into her lap, giggling and breathless, Kim realized that happiness had found its own way in. It didn't look like the crowded living room she once dreamed of, or the baby shower she never had. It looked like sticky fingers reaching for her cheek, like Dimitri's arms circling them all in a messy embrace, like the sunlight catching in her daughters' curls. Despite everything the world had taken, this small circle of love was enough. It was more than enough.

32
Renae

The invitation came on a Thursday.

An email. An invitation with her name written in looping blue font sat waiting in her inbox. Renae Burke read through it while her son chattered in the living room, his blocks clattering against the wooden floor. It announced a party in Westport for Saturday night the following week.

Renae's lips curved into a small smile. She could almost see it. Golden candles glowing in tall glass holders, music vibrating through the floorboards, glasses clinking as friends toasted under strings of lights. Normally, she would have loved it. This was just the sort of event she longed for, thrived in. She had always loved being around people. It refreshed her, gave her something to look forward to.

But her body had other plans. Her stomach twisted, and not from nerves. A dull nausea sat heavy in her belly. Pregnancy exhaustion had been hitting her hard this time, and every muscle begged her to stay put. She pressed her hand against her swollen midsection.

Her husband, Alan, walked by and glanced at her laptop screen. "Party?" Alan asked, still in his scrubs from the hospital. He washed his hands at the sink, rubbing each finger raw under the faucet.

"In Westport. Saturday night." She leaned on the counter. "I don't think I can, Alan. I feel sick all the time. This baby is wearing me out."

He glanced at her; worry etched into the corners of his face. "Then we're not going." His tone was final, protective. "You need rest right now."

Renae nodded, a little relieved.

They found out later what happened at that party. Guests brought something home besides memories. When the news came on the radio about the outbreak, Renae's hands trembled around her mug of tea.

"We dodged it," Alan said, squeezing her shoulder. "It was close, but we are safe, babe."

But her mind wandered, the pit in her stomach grew, and she shivered at the thought of what might have been.

From then on, the two became hypervigilant, scared at first because of that close call, but then deeply terrified because of just how much had changed about their lives, about the world. The news was constantly rife with new updates about the virus and its spread. Alan, being a physician, saw firsthand just how overwhelmed the hospitals were. Renae thought that in just these few months, he had aged years. The lines on his face had deepened, and the bags under his eyes never seemed to soften.

This did not at all look like the pregnancy she had imagined.

With her son Matthew, there had been baby showers, relatives dropping off casseroles, hands eager to touch her belly. This time, there was silence. Nothing. Only video calls and congratulatory text messages. However, the absence of family and friends was not the only thing that made her feel like this pregnancy was incomplete.

At doctor's appointments, she sat alone, her mask pressing against her skin, her breath hot inside it. She listened to the whoosh-whoosh of her baby's heartbeat through the monitor, but no one sat beside her to share the joy.

When she came home, she sometimes leaned against the door, eyes stinging with tears.

"Another good appointment?" Alan would call from the basement, where he had moved to protect her and the baby from any germs he might bring home from the hospital.

"Yes," she'd answer, though her voice cracked. She'd leave his dinner on the top step, knock lightly, and scurry back before he opened the door. They spoke on video calls at night, her face glowing on his screen even though he was only a floor away.

Matthew tugged at her sleeve one evening. "Why does Daddy live downstairs?"

"Because he wants to keep us safe, sweetheart," she said, brushing his hair off his forehead. But her chest ached with the loneliness of a house divided.

And the house was not just divided; it was their cell.

Renae would work on her laptop in pajama pants, taking video calls where coworkers didn't even notice her growing belly. The work-from-home policy had been welcome, and some days, she found herself almost grateful for the stillness. No rushing, no heels, no makeup. Just her and the hum of the house.

But the stillness had teeth. By evening, she sometimes sat staring at the wall, her son's laughter echoing faintly from the next room. She felt hollow, as if the world had folded in on itself, leaving her alone with her thoughts.

"Once the baby comes, maybe things will get better," she thought.

However, when the time came, in October 2020, nothing was as she had expected.

Labor came in the middle of the night. The hospital hallways smelled of disinfectant, the halls lined with masked nurses. They helped her into the bed, the mask tugging at her ears, her breath shallow.

"I can't," she whispered to Alan when he was finally allowed by her side, his own mask hiding his jaw. "I can't breathe with this thing on."

"You can," he said firmly, holding her hand tight. "Just a little longer."

Hours later, the baby's cry split the air. Renae's tears spilled as she tore the mask from her face just long enough to press her lips against her daughter's damp cheek. It was a stolen moment, fragile and fleeting, but it was hers.

After the joy of having her daughter Abigail in her arms wore off, Renae became aware of the dangers that surrounded her. Alan had been on edge from the very start, and though his daughter had created a warmth in his heart that kept him grounded and joyful, he could not ignore his instincts and training.

"We're leaving as soon as we can," Alan said once Abigail and Renae were declared stable and healthy. And they did.

Those first weeks postpartum were exhausting. Renae felt a familiar tug of darkness: the "blues," she called them. Each day, they seemed to creep closer. She knew it was worse this time, worse than it had ever been before. Before she had had a support system, friends, parties, dinners, distractions. Now, it was just her. No friends visiting, no family holding the baby while she showered, no one dropping by with a meal.

"I don't know if I can do this." The thought, the doubt, popped into her mind constantly.

But she acted. She cared for Mathew and Abigail. She reached for help. She called her doctor, admitting the heaviness pressing on her. She fought for herself, for her little ones.

And things got better. Especially once vaccines were made available and Alan was able to come out of the basement to be with his family. Together, they made it work.

They found new rituals: outdoor playdates, bundled in coats, children shrieking with laughter from opposite ends of driveways. Virtual music classes where Matthew clapped along to songs on a screen, while Abigail cooed and babbled in time with the music. FaceTime calls where grandparents watched the baby until their eyes shone with tears.

They had even turned the nearby construction site into their new playground. Matthew would press his nose against the fence for hours there, watching the cranes and trucks. Renae could see the joy clearly on his face as he did so, and she knew that no matter what, she had managed to keep her children safe and happy.

One evening, the family sat together in the living room: Abigail in her crib, Matthew playing with his blocks on the floor, Renae and Alan watching a movie. Renae leaned her head against Alan's shoulder and let herself breathe. They had been tested. They had been lonely, frightened, stretched thin. But here they were.

Stronger. Together.

33
Hailey

It was in February 2020 when Hailey learned about her pregnancy. She had been feeling waves of nausea and sickness for a while now, and her first guess was the COVID-19 virus, which had recently gotten prevalent in the air worldwide.

When she observed that she was not experiencing any other symptoms of the viral attack, she went straight to her friend who was an Obstetrician in the office where she worked as a registered nurse.

Upon completing some tests, she found out that she was pregnant. With an overwhelming wave of elation, another darkening thought loomed along.

I am pregnant when there's a virus threatening the entire world.

She had not planned any of that. She had not planned this pregnancy, let alone at a time when the world was crumbling, when hundreds of people were dying on a daily basis, when everyone was uncertain of the coming days. She did not want this baby to enter such a tense world. But now it was here, in her belly, and she could only take a deep breath, brace herself, and accept it as it was.

Her worry only grew with time, when, the next month, on March 14, 2020, the whole world was shut down under lockdown because of the constantly increasing positive cases and death toll.

Working in healthcare wasn't easy, given the gravity of the situation. Hailey feared that her being pregnant and being around infected patients wasn't a good idea for the safety of her and her baby. Hence, as soon as the lockdown was announced and the medical practice was issued a red alert, the medical office where she worked assigned her to work as a receptionist to limit her contact with patients. Hailey was grateful for their understanding and loved her work regardless.

As time passed and her baby developed inside her, the complications also increased. Hailey conceived this pregnancy at 35 years of age; hence, her pregnancy was deemed an Advanced Maternal Age pregnancy.

Both she and her husband, Justin, were obsessed with constantly cleaning and sanitizing everything. Their house now looked like a store for cleaning supplies, with Lysol bottles, scrubs, and rags kept everywhere along with sanitizer bottles. Even though she no longer had direction contact with patients, Hailey still took care to sanitize everything, remove her shoes and coat at the doorstep before entering the house, and immediately hop into the shower. She would also make sure their house was cleaned every day. Both Justin and Hailey took turns cleaning, relied solely on online delivery for groceries and necessities, and avoided going out or meeting people unless it was truly necessary.

Her complicated pregnancy made it hard for her to have peaceful nights and normal pulse rates. She would often wake up in the middle of the night, breathless, sweating, and heaving. Then, it would take her another hour to settle down into a short moment of quiet sleep. Justin was her constant backbone through it all and made sure to ease her pain as much as he could.

However, Hailey wasn't the only one who had to face the storm. It was hard for Justin to see her going to all of her obstetrical appointments and ultrasounds alone. He yearned to be there with her, to be able to hold her hand and see their baby on the monitor and to hear their baby's heartbeat together. Without all of these experiences, it all sometimes seemed to him as if it was an illusion. He often thought that he was dreaming it all. Was it even real? Did the baby really exist? Was the baby growing well?

After every medical visit, as he waited for her in his car parked in the office's lot, he wondered about what must be going on inside. How was the baby doing? What was Hailey feeling? Was she okay or not? Was the baby okay or not?

On the other hand, Hailey loved going to her doctor's visits. The office was warm and welcoming, and the people there had become her safe place. Everyone knew her by name, and their smiles, even behind the masks, radiated a familiarity she did not take for granted. In a time when the world felt cold and detached, the office was one of the few places that offered her comfort. The sound of the monitor tracing her baby's heartbeat had become her favorite melody. She would close her eyes and just listen to the steady, reassuring rhythm.

Hailey often thought that these visits were her salvation. She loved everything about them, from the machines' constant hum to the sterile scent of cleaning detergents, and the way her physician would look her in the eye and genuinely ask, "How are you doing today, Hailey?" She would always answer truthfully, sometimes smiling, sometimes tearing up, but always grateful to be asked. Even when sometimes the news wasn't what she wanted to hear, when her blood pressure spiked, or the ultrasound hinted at something uncertain, she never felt abandoned. The team there was her second family, her tribe through this storm. They were not just doctors or nurses; they were her friends, companions in a fight she hadn't chosen but was determined to face bravely.

When her obstetrician mentioned the first signs of preterm labor, Hailey felt the floor slip away from under her feet. It was too soon. She wasn't ready, and neither was the baby. Her body had begun contracting earlier than expected, subtle at first but not something she could miss. Her doctor had immediately prescribed bed rest, urging her to stay home, to do as little as possible, to let her body rest and hold on just a little longer.

At first, Hailey thought she could manage; however, it wasn't an easy task for a go-getter like her to stay idle at home. She told herself she'd use the time to read, to rest, to prepare. But the reality of being confined was far harsher than she'd imagined. She was used to movement, to working, helping others, staying busy. Lying in bed all day made her restless, and her brain whirled into overthinking. Every small ache sent her spiraling into worry. Was the baby okay? Was she doing something wrong?

Justin tried to comfort her, bringing her meals, giving her massages to calm her down, and keeping her company when he could between his remote work meetings. He'd sit beside her, laptop open, and hold her hand while typing, and make sure that she didn't feel alone.

But eventually, even that wasn't enough. When her contractions became stronger, her doctor admitted her to the Maternal Care Unit. That day, as Justin helped her pack a small overnight bag, neither of them knew she would be there for weeks.

The room was clean and softly lit, but it felt more like a box than a sanctuary. Because of the strict COVID protocols, she wasn't allowed to leave her room, not even for a brief walk down the hall. The isolation was crushing. Nurses checked in periodically, but their visits were quick and mechanical. They were kind, but cautious, staying only as long as necessary before slipping back out, leaving Hailey wrapped in silence. She understood that they had their own safety to think about, but still, the loneliness ached.

Days blurred into weeks. She watched the sunlight crawl across the same spot on the floor every morning, marking time in slow, predictable intervals. Meals came on trays wrapped in plastic. Conversations happened through screens. She kept her phone nearby at all times, the only window to the world outside. Justin called her several times a day and talked to her about mundane things to keep her mind distracted.

Her Gender Reveal Party took place over Zoom. She had dressed up for it, even put on a light layer of makeup and brushed her hair, though her hands trembled slightly as she did. She wanted to feel beautiful, radiant, like every glowing mother-to-be she had once seen in magazines. But when she looked at her reflection, pale under the white lights, hospital band snug on her wrist, it didn't feel quite real. Justin had set everything up at home, balloons and a banner in the background. Their friends and family joined in, tiny squares of faces on a laptop screen. When they announced it was a boy, everyone cheered. Hailey smiled, tears spilling freely, both from joy and longing. She wished she could hug them, could see their eyes without a screen separating them.

Her quasi-baby shower followed the same format as a virtual gathering, filled with love, laughter, and voices through microphones. Her friends played games online, sent gifts to her doorstep, and told her how beautiful she looked. She appreciated every effort, every thoughtful gesture, but deep down, she mourned what she didn't have. She missed the physical touch, the laughter shared over cake, the hugs, the group photos, the tiny moments that make memories tangible. It felt like she had been denied all the "fun stuff," as she put it, and that realization sometimes broke her heart in unfathomable ways.

Yet, in those still moments, she also began to notice things she might have otherwise missed. The tiny flutters that grew stronger each day. The way her baby responded to her voice, kicking softly when she read aloud or hummed. She started journaling, writing letters to her unborn daughter, promising her love, safety, and strength. Those letters became her lifeline and a way to connect, to hope, to look forward.

The medical team continued to monitor her closely. Every day brought a new test, a new number, a new set of possibilities. The goal was simple: keep the baby safe, keep him inside just a little longer. Each extra day felt like a small victory. Hailey held onto that, celebrating every week that passed without complication.

As the days grew shorter and her due date slowly approached, Hailey began to find a strange peace in her solitude. She no longer resisted the stillness as much. Instead, she leaned into it, letting herself rest, breathe, and trust her body despite everything. There was still fear, but there was also an underlying current of strength. She had made it this far. So had her baby.

Sometimes, late at night, when the room lights dimmed and the world seemed to hold its breath, she would rest her hands on her belly and whisper softly, "We're okay, little one. We're okay." And in those moments, with her baby's steady movements inside her, she almost believed it.

Weeks later, Hailey's son was born. The delivery was not as painful as her last trimester. Jonah came out easily, healthy, and completely fine.

Hailey's postpartum care in the hospital was also wonderful. The nurses were gentle, attentive, and kind, treating her with a level of compassion that she would remember for years. They checked on her often, offering warm blankets, soft encouragement, and reassurance during those first fragile days of recovery. Yet, despite the excellent care she received, there was an emptiness she couldn't shake, because her son was in the Neonatal Intensive Care Unit.

She had imagined holding Jonah right after delivery, feeling his tiny heartbeat against hers, breathing in his newborn scent. But instead, he was whisked away before she could even properly see him. She didn't get to hold her son for the first twenty-four hours of his life. That separation felt unbearable. She lay awake that first night, her body still in pain, her heart heavier than she could have imagined. She could hear the faint cries of other babies in the distance and longed for her own son's voice. When she finally saw Jonah, small and perfect in the incubator, surrounded by the soft beeping of machines, tears flooded her eyes.

Only one parent was allowed in the NICU at a time because of the ongoing COVID-19 restrictions. That meant she and Justin had to take turns visiting their son, handing off the baton of parenthood in carefully scheduled time slots. It was never enough. Hailey would sit beside Jonah's crib for hours, whispering softly, her fingers gently tracing the outline of his hand through the tiny opening in the incubator wall. When she was finally allowed to hold him after those first twenty-four hours, she requested skin-to-skin contact immediately. The moment his fragile body rested against her chest, all the walls she had built up to protect herself from worry came crumbling down. She cried quietly, overwhelmed by love, fear, relief, and exhaustion all at once.

But their challenges didn't end there. Hailey was discharged before her son was, forced to leave the hospital without him. Walking out of those doors without a baby in her arms was one of the hardest things she had ever done. The car seat in the back of the car sat empty, and she couldn't look at it without tears filling her eyes. Each day, she and Justin made separate visits to the NICU, rotating shifts so that Jonah would never be alone. The days were long and emotionally draining, but they clung to hope and to each other.

When they finally brought him home, life slowly began to settle into a new routine. Hailey's parents were incredibly supportive during her postpartum recovery. They stepped in without hesitation, helping with feedings, changing diapers, and offering the kind of care only grandparents can. Their presence allowed Hailey to rest, to heal, and eventually to return to work with peace of mind. Her parents became Jonah's second set of protectors, and their love wrapped around him like a shield.

Hailey and Justin were cautious, perhaps overly so, but it felt necessary. They decided not to send Jonah to daycare until he was three years old. The fear of exposing him to others, to illnesses, and to uncertainty all lingered long after the world began reopening. They built their own little bubble, finding safety in the familiar walls of their home.

Then came the hardest blow of all. Despite all their precautions, her family contracted COVID. Hailey's father, her constant source of strength and calm, didn't survive. His passing left an ache that words could never fully capture. Losing him felt like losing a piece of the foundation she had built her life upon. The grief was heavy, slow, and unrelenting. Even now, she admits that it remains one of the greatest hurdles she has ever faced.

When Hailey looks back on her pregnancy and early motherhood during the pandemic, her emotions are complex. She acknowledges how many medical complications she faced, how the stress of the pandemic only worsened everything. The isolation from both her medical restrictions and the world's lockdown blurred together until she could no longer tell where one ended and the other began. The loneliness, the seclusion, the endless uncertainty, all of it heightened her anxiety and made what should have been the happiest time of her life one of the hardest.

But time, she has learned, is a healer. Now, with the pandemic behind them, life feels lighter. She smiles more. Jonah, now full of energy and curiosity, fills their home with laughter. They take walks in the park, visit friends, and share meals without fear. They are learning to live again, to be more active, joyful, and open. She says it feels as if they are finally living life as it was before COVID, maybe even better, because they now understand just how precious it all is.

When someone asks her if she would choose to be pregnant during a pandemic again, Hailey doesn't hesitate. "A thousand percent, no," she says with a small laugh. "Never again." She means it. Despite her deep love for her son, she would never wish to endure that kind of uncertainty and fear again. Yet, as she looks at Jonah now, strong, happy, and thriving, she knows that every sleepless night, every tear, and every lonely moment was worth it.

Hailey was grateful. Grateful that life has found its way again. Grateful for her family, for the laughter that rings through their home, for the ordinary moments that once felt unreachable. She carries the weight of the past, yes, but she carries it with grace and a renewed appreciation for the beautiful, fragile, ordinary miracle of life.

34
Emily

Emily's second pregnancy was nothing less than a raging storm. She and her husband, Travis, had planned their second child after having a positive pregnancy experience. Yet, it was nothing they had imagined, even in their wildest dreams.

As the year 2020 began, it brought along with it the deadly pandemic of coronavirus. Emily was in the third month of her second pregnancy when all the local and international news channels repeated the same headlines—COVID-19, rising death toll, increasing number of positive cases, and schools and institutions being locked down.

It was all an overwhelming surge of grim and scary information that made Emily sit down on the couch and breathe in and out to calm herself down.

Soon, within a week or two, the outbreak was declared a pandemic, the world had been completely shut down, except for essential services like healthcare, all flights were canceled or postponed, stores were shut, and people were strictly advised to stay indoors.

Emily and Travis had been assigned to remote work and had no idea when they would be able to resume their normal lives. Their first child, Oliver, was just a toddler, and their second was still inside the belly, completely oblivious to the battleground the world had turned into.

One evening during the cold winter of January, she and Travis sat on the couch in their living room. The room was dimly lit with the warm street light filtering through the curtains, and they were snuggled in blankets, drinking steaming cups of hot chocolate. Despite the warm and cozy setting, both of them had frowns plastered on their faces. Emily lightly brushed her fingers through Oliver's hair as her eyes focused on the TV.

The usual news, just new numbers of positive cases and an ever-rising line on the death-toll graph. She averted her eyes from the screen and looked at Travis. His face was lit with the blue light cast from the TV, and his face held the same upset frown.

“Trav?” she whispered in a low, cautious voice.

“Yes, Emily?”

“What do you think will happen? This is all so scary.”

“Honestly, I have zero idea. The updates don’t seem too positive.”

“I am just worried about our kids. Oliver is too young to be exposed to the virus. We can’t risk his safety,” then she placed her hand gently on her belly, “and this little baby, it hasn’t even fully formed yet. It doesn’t even know that this is the world it will open its eyes to. What if something happens to it?”

Travis removed his arm from under the blanket and draped it across Emily’s shoulders, hugging her from the side and pulling her closer.

“Let’s hope for the best. For now, the best we can do is to be updated on the news and follow the healthcare guidelines. That’s the only way to keep ourselves and our kids safe.”

Emily nodded with conviction, partly making herself believe his words. At that moment, having faith in each other and God was the only thing she could do. She could not fight the virus and stop the chaos even if she wanted to, so she just closed her eyes, made a silent prayer in her heart, and took a deep breath.

With each passing day, as the number of positive cases went up, their worry also heightened. After completing their remote work, both of them cleaned the entire house with Lysol and sanitized every single thing. Travis made sure to keep enough masks and gloves around the house, in every drawer and cabinet, on the coffee table, and on the kitchen counter.

Emily did not notice it at first, but she was starting to have more sleepless nights than she did initially. It was not morning sickness nausea, because it had subsided when her third month began. She was physically fine; her obstetrical visits showed her vitals were normal and the baby was developing well, yet she could not find a reason for the breathless, sleepless nights that were becoming more frequent.

"Ms. Scott, it is normal to have a little restlessness during pregnancy," her obstetrician explained when Emily inquired for an answer.

"I think you are right," Emily agreed in a low voice, her eyes staring into a void.

"You have been through a pregnancy before. You should know. I know the situation is a little different this time, but you will be fine. Keep taking your medications on time, and eat healthy. Nothing to worry about," Dr. Moriyah said, as she placed her hand in a comforting gesture on Emily's shoulder.

"Thank you so much, Dr. Moriyah. I will make sure to follow your instructions. See you next week. Bye," she said with a half-smile.

She picked the ultrasound pictures from the doctor's table, pulled her mask up to her nose, and walked out of the room. Her feet took slow and mindless steps as she walked down the hallway. The Obstetricians office did not allow significant others, but she still kept her mask up. She looked at other patients with faces also covered behind masks, the nurses running back and forth, overworked and busy, the other pregnant ladies sitting with their hands on their protruding bellies.

Her mind plunged into an endless train of thought. These women were way ahead in their pregnancies; she still had months to go. They seemed fine and pretty healthy, but would she be able to keep her baby healthy? They all wore masks, eyes passive; she probably looked the same.

One thing common between her and the other pregnant ladies was the absence of their partners. Her eyes darted around, scanning the hallway. There were no husbands in the waiting room; all the mothers were handling it all alone. Maybe some of them were single mothers, and she could not help but feel the same.

Like all other patients' partners, Travis was not allowed to accompany her to the weekly prenatal visits. It was part of the healthcare guidelines issued amid the pandemic. She had started to feel like a single parent, like she was the only one doing it all on her own. Their first baby Oliver was definitely *theirs,* but this baby felt like just *hers.* She felt that Travis was very disconnected from this pregnancy. In the beginning, he used to wait in the car for her and show excitement for the ultrasound images. But after a couple of weeks, the signs of elation disappeared. She started to drive and go to the visits alone, and even when she brought the images to him, he would just smile and say repeated words like "yeah," "that's nice," or "thank god."

He did not question further, wasn't very curious, and that created a deep pit of loneliness in Emily's heart. She knew that part of the reason for his mental absence was the physical absence. If the situation were different, if there had been no pandemic, if he were allowed to accompany her to the visits, he would not have been so distant and disconnected.

With that consolation, she went to her car and headed for home. She stifled her thoughts deep down in her heart and entered with a happy face. Travis was there with Oliver, both of them sitting on the floor, playing with Legos.

She did not let a speck of worry show on her face as she took off her jacket and shoes by the door, sanitized her hands, and went straight to the shower.

On every prenatal visit day, she bore the same feelings, letting them wash over her again and again. After a few months passed, the loneliness and overthinking came to an end—or so she thought.

In July, it was finally time for her to go into labor and deliver her second child. From winter to summer, she had felt a whirlwind of emotions, had countless sleepless nights, and doubted every single day that she would not be able to make it. Yet, here she was, finally in labor, ready to deliver her baby. She saw all the staff covered and clad in white personal protective equipment. Travis had bought a huge amount of masks and gloves just to ensure that they were protected against the virus at all times.

Travis recommended having the baby delivered at home in a water bath. He did not trust the hospital staff to keep them safe.

"Emily, we don't know who's positive there. It's a lot of risk. I don't think that's a good idea. Maybe you should just call a midwife and deliver at home. One person from the outside is better than being in a hospital, risking exposure to COVID."

But Emily was not in favor of his idea. She immediately shook her head and refuted.

"Travis, my labor room would be on the non-COVID floor. Besides, don't you remember the first time, how I had the postpartum hemorrhage? It will be disastrous if it develops again, and I would be stuck at home with no professional help."

In the end, Travis agreed. The situation was the same as their first pregnancy, but they realized that delivering in the hospital was a better idea than to do it at home.

Emily called her parents before going to the hospital, and they wished her well.

"We are here for you, baby. We are praying for you. Stay strong," her mother's voice came through the speaker, and Emily shed a tear.

It broke her heart that she could not have her parents with her through these times of trial. This whole pregnancy, she missed her mother's warm hug to console her whenever she had an episode of overthinking. Every time she felt lonely, she needed her to say that she was here, to make her sweet ginger tea, and to tell her that everything would be alright.

The delivery experience was better than they had expected. When Emily and Travis entered the hospital, they were very skeptical. They had brought their own sanitizers along with masks and gloves. Emily was doubting every person walking in the hallway, eyeing them with scrutinizing glances, wondering if they had COVID or not.

However, no one other than the nurses and doctors entered their room. And those who did were fully masked and covered. They were very gentle and attentive during her labor and delivery.

The postpartum experience disappointed her, though. The staff was short and overworked. Nurses, even though soft and polite, were barely available. She had problems with lactation initially, which was ignored by the lactation consultant. This led to Emily visiting the hospital ER because of the development of mastitis.

As the days passed, with two babies on her arms, her loneliness started to deepen. She was on maternity leave from work, but Travis still had to be present in front of the laptop. He helped her a lot with everything, cleaning diapers, maintaining the house, sanitizing, and doing minimal chores as much as he could. Yet, the haunting feeling in her stomach, the restlessness, and the sleepless nights did not disappear.

After ten months postpartum, her parents were finally able to visit their grandchildren. They were a great support and Emily did not realize how much she had missed them during the isolated pregnancy until she touched her mother's hand for the first time in a year. Tears flooded from her eyes, and she hugged them both tightly. By that time, all of them had gotten vaccinated, so she was not as worried about the virus as she was in the beginning.

After COVID, with her toddler and her baby a bit older, Emily decided to reach out to a therapist. Her mood swings and episodes of anxiety had not calmed down; they had only been shoved under the carpet.

After a couple of sessions, her therapist, Dr. Yara, held her hands and told her the diagnosis, "You have PTSD. From the experiences you had to deal with in COVID. I want you to know that it's not your fault. Being pregnant and being responsible for another life, along with your own, especially during a pandemic, is not an ordinary task. And you did really well. You just need to let your emotions out and speak about them. That's the only way they will leave your mind and heart. And that's how you will become a healthy parent too."

Emily was not shocked to hear that. If anything, she agreed with it and decided to make amends with herself, "I am very grateful for you helping me with this. It was indeed a traumatizing era, and if it's up to me to choose, I would never willingly ever be pregnant again in a pandemic. Having another child would be nothing less than a blessing, but if there's a pandemic? Please, no," she paused and laughed.

35
Ariana

Ariana took her cup of hot chocolate, tightened her robe around, trapping her body against the cold, and sat in front of her laptop. She set her cup on the kitchen counter and settled comfortably in her chair. Her eyes stared intently at the screen as she scrolled through the news.

It was March 2020, the air was still a little chilly, the flowers were still waiting for April to bloom. Ariana could see the morning sun rising from her apartment window. Everything appeared to be absolutely normal. But… there was this little, tiny, invisible virus that was about to transform the world into something no one had ever heard of before.

The COVID-19 virus had been declared a pandemic, and the entire world was shut down in all literal and metaphorical senses. Stores and businesses were closed, schools and educational activities were halted, and people were firmly advised to stay at home unless completely necessary. Only public service workers, like healthcare and police, had to leave their homes in order to protect the rest of the population.

As Ariana's eyes scrunched and focused on the online news, she clearly remembered the day two weeks ago when the news of the lockdown was announced. She had been admitted to the hospital that day because she had developed kidney stones. She was recuperating after her operation, when she noticed the nurses rushing here and there in urgency. She was not too worried, if anything, grateful to see nurses being so caring and attentive to the COVID-positive patients. Even though they were overworked, they did not let it show. They cared for every patient the same, and it warmed Ariana's heart from the inside.

She was almost six months pregnant, so she was shifted to a room on the non-COVID floor of the hospital. There, the floor was understaffed, and she had to wait longer than usual before assistance was provided. But she did not mind it, since she understood the severity of the situation.

Her husband, Steve, on the other hand, was restless. He worried that something would happen to his wife and the unborn child. There was not a single positive answer to any of his questions, and that scared him even more. He would peek out of the small transparent square on the hospital door, looking out for a nurse and answering their queries. But for long minutes, when no one would come, he would despondently huff and sit on the small chair in the corner of the room. After a couple of hours, he had had enough and all he wanted was to take his wife home as soon as possible.

When Ariana returned home, she could not deny that she was worried too. She, too, had questions and uncertainties, but she could not panic when Steve was pulling his hair out. She knew that one of them had to maintain sanity and control of the situation.

When they had planned this baby, they had made a list of questions and found answers to them either through friends and family or through the internet. But not even in the worst of nightmares had they considered having to deliver this baby in the middle of a pandemic. When they finally conceived in October 2019, the news of the virus emerging from China had already made it to the headlines, but like most people, they thought that it was perhaps local to that city, and it would be controlled before it got out of control. From day to day, the graphs spiked, and the number of COVID-19 positive patients rose. Until it became so serious that the whole world was issued a red alert warning. Now, at six months pregnant, there was nothing much she could do except follow the healthcare guidelines and advice being issued by the government.

Ariana was innately a grateful and hopeful person. She always looked for the silver lining among the dark clouds. So, when such a fatal pandemic arrived during the happiest time of her life, she focused her mind on looking for hidden good parts. She was not escaping or trying to hide away from reality; she was just trying to survive this dark memory with a good heart.

The first thing she was instantly grateful for was working completely from home. She saw the police officers, nurses, firemen, and people who had to be there in person for their jobs, and could not help but feel thankful that she had the convenience of staying safe and working from the comfort of her home.

She sipped the hot chocolate from her cup, savoring in the warmth, whispering words of gratitude inside in her heart. Her fingers moved over the trackpad on her laptop as she shut down the news channel's website and opened up her work portal. The remote work did not require set hours; she could do it and submit her work at her own discretion before 6 PM any time. Yet, being an early bird by nature, she liked to wake up with the sun, get her work done, and set aside the rest of the day for herself. She focused on cleaning her house and spraying everything with sanitizer and Lysol. That was the least she could do with the COVID situation worsening day by day.

One thing that bothered her, even after being very optimistic about the situation, was that she could not go outside and see real people. She knew that she had to find a way for that while making sure to maintain a six-foot social distance and avoid skin-to-skin touch with anyone.

That day, she completed her work in a few hours, submitted it, and by the time she was in the kitchen about to cook herself a quick lunch, a brilliant solution had already popped up in her mind.

A dog!

She knew that if she got a dog, she would have to take it outside for a walk at least two times daily, and that would also give her the opportunity to be out in the fresh air and see the people, birds, the blue sky, and feel it all in real life, and not from her living room window only.

Moreover, she thought that there could be no better time than this to get a dog. She was at home 24/7 except for the weekly prenatal appointments, everything was on hold and she had free time to train and take care of a dog.

So, after pitching her idea to Steve, Ariana arranged to get a cute little golden retriever pup. She took her out for a walk once in the morning before she sat down for work and once in the evening before sunset. She would make sure to wear her mask whenever she left the the house, and wash and sanitize her hands right after she came back.

She would pull her mask down slightly and breathe in the fresh air, which carried signs of the spring season. She could smell it in the air. It was warmer, fresher, and lovelier. The flowers in her garden were starting to bloom, there were more birds on the branches, and more animals out of their hideouts since there were fewer humans on the streets.

Apart from the rapidly growing number of people becoming victims of COVID in the outer world, everything seemed to have halted and taken a step back. Even in her personal life, Ariana was enjoying the laid-back routine, the pause, and the freedom of time. She was enjoying it as long as the baby inside her was growing well.

However, the same thing could not be said about Steve. He was quite the opposite of Ariana. He noticed every growing number on the charts, took extra care with cleaning and sanitization, and asked a million questions to Ariana's obstetrician.

When April began, and the situation around COVID only spiked and worsened, Dr. Hoffman, in accordance with the healthcare guidelines, did not allow Steve to accompany Ariana to the weekly prenatal visits. That was a blow at Steve's already haywire brain. The weeks following that, he would see Ariana entering home with ultrasound pictures and her case files in hand and he would have a gazillion questions to blurt out at her but first, he let her change and shower before she could sit beside him and answer every question in detail:

"What did the doctor say?"

"Is the baby fine?"

"Did you get your COVID-19 screening done? You are not positive, are you?"

"How's the baby growing? Is the movement fine?"

And on and on and on he would go, and Ariana would answer every question in detail, and calmed him down with positive feedback from the doctor. She was his comfort, his silver lining among the dark storm, and his warmth against the cold.

Yet even after all her comforting replies, Steve had a little feeling of disconnect with his unborn child. He could not be there in person to see the baby move on the little monitor, to feel the kicks and hear the heartbeat. He could only look at the black and white pictures and believe that his child was fine.

Not only Steve, but Ariana's family also held the same worries. They would call her multiple times a week and ask the same questions about her and the baby's health. Ariana would always repeat the same answers and tried to comfort them as she would with Steve. She would tell her mother each and every daily update about the baby; how many times he kicked in a day, how his movements were, how well she was eating, everything.

Ariana's mother worked in a pharmacy, so everyone in the family, including Ariana, had to maintain a distance from her for everyone's safety. It was upsetting for her, too, that she could not have her family by her side, but overall, she was happy that even if she could not meet them, they were at least safe.

It was in early May when Ariana's grandmother contracted COVID and succumbed to it before doctors could take extreme measures to save her. Her old age made it easy for the virus to attack her and become the cause of her demise. Ariana's mother was the most heartbroken, and it upset Ariana even more that her baby could not meet her grandmother before her death. No matter how much she wanted to comfort her mother in her time of need, the COVID virus prevented her from doing that.

What couls she do except blame the damned invisible virus, which took not only her grandmother's life, but also the lives of hundreds and thousands across the world. This realization overwhelmed Ariana with empathy and compassion for all humanity and made her feel more grounded and grateful for the safety of her unborn child.

In June 2020, Ariana delivered her daughter Charlotte in a small white hospital room. The experience was smooth and comfortable. Aside from the painful and exhausting process of labor and delivery, everything else, including the hospital staff and the care they provided, was excellent. Ariana noticed that the staff was overworked and the hospital was crowded, but all her needs were met. The safety of her and her baby were prioritized, and no visitors were allowed in her room. Even the nurses were limited in number and all wore protective gear, including masks and gloves. She was grateful for not having visitors, for not having to wear a mask during delivery, and for having alone time with Charlotte and her husband, who had to wear gloves and a mask too.

When Ariana's postpartum period started, that's when she felt the burden of isolation, the negative side of the pandemic. She missed her mother, and how she was always there to support her whenever she needed her. Every time she changed the diapers, or had problems with lactation, or was just tired from carrying the Charlotte around and rocking her to sleep, she missed her mother a little more.

She would sit with her laptop on the couch; her daughter cradled in one arm and her other hand busy with work. Her coffee would turn cold because she would forget about it amid work and cradling her daughter.

Steve would help her when he was home; he would make sure that Ariana got enough rest and sleep while he took the night shift with Charlotte. He would rock her to sleep and change her diaper if needed.

Ariana was grateful for that too. She was extremely grateful that even after all the uncertainties and hardships that she had to face during her pregnancy in the pandemic, she did not have to go out for work; she and her family were safe, her husband was supportive, and she could stay home and rest whenever she wanted.

Even if someone asked her if she would get pregnant in a pandemic again, she never doubted it. She said it with conviction that she was extremely thankful for the time and experience she had, and that if she and her husband wanted it, they would plan another baby regardless of the pandemic.

36
Meredith

I am a mom of two, and I can say that I am pretty experienced with this thing, but this third child made me feel like a nervous-nelly first-time mom. Honestly, I am very pleased and blessed to be a mom of three beautiful kids, and I was also very sure and elated to plan and conceive the third one. However, I had no idea that it would end in such a disaster.

So, in March of 2020, I was ready to deliver my daughter, my third child. I had prepared almost everything, but then COVID-19 struck, and suddenly the whole world was under a lockdown. My first thought was, 'What should I do?' and then my second thought was to hoard all the supplies I would need during postpartum. Once I knew that the grocery stores would be shutting down and there would be a potential shortage of cleaning supplies, I almost sprinted to Walmart and grabbed as many postpartum supplies as possible.

My husband, Ryan, had also broken his leg right before the lockdown, so I had to do it all alone. I bought as many diapers as my cart could hold, lotions, baby care, and then we heard that sanitizers were suddenly a household staple, so I had to buy them too. The stores were out of hand sanitizers, and that shocked me.

After two weeks, I was admitted to the hospital in labor. The hospital was swamped with patients, almost everyone was masked, and no one could guess which one of them carried COVID and who didn't.

Inside my room, I was tested for COVID before I was handed a mask to wear during labor. I took the mask with hesitation since I did not know if it would be easy for me to deliver with a mask to stifle my screams. When I was about to receive my epidural anesthesia, I noticed that the nurses made Ryan stand behind the hospital curtains because he was not wearing a mask.

I did not know what to feel about it. The hospital had run out of protective gear, so they did not have any more masks left to give to Ryan. Not only Ryan, but some of the nurses entering my room were also not wearing masks or any protective gear. It had only been two weeks since the lockdown began, so I did not know how to respond to things. I did not even know the right questions to ask the healthcare staff. It was actually funny to see him hiding behind the curtains, standing there with a broken leg.

While the nurse told me to practice breathing exercises, I saw that my husband was moved from behind the curtains to the area that used to be the waiting room before the COVID lockdown. I asked the nurse if my husband would be able to be there with me during my delivery. But the nurse was unsure at that time.

I'd been through labor and delivery twice before with Mason and Harper. It was not new to me. What was new was the anxiety this time. I knew that this hospital also catered to a hundred COVID-19 patients, that this same nursing staff took care of them too, that when I delivered my baby, it would open its eyes to a virus.

I had also heard the virus was disproportionately affecting infants and the elderly because of their weak immune system. That thought piqued my worries even more. I did not want any unmasked nurses to enter my room; I didn't want anyone to touch my newborn daughter, Emma. All I wanted was to take her straight home and hide her away from it all.

Since I was furloughed from my job, I was homebound until I found a new one. Ryan was also working remotely for his firm, which made it easier for both of us to stay home and focus on our children.

After I got home with my daughter Emma, things felt both strangely calm and wildly chaotic. Outside, the world was spinning out of control, with everyone panicking, news channels filled with climbing death toll numbers, and stores closing. Neighbors disappeared into their houses like shadows. But inside my little bubble, everything almost felt safe. Ryan was on leave with his broken leg, and my mom, my saving grace, was in my COVID bubble with me.

That bubble became my world. Mom had helped me after my first two deliveries, and she was always the strong, loving hand that kept everything from falling apart. I remember calling her a few days before delivery, worried that she might not be able to come because of lockdowns. She just said, "Don't worry, honey, we'll figure it out," and she did. She quarantined, stayed put, and when I came home with the baby, she was right there waiting on the porch, mask on, gloved up, ready to hold her granddaughter. I don't think I've ever been so grateful for another person in my life.

Her being in my COVID bubble meant I could breathe a little easier. She took over diaper duty when I couldn't get up, helped Mason and Harper with their remote schoolwork, and somehow still managed to make dinner while singing lullabies. I truly felt supported. For a while, it didn't feel like the world was in the middle of a pandemic; it felt more like a pause from nature. Home was the only place that mattered.

Still, there was something different about this postpartum period. I had been through it twice before, but this time, it all felt new and uncertain again, like I was a first-time mom all over. The fear of the virus loomed over every little decision. I made everyone who stepped into the house wash their hands for a full twenty seconds. Masks were non-negotiable. Even my mom, who technically lived with us, would put one on whenever she held Emma, and I found myself checking to make sure it was properly covering her nose.

I would laugh about it later, how neurotic I must have seemed, but at the time, it didn't feel funny. It felt like survival. I was terrified that this invisible thing could harm Emma. I had heard all those stories about infants getting sick, and the idea of taking my fragile baby into a pediatrician's office filled with COVID patients was something that haunted me. I was determined not to let anything happen to her.

Ryan and I spent long days together at home. He was hobbling around on crutches, trying to be helpful despite his leg, and I appreciated every bit of effort he made. Since he couldn't go back to work yet, he took over some of the household duties, mostly sitting at his laptop and making grocery orders or managing the kids' online school schedules. We made a good team, even if we were both a little anxious. There were moments when the pessimistic thoughts won, when the walls of the house seemed to close in, and I'd find myself staring out the window, missing things I had never thought I'd miss, like the grocery store aisles, the chatter of coworkers, the feeling of normalcy.

Getting laid off two weeks before delivery was its own heartbreak. I remember the email. It was short, cold, and full of phrases like "due to unforeseen circumstances" and "economic downturn." It hit me like a punch. I had been loyal to that company for years, and suddenly, in the middle of a pandemic and right before giving birth, I was unemployed. It was one of those moments where you just sit there, numb, thinking, *what now?* But the weirdest thing was that after the shock faded, I also felt a strange sense of peace. I knew I had to focus on bringing this baby into the world, on staying healthy, on keeping my family safe. The job could wait. Life couldn't.

After my delivery, I told myself I'd start looking for work again once things calmed down — though I had no idea when that would be. Ryan's job was stable, even though he was on temporary leave, and we were confident that we'd make it through. Somehow, amidst all the uncertainty, we both believed that things would eventually fall into place. Maybe it was blind faith, or maybe it was the necessity of hope, but that belief kept us going.

Postpartum hormones, though, were no joke. There were days I would sit on the couch, holding my daughter close, tears streaming down my face for no apparent reason. I'd watch the news and feel this mix of gratitude and guilt. Gratitude that we were safe, and guilt that so many others weren't. My emotions were like waves, unpredictable and consuming. Ryan tried to comfort me, but sometimes, I just needed to cry it out.

My older kids, Mason and Harper, adjusted surprisingly well. They adored their little sister. Since schools were closed, they were home all day. They played a lot, running around, laughing, fighting over snacks, and then suddenly turning into babysitters when their sister cried.

Having them home all the time was exhausting, yes, but also beautiful in a way. We were all together in a way we hadn't been before.

But the isolation crept in, too. Friends couldn't visit. There were no baby showers, no relatives visiting, no friends stopping in with gifts or hugs. Everything happened over video calls. My mom was the only person outside our immediate family who saw Emma in those early weeks. Sometimes I'd sit in the nursery, rocking the baby, scrolling through my phone, watching videos of "normal" life from before, and it felt like another lifetime.

Still, I tried to focus on the small joys. Emma's first smile. The smell of her hair after a bath. I held on to those moments tightly because they reminded me that even in chaos, there was love, and that love was enough to keep us grounded.

When I think back on that time now, I realize how much resilience we found in ourselves without even knowing it. The uncertainty, the fear, the constant adaptation, all of it became part of our story. We learned to live differently. We learned patience, teamwork, and the art of letting go of what we couldn't control.

Looking for a new job after maternity leave wasn't easy, especially with a baby at home and two other kids doing remote schooling. But by then, I had learned to take things one step at a time. COVID had forced us all to slow down, to focus on what truly mattered. My priorities shifted. Now, it wasn't just about having a career anymore. I focused more on building a life that felt safe and meaningful, no matter how uncertain the world outside was.

If there's one thing that the whole experience taught me, it's that motherhood, especially in the middle of a pandemic, is equal parts strength and surrender. You prepare for everything you can, and then you just have to trust yourself to get through the rest.

Looking back now, when I think about what COVID really meant for me and my family, I can honestly say that we were fortunate. I know so many others faced loss, sickness, separation, and somehow, we were spared most of that. It wasn't an overly negative experience for us, though it was far from easy. I think that's what I've come to realize: two things can be true at once. You can feel blessed and still be deeply anxious.

I was, without a doubt, anxious. The anxiety that sits heavy in your chest and doesn't quite let up, even on good days. Every cough from the kids sent me spiraling. Every trip to the grocery store felt like stepping into danger. I remember wiping down groceries, sanitizing the mail, and washing my hands so often they cracked. I was grateful, yes, but also constantly on edge.

Still, in a strange twist of fate, being laid off turned out to be something of a blessing. At first, it felt like the world was ending, losing my job right before giving birth, in the middle of a pandemic. But then came the Federal Funding assistance, and that helped more than I could ever have imagined. My industry had basically come to a standstill, so even if I'd wanted to work, there wasn't much out there. But that time, that pause, gave me a chance to just *be*. To focus on my newborn, to recover, and to adapt to this new view of motherhood.

Ryan's insurance also turned out to be a huge relief. We didn't have to worry about Emma's medical care or the mounting bills that so many other families were struggling with. Knowing that we had that safety net gave me one less thing to lose sleep over, though believe me, sleep was already hard to come by with a newborn in the house.

The hardest part, beyond the daily anxieties, was the uncertainty about the future — especially when it came to work. I knew I'd have to start job hunting eventually, but the thought of trying to find employment in the middle of a global shutdown was terrifying. Who was hiring? Who would even consider a mom of three with a baby just months old? I remember sitting at my computer during nap times, scrolling through job postings one after another. It felt impossible. Almost.

Five months into postpartum, I got an offer. I almost cried, partly from relief, partly from pride. Somehow, against all odds, I had done it.

Even though that period was riddled with anxiety, I can't deny that it also gave us something incredibly precious: time. Family time. For once, we weren't rushing out the door in the mornings, juggling commutes, and missing dinner together. We had slow mornings with pancakes, movie nights with all three kids piled on the couch, and calm afternoons where Ryan and I just sat and watched Emma sleep. Those moments, in the middle of all the chaos, were pure gold.

If you asked me whether I'd want to be pregnant during a pandemic again, I'd probably say no. There's never a perfect time to be pregnant. That much I've learned, but a world-wide health emergency certainly doesn't make it easier. I was lucky that our timing was what it was, that Ryan was still able to be there when our daughter was born, and to attend every antenatal appointment with me. I can't imagine going through that without him.

If the restrictions had been any stricter, if he hadn't been allowed in the delivery room or to attend ultrasounds, it would have broken my heart. Those are moments you can't get back. Knowing that there were mothers who went through all of that alone still makes me ache for them. I don't know if I'd willingly go through pregnancy during another pandemic, not because I regret any part of having my daughter, but because I'd want a different kind of experience. One without masks and fear and isolation.

At the same time, I have to acknowledge what the experience taught me. It taught me how strong I am, how adaptable my family can be, and how love can thrive even in isolation. It reminded me that life doesn't pause for pandemics. Babies are born, families grow, and hope continues. So, while I might not choose to be pregnant during another world crisis, I can say that surviving this one has left me stronger, more grateful, and more aware of what truly matters.

Conclusion

Considering the chaos and uncertainty that defined early 2020, it is remarkable that most of the pregnancies documented in this book were not only successful but also, in many cases, ultimately joyful and healthy experiences for the women, their families, and their newborns. Despite the unique set of challenges brought on by the pandemic, the majority of participants I interviewed carried their pregnancies to safe outcomes. They described facing "bumps and hurdles" throughout their antepartum, delivery, and postpartum journeys, yet they persisted with resilience and determination, choosing to nurture their families.

The majority of women interviewed had planned pregnancies, but none who delivered in the early months of COVID-19 anticipated the pandemic. For those whose pregnancies were unplanned, most still embraced the experience and found it to be a source of unexpected strength and joy. In fact, a few women even chose to pursue a second pregnancy during the pandemic. Their decision displays how the desire to grow and sustain family life can often outweigh perceived anxieties and disadvantages.

While celebrating the positives seen through this research is warranted, it is equally essential to acknowledge the lived experiences and very real difficulties that families faced during COVID.

Expectant and postpartum women were particularly vulnerable to the isolation, disrupted care, and heightened uncertainty caused by the pandemic. Their experiences underscore the critical role that accessible resources, strong support systems, and compassionate care play during such unprecedented periods, as well as in everyday life. While many families found ways to adapt and cope, the lessons from this time period show us that much more could have been done to support them.

This book, through its collection of real voices and lived experiences, not only documents what women and families went through but also highlights what worked well, where systems fell short, and how we might better prepare for the future. By capturing these stories through qualitative research, the aim is not only to record history but also to offer insights that can guide more resilient, empathetic, and effective care for mothers and families, both in times of crisis and in the in everyday life moving forward.

There were a number of significant changes that families had to adapt to during the pandemic, and parents, in particular, carried much of that responsibility. Expectant mothers and fathers had to learn not only how to protect themselves but also how to safeguard their newborns in a climate of fear and uncertainty. They were required to process constantly shifting information and integrate evolving medical protocols into their pregnancy and newborn care. They were often forced to make difficult decisions without precedent to guide them. Those who delivered during the very earliest months of the pandemic had virtually no time to prepare or even understand protective measures. As one mother expressed, they simply "had to do it." They tried to follow the most recent, but frequently changing, guidelines, even when those rules became confusing, contradictory, or disheartening. Fear of COVID-19 was ever-present, but despite this anxiety, these families did all they could to protect one another.

Across many of the interviews, women emphasized that family and social support were among the most essential reasons they were able to stay positive. Family has always held a central place in our society, but COVID highlighted its importance in new ways.

For many, the shift to remote work was a transformative experience. Partners who might otherwise have been absent due to professional obligations found themselves at home, able to both maintain their jobs and actively participate in caring for their children. This change not only offered much-needed practical support but also revealed the rewards of being fully present in family life. Parents learned that they could balance careers with "active parenting," often in creative and resourceful ways. Many expressed that, despite the hardships, this was one of the most positive aspects of having a baby during the pandemic. Fathers in particular valued the time they were able to spend with their newborns.

Although physical interactions with extended family and friends were limited, technology greatly aided in parents' ability to stay connected and not feel isolated. Zoom and FaceTime allowed people to stay connected. Families celebrated milestones, maintained relationships, and, in some cases, even met newborns for the first time through a screen. While not a perfect substitute, these digital gatherings demonstrated that humanity will do all they can to achieve the human need for connection.

For the women whose pregnancies unfolded during the earliest months of the pandemic, one of the most difficult realities was the feeling of "being pregnant alone." Restrictions meant that partners, family members, and loved ones could not accompany them to routine check-ups or participate in the intimate journey of antepartum care. What is typically a shared experience, hearing a heartbeat together, seeing an ultrasound image for the first time, asking questions as a family, was suddenly stripped down to solitary visits. These women alone were permitted to sit in waiting rooms, meet with their physicians, and receive updates about their babies. But despite the absence of their support networks, they persevered.

This situation was, of course, worsened because hospitals were overwhelmed with COVID cases, and access to care was complicated by fear of exposure, staff shortages, and the constant reorganization of medical services. In many cases, in-person visits were minimized or replaced entirely with telemedicine, a practice that was unfamiliar to most expectant mothers at the time. For some, online consultations felt impersonal or inadequate compared to the reassurance of face-to-face care; others greatly appreciated the option and felt that it allowed for faster responses from their providers, especially since leaving home seemed too risky.

What these stories revealed most clearly was the power and resilience of these determined women. Without the physical presence of loved ones, many learned to carry the weight of medical decisions on their own, to advocate for themselves in uncertain circumstances, and to adapt to new ways of receiving care. The emotional toll was heavy; feelings of loneliness, anxiety, and disconnection were common, but so too was a sense of strength and self-reliance. Their ability to protect both themselves and their unborn children is well worth acknowledging and celebrating.

The collapse of the healthcare system is perhaps the most important effect of COVID to be understood and learned from. At times, women were seen through televisits, other times, they were able to attend in-person appointments. When emergent needs arose, however, they were required to present to the emergency room entirely on their own. Hospitals, overwhelmed and striving to reduce the spread of infection, maintained strict social distancing protocols. As a result, only patients were permitted inside emergency rooms, leaving many women to face urgent and frightening situations without the immediate comfort of their loved ones by their side.

During the early months of the pandemic, even the medical community was grappling with uncertainty. Providers were learning in real time how best to protect the health of their patients while protecting themselves and their own families. Expectant parents, in turn, placed their trust in these providers, attempting to follow their guidance and adopt careful patterns of "pandemic living." Those who delivered during this period often encountered the reality of limited personal protective equipment (PPE) in hospitals. They were acutely aware of the anxiety that healthcare workers carried, balancing their duty to care for patients with their own vulnerability and fears. In fact, quite a few of those interviewed were either healthcare workers or their spouses, offering a unique view into what it was like for a provider to be expecting a child during this time. Mask-wearing and social distancing were taken seriously by both patients and providers, though these measures could not entirely shield mothers from the strain of navigating childbirth in such conditions.

Another challenge that surfaced repeatedly was the difficulty of establishing effective breastfeeding practices. Several women described struggling to develop good techniques, and while the causes cannot be pinpointed with certainty, a few contributing factors stood out. Some mothers were discharged from the hospital sooner than usual to reduce potential exposure, leaving less time for in-hospital support. In addition, many experienced lactation consultants retired during COVID, leading to a reduction in hands-on guidance. As a result, complications such as mastitis became more common. Some women sought help through tele-visits, while others required in-person evaluation in emergency rooms. These stories highlight not only the gaps created by the pandemic but also the ways in which families and healthcare providers alike attempted to adapt to extraordinary limitations.

Women who were pregnant during the later months of 2020 and into early 2021 continued to follow careful protocols, but their experiences were notably different from those who delivered at the very start of the pandemic. By this time, they were aware that vaccines were in development and that mortality rates were beginning to decline. Although they still could not share their antepartum care with partners, family, or friends, many women described feeling that there was "light on the horizon." They lived with caution, but with less fear of the disease process than their counterparts in early 2020.

Much more information about COVID-19 and pregnancy was available, though it was not always consistent. Many of the women I interviewed spoke about the challenge of sorting through contradictory advice and choosing what they believed to be the safest path for themselves and their families. Social distancing remained a central practice, and most families continued to limit visitors. At the same time, many parents found creative ways to balance safety with connection, forming "pods" or "bubbles" that allowed them to see a few trusted individuals, often grandparents, so that their newborns could still be introduced to family.

By a year into the pandemic, women reported that they felt more confident about managing pregnancy in this new reality. They had learned how to adapt their daily lives, protect their health, and keep their newborns safe. Many reflected on how much progress had been made in just a year and expressed gratitude for the tireless work of scientists, healthcare providers, and public health experts. What once felt unimaginable in early 2020, carrying and delivering a healthy baby in the midst of a global pandemic, had become something they not only managed but also mastered. Hospitals and providers also reported feeling more prepared and equipped to protect both themselves and their patients, further reinforcing this growing sense of stability.

One of the most significant turning points of the pandemic came with the development of vaccines in early 2021. Looking back, it is clear how fortunate we are to have access to safe and effective protection against COVID-19. The Centers for Disease Control and Prevention (CDC) strongly recommends vaccination for women who are pregnant, postpartum, planning pregnancy, or breastfeeding.[7] Evidence shows that women who receive the vaccine during

---

[7] Centers for Disease Control and Prevention. "COVID-19 Vaccination for Women Who Are Pregnant or Breastfeeding." Last modified September 10, 2024. https://www.cdc.gov/covid/vaccines/pregnant-or-breastfeeding.html.

pregnancy pass high levels of antibodies to their babies, both in utero and through breastmilk.[8] Research has demonstrated that vaccination reduces the risk of stillbirth by 15% and decreases the likelihood of infants contracting COVID-19 in their first six months of life.[9] [10] For mothers themselves, vaccination offers remarkable protection: 96% against infection, 97% against symptomatic illness, and 89% against hospitalization.[11]

Despite these benefits, hesitancy among pregnant women was common in the early rollout of vaccines. Many were understandably uncomfortable with the idea of vaccination while pregnant, largely due to the limited information initially available. However, as more data emerged, particularly the finding that vaccination during pregnancy not only protected mothers but also their unborn children, many women were persuaded to receive the vaccine. For them, the knowledge that they could safeguard their babies was the decisive factor.

For pregnant families, the possibility of protection was life-changing, offering both relief and hope that the end of the pandemic might finally be within reach.

What COVID-19 Taught Us About Pregnancy and Parenthood

I am proud to share that most of the women I interviewed reflected on their pregnancies during COVID with positivity and strength. Despite the uncertainty of the times, many spoke emphatically about how much they learned about themselves through the experience. They discovered resilience they had not known they possessed,

---

[8] Ibid.

[9] Schwartz, David A., Sarah B. Mulkey, and Drucilla J. Roberts. "SARS-CoV-2 placentitis, stillbirth, and maternal COVID-19 vaccination: clinical–pathologic correlations." *American journal of obstetrics and gynecology* 228, no. 3 (2023): 261-269.

[10] Centers for Disease Control and Prevention. "Effectiveness of Maternal Vaccination with mRNA COVID-19 Vaccine During Pregnancy Against COVID-19–Associated Hospitalization in Infants Aged < 6 Months — 17 States, July 2021–January 2022." *Morbidity and Mortality Weekly Report* 71, no. 7 (February 18, 2022). https://www.cdc.gov/mmwr/volumes/71/wr/mm7107e3.htm.

[11] Dagan, Noa, Noam Barda, Tal Biron-Shental, Maya Makov-Assif, Calanit Key, Isaac S. Kohane, Miguel A. Hernán et al. "Effectiveness of the BNT162b2 mRNA COVID-19 vaccine in pregnancy." *Nature medicine* 27, no. 10 (2021): 1693-1695.

realizing that they could face difficult circumstances and find creative ways to overcome them. Several described feeling genuinely "proud" of having navigated such an extraordinary time while still accomplishing what mattered most, bringing healthy babies into the world.

Some parents were even inspired to pursue another pregnancy during the pandemic. They found that being more present for their children, combined with the shift toward remote work, created an environment in which expanding their families felt both possible and deeply meaningful. The isolation of lockdown was not without its difficulties, but many families spoke about how they still managed to find connection, community, and love. Online forums and virtual support groups became important spaces where mothers could share their stories, listen to others, and feel less alone in their experiences.

Although some of the information circulating online was unreliable, and in some cases gave way to misinformation or even extremism, many women recognized that the widespread conversations reflected a shared sense of concern. They valued the genuine attempts people made to support each other, however imperfect, and drew comfort from the fact that they were part of a broader community navigating the same uncertainties.

Reflecting on this time, it is clear that COVID-19 changed how we think about pregnancy, parenting, and family life. While the challenges were immense, what emerged was a powerful set of lessons that can help guide us moving forward.

One of the most important lessons was about the adaptability of healthcare. Telemedicine became a lifeline for many expectant parents, showing us that care can be delivered in more flexible ways. Even though online visits sometimes felt less personal, they provided access and continuity in moments when leaving home was unsafe. These innovations remind us that hybrid models of care have the potential to support families well beyond times of crisis.

Mental health also became impossible to ignore. The isolation and uncertainty of pregnancy during COVID brought stress, anxiety, and loneliness to the surface. Families learned that caring for mental health is just as essential as physical health, and healthcare systems must build in stronger supports for emotional well-being, especially for pregnant and postpartum women.

Another truth that surfaced was the enduring importance of community. Even when in-person contact was limited, families sought out connection through neighborhood "bubbles," online forums, or video calls. These creative solutions highlighted that no parent should feel alone, and that support networks, whether physical or virtual, are vital for the health of families.

At the same time, the pandemic exposed inequities. While some families could adjust to remote work and stable income, others faced compounded struggles due to lack of access, financial strain, or limited childcare. These disparities make it clear that we need more equitable systems of support so that all families, regardless of their circumstances, can thrive.

Taken together, these lessons suggest that pregnancy and parenting are not fragile experiences, but ones that can flourish with the right support. The pandemic forced us to reimagine care, community, and work-life balance in new ways. It showed us not only what needs to change but also what is possible, and it is our responsibility to carry those lessons forward for the sake of families, children, and future generations.

Reflecting on this period, it is clear that COVID-19 deeply affected all of us, and pregnancies in particular. Yet because of the adaptability and resourcefulness of expectant and new parents, the disruptions were relatively short-lived. By embracing lifestyle changes and prioritizing safety, families were able to continue growing in spite of the pandemic. My interviews underscored a timeless truth: the desire to become parents and nurture families remains a powerful and enduring part of our society.

www.ingramcontent.com/pod-product-compliance
Lightning Source LLC
LaVergne TN
LVHW050909210926
848482LV00012B/385

ACCA F2: Management Accounting

ACCA

Dr. M. Imran Ahsan

Published by M. Imran Ahsan, 2025.

ACCA F2: MANAGEMENT ACCOUNTING

First edition. August 10, 2025.

ISBN: 979-8231339563

Written by Dr. M. Imran Ahsan.

Also by Dr. M. Imran Ahsan

ACCA

ACCA F2: Management Accounting

To all smart learners,

"Numbers tell a story — and management accounting teaches us how to read it."

Preface

This book, *F2 Management Accounting*, has been developed as a concise yet comprehensive resource for students and professionals seeking a clear understanding of the principles and practices of management accounting. It is aligned with the ACCA F2 (MA) syllabus and aims to deliver key concepts in a simplified and structured manner.

Completed within the span of one week, this work is the result of focused effort, practical experience, and a commitment to making financial learning accessible. The fast-track completion was driven by a desire to provide learners with an efficient study tool that balances depth with clarity, especially for those preparing for professional exams under time constraints.

This book is particularly designed to support self-study, revision, and classroom use. Complex topics are broken down into manageable sections, supported by examples, summaries, where applicable.

I hope this book serves as a valuable companion on your learning journey in management accounting. Constructive feedback is always welcome for future improvements.

Dr. Imran Ahsan

Ch.ImranAhsen@gmail.com

WhatsApp # 00923465006818

Chapter 1: The nature and purpose of Management accounting

1. Data and information

Data consists of raw facts – including numbers, letters, symbols, events, transactions, and recorded details – that have not yet been processed into a usable form.

Information emerges when this data is purposefully organized to support decision-making. It becomes valuable by distilling complex details into clearer, simplified summaries tailored to the user's needs.

2. Qualities of high-quality information

Management relies on information to aid in planning, controlling, and decision-making.

The information must be ACCURATE to be high quality: Accuracy, Completeness, cost effective, understandable, Relevance, Accessibility, Timeliness, and Ease of use.

Accurate: Data needs to reflect reality and be devoid of mistakes accurately.

Completeness: The information should be comprehensive enough to answer the query or cover the subject.

Cost-Effective: Weighing the advantages of the information against the expenses of acquiring and utilizing it is crucial.

Understandable: Simplify your language and avoid using technical phrases to be understood with a reasonable level of accounting knowledge.

Relevance: The data must be directly relevant to the problem at hand.

Accessibility: The data must be readily available and easy to comprehend for the people using it.

Timeliness: The information should be timely to related parties (i.e., managers) to make informed decisions.

Easy to use: The information should be easily usable by users without much effort.

3. Process of decision making and control

Planning and decision-making are the main jobs of the managers.

3.1 Planning:

Organizations must establish objectives and devise strategies to achieve these objectives. It enables them to make intelligent decisions. Usually, past performances and decisions lead organizations to make better future decisions. For example, historical sales data in a specific time of the year can be used to predict future sales in that season. This helps in planning strategically (with long-term objectives) and tactically (emphasizing the short term).

3.2 Decision making:

Decision-making means choosing between options using the information you have. Good decisions require accurate information to understand the risks and benefits of each choice. The decision-making process involves two main parts: planning what to do and controlling how it is done.

3.3 Control

Managers get reports on how the company is · doing. They use this information to make corrections and adjust their plans or budgets. This feedback, used for control, comes from inside the company."

4. Mission statements

Before any planning, a business needs a mission. A mission statement is a simple document that explains the company's primary purpose.

4.1 Elements of a good mission statement

Purpose: What is our reason for existing, and whom are we co-fitted to support?

Approach/strategy: What are the business's key activities, what goods/ services does it provide, and how does it provide them?

Policies: How does the business organization expect its staff to behave?

Principles/values: What fundamental beliefs guide this business's decisions and actions?

The mission statement gives the big picture, and all goals and plans should support it.

5. Levels of planning

Good business planning follows a clear system, starting with the company's mission.

The mission statement should support every plan.

Business's objectives should be S ART:

- **Specific:** Clear and straightforward.
- **Measurable:** Objectives should be measurable.
- **Attainable:** Objectives should be achievable.
- **Relevant:** They matter to the mission statement.
- **Timed:** Missions with deadlines.

5.1 Three Planning Levels:

- **Strategic (Long-Term):** Big picture, 5+ years, set by top leaders for the whole company.
- **Tactical (medium-term):** Breaking down the big plan into smaller, yearly plans for different departments, handled by middle managers.
- **Operational (Short-Term):** Daily decisions and problem-solving are handled by all managers."

6. Centres of cost, centers of profit, centers of investment,

6.1 Responsibility Accounting

There are different parts of a business that are responsible for different managers. This is what responsibility accounting is based on.

A responsibility center is part of a business whose boss is personally responsible for how well it does its job. The main centers of responsibility are:

- cost centre • Revenue centre • Profit centre and Investment centre

6.2 Cost centers

A cost center is a production or service place, function, item, activity, or equipment whose costs are identified and recorded.

• For Car manufacturing Companies, Cost Centers can be

- Production Department:
- Quality Control Department:
- Research and Development(R&D) Department:
- Maintenance Department:
- Information Technology (IT) Department:
- Logistics and Supply Chain Management:
-

For an accountancy firm, most centers can be

Administrative Department, Human Resources (HR) Department, Information Technology (IT) Department, Marketing and Business Development, Training, Audit, Building Security, etc.

The people in charge of most centers need to know about the costs that are paid for and billed to those centers. Assessing how well a cost center manager meets most goals is a key part of their job.

6.3 Revenue centers:

A revenue center is a part of a company that earns money through sales. Unlike most centers, which spend money, revenue centers focus on bringing it in. Think of it as a sales department. For example, a regional sales manager runs a revenue center. They have sales targets and are judged on how well they meet them. The company tracks sales back to each region to see how each manager performs."

6.4 Profit centres

"A profit center is a part of a business where we track costs and earnings.

- Large Companies often divide into profit centers, treating each department like a mini-business.
- Each profit center can have smaller cost and revenue centers within it.
- A manager's performance is judged by how much profit their center generates.
- The manager controls both the spending and the earnings.
- Accurate cost and revenue data must be collected and reported for each profit center."

6.5 Centres of investment

Investment center managers handle investments, and I track both costs and profits.

- They are accountable for how well they use company money and how much profit they generate.
- Their performance is measured by how much profit they create relative to the money they invest, which is called return on capital employed (ROCE)."

ROCE = Profit / Capital Used.

1. Financial, Cost, and Management Accounting

7.1 Financial Accounting

Financial accounting tracks a company's finances and creates standard reports for outsiders to understand its finances.

- Financial accountants maintain accurate records and produce legal financial statements.
- However, these standard reports do not always give managers enough detail for making internal decisions."

7.2 Cost Accounting

Managers need detailed cost and revenue information for each product or service. Cost and Management accounting provides this.

- Cost accounting tracks the expenses of producing goods or services and identifies the costs of specific tasks or departments.
- It analyzes how the business uses its resources.
- It provides financial data to help managers understand current performance and plan for the future.
- Often, "most accounting" and" Management accounting" are used interchangeably."

7.3 Management Accounting

Cost accounting is one of the most important parts of Management accounting.

7.4 Financial Accounting vs. Management Accounting

Audience:

Financial Accounting: This is mainly for those outside the company, such as investors, creditors, lenders, and regulatory agencies, to judge its financial health.

Management Accounting: This is mainly for those who work at the firm, such as managers and employees. It gives the company the information to plan, make choices, and monitor its actions. Gives everyone in the firm the information they need to make decisions, plan, and run the business.

Purpose:

- **Financial Accounting:**
  - To provide a standardized and reliable view of the company's financial performance and position.
  - Focuses on historical data to report on past performance.
- **Management Accounting:**
  - To provide information for internal decision-making, such as budgeting, forecasting, and performance evaluation.
  - Focuses on both historical and future data to support planning and control.

Reporting Standards:

- **Financial Accounting:**
  - Must adhere to generally accepted accounting principles (GAAP) or International Financial Reporting Standards (IFRS).
  - Subject to strict regulations and external audits.
- **Management Accounting:**
  - Not bound by strict regulations or standards.
  - Reports are customized to meet the specific needs of Management.

Time Horizon:

- **Financial Accounting:**
    - Primarily focuses on historical data.
    - Reports are typically prepared for specific periods, such as quarterly or annually.

- **Management Accounting:**
    - It uses both historical and future data.
    - Reports can be prepared as needed, focusing on providing Timely information for decision-making.

Information Type:

- **Financial Accounting:**
    - Primarily focuses on monetary data.
    - Summarizes financial transactions into standardized financial statements.

- **Management Accounting:**
    - It uses both monetary and non-monetary data.
    - Provides detailed information, including cost analysis, performance metrics, and forecasts.

Financial accounting provides a snapshot of the company's financial health for external stakeholders, while Management accounting provides the internal information needed to guide the company's operations and strategy.

Aspect	Financial Accounting	Management Accounting
Audience	External stakeholders	Internal managers
Focus	Past performance	Future decisions
Regulations	GAAP/IFRS required	No formal standards
Data Type	Monetary, summarized	Monetary + non-monetary
Frequency	Quarterly/annual	As needed

1. The role of Management accounting within an organization's Management information system

Management accounting helps managers make decisions by providing key reports. These reports include budgets, profit analysis, cash flow forecasts, investment reviews, cost control, and tax filings. Managers get this information through regular reports or when they ask for it.

9. The limitations of Management information

Management accounting information can fail to help managers for several reasons:

9.1 Useless Information:

- **Inaccuracy:** Wrong cost or sales estimates lead to bad decisions.
- **Untimely:** Late information means missed opportunities and wasted resources.
- **Unclear:** Complex data that managers do not understand is ignored. d.

9.2 Irrelevant Costs and Revenues:

- Accounting data is not always decision-ready.
- Managers need information that will change based on their choices:
    - **Future:** Only future costs and revenues matter. Past costs are irrelevant.
    - **Incremental:** Focus on the extra costs or income from a decision.
    - **Cash Flows:** Use actual cash, not just accounting figures.

9.3 Non-Financial Information:

- Managers consider more than just numbers. They examine the qualitative, behavioral, motivational, and environmental impact. These factors are complex and important to measure.

9.4 External Information:

- Businesses are affected by outside factors like government policies, competitors, and customer trends.
- Traditional accounting focuses on internal data, but managers also need external information.

- This is called environmental analysis.
- Accounting systems might include information about the world outside the company."

Chapter 2 Sources of Data

1. Information from inside the company

Companies get internal information from several sources:

1.1 Record Keeping:

- Bills, timesheets, and journals provide raw data.
- This data is organized by cost type, department, manager, and project.
- Regular reports show costs compared to budgets, helping with planning and control.
- On-de and reports support quick decision-making.
- **Examples:**
    - Sales data helps predict and plan production.
    - Production data helps estimate material, labor, and machine needs.
    - Cost data helps set product prices and control budgets.
    - Sales trends inform long-term product strategies.
    - Accounts reports help manage debt collection.
    - Waste data helps me prove product quality.

1.2 Payroll System:

- Provides detailed labor cost information.
- Tracks work vs. non-work hours (training, sick leave, etc.).
- Shows employee turnover rates, helping evaluate HR strategies.

1.3 Strategic Planning System:

- Contains information on company goals and objectives.
- Includes assume pitons about external factors.
- Details of financial investments and new product plans.
- Some information is confidential and restricted to top Management.

1.4 Advantages of Internal Information:

- Easily accessible.
- Easy to organize and analyze.
- Reports can be generated quickly.
- Directly relevant to the company.

1.5 Disadvantages of Internal Information:

- This data may need to be further analyzed for management usage.

2. External sources of information

Businesses must pay attention to the outside world to survive. Management accountants are increasingly responsible for 'environmental scanning' – gathering information from inside and outside the company to help managers make decisions.

2.1 Key External Information Sources:

- Government data
- Business partners (suppliers, customers)
- Industry groups and publications
- News and financial media

2.2 Government Data:

- Governments release statistics on the economy y, population, trade, and prices.
- This data helps governments and businesses plan for things like investments and hiring.
- The information is usually general, covering entire industries or regions.

2.3 Contacts for business

Government data is broad. For specific information, businesses can talk to their customers and suppliers. This information is often free.

2.3.1 Customers tell you about:

- Their exact needs.
- Quality expectations.
- Delivery schedules.
- Packaging and shipping preferences.
- Feedback on products and services.

2.3.2 Suppliers tell you about:

- Discounts and refunds.
- Current products and services.
- Potential future products and services.
- Product specifications and how they work."

2.4 Industry groups

Most industries have trade groups that support their members. These groups:

- Represent businesses in legal and other issues.
- Offer quality testing programs.
- Set industry standards.
- Publish magazines and resources for business owners.

Examples (UK):

- Confederation of Agricultural Industries
- Association of Airport Operators
- Association for Pay Ent Clearing Services
- And any more.

These groups and other publishers release trade magazines with industry news and information. For Example, "The Grocer" is a well-known UK magazine for the food industry."

2.5 The business press, financial press, and other news sources

Newspapers and financial publications, like The Financial Times and The Guardian, provide business news, financial data, and economic analysis. They also report on market indexes like the FTSE 100.

This information is readily available online and through business news channels like Bloom Berg TV.

2.6 Pros and Cons of External Information:

- Internal data flaws are known because the company creates them.
- External data quality can be uncertain because the company does not control it.

2.6.1 Benefits and limitations of data from an external source

Pros of External Information:

- "Lots of information available."
- "Easy to find, especially online."
- "Provides broad industry and market insights."
- "You can find specific details you require."

Cons of External Information:

- "Information might be inaccurate."
- "Finding the correct information can take time.

2.7 The general state of the economy

The economy affects a company's profits and costs.

- Strong economy: People spend more, businesses can raise prices, and profits increase. Costs may rise due to supplier price increases.
- Weak economy: People spend less, sales drop, prices might stay high, profits decrease."

3. Sampling Basics

"Sapling studies an s all part (sample) of a larger group (population) to understand the whole.

- Population: All things being studied (people, objects, etc.).
- Examples: Polling TV viewers to test product quality.
- Why sample? The population may be unknown; the complete study is mostly/time-consuming, and testing may destroy it.
- To be accurate, the Sample must be large enough and representative."

4. Sampling methods:

- **Random Sampling:** Every item has an equal chance.
  - Example: Numbering bills for an audit.

- **Systematic Sampling:** Select every nth item.
  - Example: Choosing every 100th item.
  - Caution: It cannot be very objective with repeating patterns.
- **Stratified Sampling: Sample** proportionally from subgroups (strata).
  - Example: Sapling age groups for a survey.
  - Ensures representation of all groups.
- **Multi-Stage Sampling:** Divide the population into levels (regions, towns, streets, houses) and sample at each level.
  - Example: National opinion polls.
- **Cluster Sampling:** Sample entire groups (clusters).
  - Example: Surveying all houses in selected neighborhoods.
- **Quota Sampling:** Select specific types of people until quotas are met.
  - Example: Interviewing specific demographics.
  - Caution: Can be biased by interviewer choice.

5. Comparing Sampling Methods:

A sample should represent the whole population

- Random sampling is ideal but expensive.
- Other methods balance cost and accuracy.
- Choose methods carefully: Systematic sampling is bad for repeating patterns, and quota sampling can be biased.

Chapter 3: Presenting information

1. The Essence of Management Accounting Information

Management accounting revolves around transforming data into actionable insights. While prior chapters covered *data collection* (the input), this chapter explores how the management accounting department processes and presents this information to decision-makers.

Historically, management reports were criticized for being overly complex, alienating non-expert users. Today, clarity and accessibility are prioritized, ensuring stakeholders with basic financial literacy can grasp key insights—often aided by visual tools like charts and graphs.

2. Crafting Effective Reports

Reports bridge data and decisions. Follow this streamlined four-step process:

2.1 Prepare

- ◈ **Define format**: Memo, formal report, or presentation notes?
- ◈ **Identify users**: Tailor language and depth to the audience's expertise.
- ◈ **Clarify purpose**: Most reports exist to inform strategic choices.

2.2 Plan

- ◈ **Analyze data**: Summarize, interpret, and convert raw data into insights using management accounting techniques.

- ◈ **Structure logically**: Organize findings for coherent storytelling.

2.3 Write

- ◈ **Adopt clear style**: Avoid jargon. Prioritize precision and simplicity.

- ◈ **Refine readability**: Ensure sentences flow logically; check grammar and tone.

2.4 Review

◈ **Proofread**: Eliminate errors.

◈ **Validate**: Ensure completeness, compliance with guidelines, and ease of understanding.

2.5 Standard Report Structure

1. **Title**: Date, recipient, and subject.
2. **Introduction**: Scope, methodology, and findings overview.
3. **Analysis**: Breakdown of data into digestible segments.
4. **Conclusion**: Summary and recommendations (*no new information*).
5. **Appendices**: Supporting data, calculations, or references.

Tip: Use numbered headings and cross-references for navigability.

2.6 Language Guidelines

◈ **Simplify**: Prefer short words and sentences.

◈ **Avoid**: Slang, clichés, puns, or unexplained acronyms (e.g., *ACCA* on first use).

◈ **Polish**: Check spelling and syntax rigorously.

3. Presenting Data: Tables

Tables organize data into rows/columns, enhancing clarity and reducing cognitive load.

3.1 Table Design Principles

Element	Guideline
Title	Clear, descriptive.
Source	Cite data origins.
Units	Specify measurements (e.g., "$000s").
Headings	Concise column/row labels.
Totals	Include subtotals/totals where relevant.
Percentages	Add ratios with calculation notes.

3.2 Layout Optimization

1. Fit content onto one page.
2. Group related columns adjacently.
3. Order rows logically (e.g., chronologically).

4. Visualizing Data: Charts & Graphs

Diagrams transform numbers into intuitive visuals. All should be **self-explanatory**, featuring:

- A descriptive title
- Data sources
- Measurement units
- Scale indicators
- Aesthetic consistency
- Keys/legends

4.1 Bar Charts

Use Case: Comparing discrete categories.

- **Simple**: Single variable (e.g., annual wheat production). Bar height = value.

- **Component**: Shows parts of a whole (e.g., grain types within annual totals).

- **Percentage Component**: Illustrates proportional composition (all bars = 100%).

◈ **Multiple**: Compares sub-categories side-by-side (e.g., sales vs. costs over years).

4.2 Line Graphs

Use Case: Tracking trends over time.

◈ **Axes**: Independent variable (e.g., time) on x-axis; dependent variable (e.g., sales) on y-axis.

◈ **Scale**: Start at zero; use scale breaks (◈) if needed.

◈ **Multi-line**: Use colors/dashes to distinguish datasets (e.g., division costs).

4.3 Scatter Diagrams

Use Case: Revealing relationships between two variables (e.g., output vs. cost).

◈ **Plot**: Each point = a data pair.

◈ **Trend Line**: Add a "line of best fit" to indicate correlation strength.

◈ **Interpretation**: Clustered points suggest strong relationships; scattered points imply weak links.

4.4 Pie Charts

Use Case: Displaying proportional contributions to a whole.

Steps:

1. Calculate total value.
2. Convert each item to degrees: (Item Value / Total) × 360°.
3. Draw segments accordingly.

Note: Label segments with percentages/values for clarity.

5. Interpreting & Communicating Insights

Well-designed visuals minimize explanatory text. However, management accountants must often:

- ◈ **Highlight key trends** (e.g., "Division B's costs are rising faster than Division A's").
- ◈ **Draw actionable conclusions** ("Optimize delivery routes to reduce van costs").
- ◈ **Advise strategically** ("Reallocate budget to high-growth products").

Goal: Transform data into decisions—not just present numbers.

Key Takeaways

- ◈ **Reports**: Structured, audience-focused, and jargon-free.
- ◈ **Tables**: Organized, annotated, and logically ordered.
- ◈ **Visuals**: Self-sufficient, accurate, and purpose-driven.
- ◈ **Insights**: Clear, contextualized, and decision-oriented.

Chapter 4: Different kinds of costs and cost behavior

1. Introduction

Management will need different types of reports, such as: Costs for a particular product, per unit cost, cost of external financial resources, costs for a particular area (most centers), planning cost and others.

2. Different types of costs;

The price of a good or service, the cost of running a department, or the cost of running a regional office.

2.1 Units of cost: A cost unit is the amount of a good or service used to determine the cost.

A cost center is where goods or services are made or provided, a function, an action, or a piece of equipment for which prices can be found.

2.2.1 Examples of Cost Centers

A department, a machine, a project, or a hospital ward.

3. Types of Costs

There are several ways to group costs.

• Element: Prices can be divided into three groups: material, labor, and expenses.

• Function: Costs can be broken down into production costs and non-production costs.

Nature: Because of their nature, costs can be either direct or indirect.

Behavior: Depending on their behavior, costs can be fixed, changeable, semi-variable, or stepped fixed.

4. Classification by elements

To classify the cost with respect to element, we need to divide them into material, labor and or expense.

• Materials: All the costs of buying things that are used in production or activities that are not production. Like raw materials, parts, cleaning, upkeep, and office supplies.

• Labor: All the costs of paying workers who work for the company.

• Expenses are all the costs unrelated to goods or labor. This covers all services bought, like rent, phone, subcontractors, and costs like the wear and tear on tools.

5. Classification of cost with respect to function

5.1 Costs of production

The costs that come up when raw materials are turned into finished goods and finished parts of goods are called production costs.

In order to figure out how much an item is worth, you have to add up its direct materials, direct labor, direct spending, and production overhead costs.

5.2 Non-production Cost

In business, non-production costs are not directly linked to buying the goods or services the business sells. Costs like selling, administration, and financing are non-production costs and are entered into the income statement as expenses. Do not use non-production cost to determine how much an item is worth.

6. Classification based on nature

6.1 Direct cost/Prime cost

Costs that can be linked directly to a specific cost centers are called direct costs. Direct costs come in three main types:

• Direct materials cost, like leather for shoes.

• Direct labor, like the payments to labors who make shoes.

• Direct expenses, other costs directly related to the production of goods and services like such as ink, lubricant, and software services. Total cost is the sum of all the direct costs.

6.2 Indirect costs

Costs that cannot be linked directly to a specific cost centers are indirect.

Examples of indirect costs:

• Indirect materials: These things cannot be linked to a specific item, like cleaning fluids.

• Indirect labor, like maintenance staff, quality control personnel.

• Indirect expense: like expenses that support the overall operations of a business but cannot be directly linked to a specific product, like rent, insurance, etc. Overheads are the sum of all the secondary costs.

7. Classification based on behavior

7.1 Variable cost: It is the cost which changes with the change in production level. For example cost of raw material. When we produce more units of shoes we need more leather so the cost of leather increases (so it is variable cost).

7.2 Fixed cost: It is the cost which does not change as the production level changes. This is

True up to some extent for example rent of factory building. Owner of the factory has to

Pay a fixed amount of rent regardless he produces 1 unit or 100 units.

7.3 Stepped cost: That remains fixed for a certain level of output range and changes when that range is exceeded. For example, if a company produces up to 100000 shoes, it needs one factory space, and after 100000 units, it needs more space, so the rent for space in this case is a specific cost.

• The total cost may be the same for a certain amount of activity, but the cost per unit decreases as activity increases.

Total cost = variable cost + fixed cost

Key Formulas:

Average cost = Total cost/output

Average variable cost = variable cost/output

Average fixed cost = Fixed cost/output

Chapter 5 Accounting for inventory

1. Ordering, receiving, and distributing Inventory

Material purchased for manufacturing must be carefully used for the purpose for which it is purchased, as it could be the biggest cost in the manufacturing business. The raw material must be received, stored, and issued in proper order to avoid wastage. A proper internal control (including documentation and authorization) must be in place to do that.

To maintain purchasing control, it is essential to acquire:

We purchase only what is absolutely necessary.

Orders are placed with the most suitable provider based on pricing and delivery information.

The quantity and quality of the items received correspond to the order.

Once the order was placed, make sure it was based on a consensus price. A strong internal check must be in place for the above procedure.

2. Inventory holding and ordering procedures

Determining the optimal type and quantity of stored assets presents a fundamental challenge for all businesses.

2.1 Core Functions of Inventory Reserves:

Maintaining inventory serves several key strategic purposes:

◈ **Buffering Demand Fluctuations:** Mitigating the impact of unexpected surges in consumption.

◈ **Securing Volume Discounts:** Achieving cost savings through bulk procurement.

◈ **Capitalizing on Seasonal Pricing:** Exploiting predictable cost variations by purchasing during low-demand periods (e.g., off-season commodities).

◈ **Ensuring Operational Continuity:** Preventing production disruptions by guaranteeing the consistent availability of necessary components.

◈ **Meeting Mandatory Requirements:** Maintaining necessary holdings due to technical, safety, or regulatory imperatives (e.g., safety stock for critical items).

2.2 Optimizing Inventory Management

Effective management of immobilized resources presents a core strategic equilibrium: balancing the expenditures associated with acquiring and retaining inventory against the targeted service level performance.

2.2.1 Comprehensive Retention Expenditures

The total cost of maintaining inventory reserves encompasses several key components:

1. **Inventory Acquisition Cost:** The initial purchase price per unit.

2. **Static Retention Expenses (Holding Costs):** Ongoing costs incurred while inventory held in reserve.

o **Opportunity cost of Capital Commitment:** The primary cost represents capital immobilized in the reserve inventory.

o Insurance coverage costs.

o **Asset Degradation:** Losses due to spoilage, damage, or expiration.

o **Value Erosion:** Depreciation from technological or market obsolescence.

o **Controllable Losses:** Shrinkage due to theft or administrative error.

o Costs for storage space, maintenance, and utilities.

o **Administrative Allocation:** Labor and overhead costs for reserve management.

Static retention expenses manifest as either:

o **Capacity-Linked Costs:** Fixed expenses like dedicated storage leases or base insurance premiums. These costs often increase in discrete increments when reserve volumes exceed designated capacity thresholds.

o **Volume-Linked Costs:** Variable expenses, notably the financing cost (opportunity cost or interest) on the capital value immobilized within the reserves. Higher reserve volumes directly increase this capital commitment cost.

Calculating Annual holding cost:

Annual Holding Cost = (Cost per Unit per Year) × (Average Reserve Level)

Where Average Reserve Level ≈ (Order Volume / 2)

3. **Ordering Costs:** Costs incurred per procurement event.

o **Procurement Processing:** Administrative and clerical costs per order.

o **Logistics cost:** Transportation and handling fees.

Calculating Annual Acquisition Transaction Expense:

Annual Ordering Cost = (Cost per Order) × (Annual Demand / Order Volume)

4. **Supply Discontinuity costs (Stock out Costs):** Costs arising from reserve depletion of critical items.

o Lost sales and associated profit margins.

o Damage to customer relationships and brand equity.

o **Operational Disruption:** Production halts caused by material unavailability.

o **Expedited Procurement Premiums:** Higher costs for emergency buying.

5. **Reserve Monitoring System:** The framework for tracking reserve status (e.g., through regular audits of perpetual inventory records).

2.2.2 **Total annual cost for inventory** calculation

1. Total annual cost for inventory management combines:Acquisition expenditure (Unit Cost × Annual Volume)

2. Procurement processing fees (Order Cost × Annual Volume / Order Quantity)

3. Storage carrying charges (Holding Cost × Order Quantity / 2)

Annual Resource Allocation Equation:
Total Annual Inventory Cost =
(Unit Purchase Price × Annual Demand Quantity)
+
(Order Processing Cost × [Annual Demand Quantity ÷ Order Quantity])
+
(Annual Holding Cost per Unit × [Order Quantity ÷ 2])

2.3 Inventory Control Protocols

2.3.1 Replenishment Trigger Mechanism

The replenishment/reordering threshold indicates when to initiate new orders, determined by:

* Supply chain delay (lead time)
* Anticipated consumption patterns

Under stable demand and fixed lead times:

Replenishment Point (reordering) = Daily Consumption Rate × Lead Duration (days)

2.3.2 Economic Order Quantity (EOQ)

Economic Order Quantity (EOQ) is a formula used in inventory management to calculate the ideal order amount that minimizes overall inventory costs, which include both holding and ordering costs.

EOQ = √[(2DS)/H]

Where:

* EOQ is the Economic Order Quantity
* D is the Annual Demand
* S is the Ordering Cost per order
* H is the Holding Cost per unit per year

2.3.2.1 EOQ Assumptions

A steady and expected demand, a constant wait time, instant restocking, no stock-outs, and a constant cost for buying and keeping.

2.3.2.2 EOQ with Discounts

Bulk orders often allow for a quantity reduction on the purchasing price.

* Accepting a quantity discount will have the following effects:
* Annual purchasing price will be reduced.
* The annual holding cost will rise.
* Annual ordering will most likely be reduced.

To determine whether to accept the discount, perform the following calculations:

1. Determine the EOQ without discounts: In the event that discounts are unavailable, the optimal inventory can be determined using the standard EOQ.
2. Determine the total cost of the EOQ: Utilize the EOQ to determine the total cost of the inventory, which encompasses ordering, carrying, and purchasing (without discount).
3. Calculate the total cost using the higher ordering quantity to secure the discount.
4. Select and choose: Select the order number that has the lowest total cost.
5. To ascertain the optimal total order number, repeat steps 2–5 in the event that there are numerous discount levels.

2.3.3 Gradual Replenishment of Inventory

So far, we have looked at cases where inventory levels were replenished quickly when organizations purchased goods from vendors. Similar issues are encountered by organizations that progressively rebuild inventory levels by manufacturing their items internally.

* Organizations that manufacture their products must choose between producing huge batches at lengthy intervals and producing all batches at short intervals.

* The amended EOQ model, called the EBQ (economic batch quantity model), is used for businesses that operate on gradual inventory replenishment.

* A machine configuration is typically used while producing items. This replaces the EOQ's ordering column.

* EOQ replenishes Inventory instantly, but this method replenishes it gradually.

* A portion of the batch may be sold or used while the remainder is still being created, depending on demand and rate.

* The average Inventory retained in the EOQ model (Q/2) is higher than the average for the same batch size (Q)

2.3.3.1 The EBQ

The EBQ model is primarily concerned with determining the number of items that should be produced in a batch (in comparison to the amount of an order with the EOQ).

The formula for EBQ is as follows:

$$EBQ = \sqrt{(2 * D * S) / (H * (1 - D/P))}$$

Where:

* D: Annual demand
* S: Setup cost per batch (the cost of preparing for a production run)
* H: Annual holding cost per unit
* P: Annual production capacity

3. Control Techniques to Minimize Inconsistencies and Losses

The amount invested in inventory and the labor costs related to its management and oversight are considerable in any organization. Consequently, organizations need to implement control mechanisms to reduce disparities and losses.

3.1 Stocktaking

The process of stocktaking entails assessing the physical quantity of Inventory held on a specific date and then comparing this balance to the

Balances on Store's ledger (record) cards are also called bin cards. Stocktaking can be done on an interval basis (periodic or continual).

* **Periodic stocktaking** involves checking inventory balances on a specific date, usually following the end of an accounting month.

* **Continuous stocktaking** entails counting and valuing inventory items on a rotating/daily basis.

* It is important to investigate the differences between the recorded 'book' inventory and the actual physical inventory. Discrepancies in the ledger or bin card may arise from errors in recording.

* Once the discrepancy is identified, update the ledger card to show the accurate physical inventory total.

* Recognize any items that are slow or outdated. This requires immediate attention from Management.

* Management will determine whether these items should be expensed on the income statement.

* **Gradual Inventory** consists of items that are slow to diminish.

* **Obsolete inventory** items are no longer needed and are outdated.

3.2 Valuing Inventory

3.2.1 Perpetual Inventory

Perpetual Inventory involves the ongoing documentation of receipts, issues, and resulting balances of specific inventory items in terms of amount, quantity, or value. Inventory records are maintained using the Store's ledger cards and bin cards. Bin cards, similar to ledger cards, show materials acquired through purchases and returns, as well as those distributed from requisitions.

3.2.2 Valuation Methods

The value of inventory is essential for financial reporting and must be included in a business's financial statements. And to determine product pricing based on inventory levels.

To charge the cost of production or cost of sales, the company will use the following methods:

* **FIFO (First In, First Out) basis:**

* In this method oldest goods that are purchased/manufactured are sold first while the newest goods purchased or manufactured remain in inventory.

* So, the ending inventory would include the most recent purchases.

* **Weighted Average Cost (AVCO/WACO) method:**

* In this method, the average costs of goods available for sale are assigned to the units sold and the units remaining in inventory.

* **Last In, First Out (LIFO) method:**

* This method is only allowed under US GAAP, but IFRS does not permit it.

* Under this method, the newest goods that are purchased/manufactured are sold first, while the oldest goods purchased/manufactured remain in inventory.

* So, the costs of the newest items purchased will flow into the costs of goods sold first.

Chapter 6 Accounting for labour

1. Direct and Indirect Labor Costs

One of the most important aspects of a firm is its employees. The distinction between direct and indirect labor costs is one of the most critical aspects to understand.

◈ Direct workers play a role in producing products.

◈ Indirect workers, such as maintenance personnel, plant leaders, and culinary workers, do not produce the items themselves. The pay of indirect workers is included in the indirect labor costs, which are part of the overhead costs.

2. Additional Pay for Overtime and Shift Work

People will be compensated for overtime if they are eligible to work more hours than they were employed for. Employees who work additional hours are compensated with a bonus in addition to their usual pay. Additional pay must be divided into direct and indirect labor costs.

◈ For persons who undertake direct labor, basic pay is always considered direct labor, regardless of whether it is for additional or regular work hours.

◈ Extra hours are often considered indirect labor, but they might be considered direct labor if the client requests them because the task must be completed quickly. Employees working night shifts or other unsocial hours may be eligible for a shift stipend or premium. Overtime and shift premiums are based on the belief that the additional money paid on top of the standard rate represents an indirect labor cost.

3. Determining Labor Input for Products and Services

Work sheets; • timesheets; and • timecards. They are used to determine how much labor goes into direct costs and how much goes into indirect costs.

- The payroll department is in charge of responsibilities that relate to the amount of labor used to complete the job.

- The payroll department calculates gross earnings using time and activity data as part of the payroll process.

- They also calculate net wages, which are wages after payroll deductions. The payroll department also considers the amount of cash required to pay employees and their direct and indirect compensation.

4. Accounting for Labor Costs

Labor costs are recorded in the accounting system. The money that an organization spends on labor is put into the labor account. The overall labor cost is divided into direct and indirect labor components.

- The labor account is **credited**, and the work in process account is **debited** for direct labor cost.

- Indirect labor cost is **credited** from the labor account and **debited** to the production overhead account.

- **Bank (1)**: Money used for wages is removed from the bank before it is recorded in the labor account.

- **(2) Direct Labor**: The majority of a manufacturing company's labor costs are direct labor costs. Direct labor costs are associated with production and are transferred from the labor account to the work-in-progress account via a credit to labor and debit to WIP.

◈ (3) **Indirect Labor**: Indirect labor costs include salary for indirect labor workers, overtime pay (unless the client requests it), shift pay, sick pay, and downtime. These indirect labor costs are totaled and applied to the production overhead account. They are deposited there by transferring funds from the labor account (credit) to the production overhead account (debit).

5. Remuneration Methods

There are two primary ways to establish pay: time-based and output-based.

5.1 Time-Based Pay

◈ The most common method for compensating employees based on their working hours.

◈ Workers are paid at a rate per hour, day, week, or month.

◈ Time-based systems do not motivate workers to be productive, requiring tight supervision most of the time.

5.2 Output-Based Pay (Piecework)

◈ Workers get paid the same amount for each item they make.

◈ Total wages = number of units produced multiplied by the rate of pay per unit.

◈ Because of minimum wage legislation, a guaranteed minimum wage is sometimes required.

5.3 Bonus Schemes

There are other ways to motivate employees to work harder but before they are implemented, managers and employees must agree on them. They should be easy to comprehend and utilize. They must benefit all employees involved in the scheme.

◈ The average pay for most bonus programs is based on time worked plus a portion of time saved. These are referred to as "premium bonus plans." Halsey and Rowan provide examples of this kind of plan.

◈ **Halsey Bonus**: The worker receives half of the value of the time saved.

o Total Earnings = (Hourly Rate * Time Taken) + (50% * Time Saved * Hourly Rate)

◈ **Rowan Bonus**: The employee gets paid a bonus depending on how much time they utilized compared to how much time they were allocated (time saved).

o Bonus = (Time Taken ÷ Time Allowed) * Time Saved * Hourly Rate

◈ **Measured Day Work**: This method aims to pay a high hourly rate, but the rate is determined by how well the worker has performed. At first, the work is measured to determine how much time is allocated for each unit (standard time). This allotted time is compared to how long the employee has previously taken, and if the actual time is less than the standard time, a higher base rate is paid.

5.4 Value Added / Gain Sharing

◈ Worker and management authorities must agree on a consistent method for calculating value added for remuneration to implement share of production plans.

◈ In this case, all value increases added—whether from more production or cheaper costs—are shared by all workers.

6. Labor Turnover

⟐ Labor turnover is the ratio of persons who quit their employment to the average number of employees.

⟐ If employee turnover is excessively high, management may want to monitor it and consider ways to reduce it.

⟐ Employee Turnover Rate = (Number of Employee Departures / Average Number of Employees) x 100

7. Labor Performance Ratios

7.1 Labor Efficiency Ratio

⟐ Compares the standard time allowed for the actual output achieved to the actual time taken.

⟐ A higher ratio indicates better efficiency.

⟐ Labor Efficiency Ratio = (Standard Hours for Actual Output / Actual Hours Worked) * 100%

7.2 Labor Idle Time Ratio

⟐ Indicates the percentage of paid labor hours that are unproductive (not due to the employee, e.g., machine breakdown).

⟐ Essential for evaluating labor efficiency and pinpointing areas for enhancement.

⟐ Labor Idle Time Ratio = (Total Idle Time / Total Paid Labor Hours) * 100

7.3 Labor Capacity Ratio

◈ Measures the actual hours worked as a percentage of the total budgeted hours available for work.

◈ Shows if a company is functioning at, beneath, or beyond its intended labor capacity.

◈ A ratio over 100% indicates surpassing budgeted hours; under 100% shows underutilization.

◈ Labor Capacity Ratio = (Actual Hours Worked / Budgeted Hours) x 100

7.4 Labor Production Volume Ratio (Activity Ratio)

◈ Compares the standard hours required for the actual output achieved to the budgeted hours for planned production.

◈ Measures the efficiency of using budgeted capacity for output. Exceeding 100% suggests effective utilization.

◈ Labor Production Volume Ratio = (Standard Hours for Actual Output / Budgeted Hours for Production) * 100

Chapter 7 Accounting for overheads

1. Direct and Indirect Expenditures

Direct expenditures are directly associated with a particular cost unit or cost center. Direct expenditures are included in the price of a product.

Indirect expenditures cannot be readily linked to a single cost unit or cost center. For instance, renting a factory space for a leather processing unit is an indirect cost since it might not only be linked with shoe making but also with other products like tyres and leather jackets being produced in the same facility. Indirect expenditures are referred to as overheads.

2. Fixed Production Overheads

Fixed production overheads

Production overheads are the sum of indirect production costs:

Fixed manufacturing overheads = indirect materials + indirect labor + indirect costs.

Fixed production overheads typically comprise the following costs:

- Heat the plant.
- Lighting the factory.
- Rent the factory.

  The entire cost of a product includes fixed manufacturing overheads. Organizations often cover fixed production overheads by including a defined amount in each product (fixed absorption costing).

3. Fixed Absorption Costing

Fixed absorption costing

Production overheads are recovered by absorbing them into the cost of a product, a process known as absorption costing. The goal of absorption costing is to recover overhead costs in a way that accurately represents the time and effort invested in creating a product or service.

3.1 Absorption Costing Stages:

Absorption costing stages:

- Allocation and distribution of overheads across several centers.

- Transfer non-production service center overheads to production centers.
- Overheads are absorbed into goods.

3.2 Allocation and Distribution

Allocation and distribution

Allocation of overheads to particular areas (production and service). Overheads for many departments must be divided via an apportionment process. Equitably distribute overheads across production and service divisions.

3.2.1 Bases of Distribution

Bases of distribution

There are no hard and fast criteria for determining which basis of apportionment to utilize, the method used to allocate overheads must be fair. Possible basis of apportionment include the following:

- Floor space for rent, tariffs, and overheads.
- Holding non-current assets for machinery depreciation and insurance purposes.
- Number of employees needed for a centre.

3.3 Reassign Service Centers to Production Cost Centers

Reassign service centers to production cost centers

Reassigning/reproportionment

Because service centers (departments) are not directly engaged in product manufacturing, their fixed production overheads must be shared with production centers (departments) on a reasonable basis.

- Here are some examples of service centers:

  - Store
  - Maintenance department
  - Mechanic centers

3.3.1 Basic Reapportionment

Basic reapportionment

The reapportionment method is employed when one service department serves many departments, including production. For instance, the maintenance center provides to all the firm`s departments.

The time spent (in percentage) servicing equipment provides a suitable basis for distributing maintenance costs.

3.3.2 Reciprocal Reapportionment

Reapportion maintenance

A technique for distributing costs that takes into account the interrelated services offered among service cost centers. This approach acknowledges that service departments can both receive and provide services to one another, necessitating a more intricate calculation for precise cost distribution. The simultaneous equations model is used to determine the actual cost of each service department. On the other hand, continuous re-apportionment is used until all of the service departments' overheads have been reapportioned to the production departments.

3.4 Absorption of Overheads

Absorption of overheads

After assigning, apportioning, and reapportioning overheads to the production divisions, they need to be linked to or absorbed by the product units. Overheads can be allocated to cost units on the following absorption bases:

- Units manufactured.
- Machine per hour rate (for machine-intensive manufacturing).
- Labor-hour rate (for labor-intensive manufacturing).
- Percentage of direct material
- Percentage of direct labor cost

Production overheads are often determined at the start of an accounting period to determine how much to allocate to a unit before determining the selling price. To determine the overhead absorption rate (OAR), formula;
OAR = Budgeted Overhead Cost / The budgeted sum for the absorption basis

3.4.1 Departmental OARs

Departmental OARs

If more than one department is involved in the manufacturing process, each department will charge OAR on its own basis. For instance, a labor-intensive department may use labor hours basis while a capital-intensive department can use machine hours basis.

3.5 Under-and Over-Absorption of Overheads

Under-and over-absorption of overheads.

If the estimated budgeted overheads and/or planned level of activity deviate from the actual outcomes for the year, one of the following can occur:

- Under absorption.
- Over absorption.

3.5.1 Calculate an Under- or Over-Absorption

Calculate an under- or over-absorption.

There is a three-step process:

Step 1: Calculate the OAR (depending on budget).

Overhead Absorption Rate = Budgeted Overhead Costs / Budgeted Level of Activity.

Step 2: Determine the overhead consumed by the actual action.

Overheads absorbed = predetermined OAR times the actual amount of activity.

Step 3: Compare absorbed to real

If the overheads absorbed after this time exceed the real overheads, then overheads have been over absorbed.

If the absorbed overheads are fewer than the real overheads, there has been under-absorption of overheads.

4. Journal and Ledger Entries for Manufacturing Overheads

Journal and ledger entries for manufacturing overheads.

Indirect production costs are charged (debited) to the production overhead account. Production overheads are credited to the production overheads account and deducted from the work in progress (WIP) account. The discrepancy between actual and absorbed overheads is called under- or over-absorbed overhead and is reported on the income statement at the end of the accounting period.

Non-production overheads are charged to one of the following:

- Administrative overheads account.
- Selling overhead account.
- Distribution overheads account.
- Account for finances and overheads.

Chapter 8 Marginal and Absorption Costing

1. Inventory Valuation

There are two methods for determining how many items have been sold and how many remain in stock: marginal costing and absorption costing. Fixed overhead costs are regarded as product costs in absorption costing, with each unit receiving a specific amount. Fixed overhead costs are considered period costs in marginal costing and are subtracted entirely from the period's earnings.

2. Marginal Costing

The marginal cost of inventory includes all variable costs associated with its production. This covers direct materials, direct labor, direct costs, and variable overheads.

Marginal costing = Direct materials + Direct labor+ Direct costs + Variable overheads

The value of inventory does not include fixed expenditures; rather, these expenses are recouped in full from the income statement at a later stage. Marginal cost is the cost of producing one extra unit of output. Marginal cost is one of the main components in managerial decision-making process.

2.1 The Concept of Contribution

Contribution indicates how much "money" you may provide to assist in paying for fixed cost.

Contribution = Price of products sold – variable costs

The concept of profit appears unhelpful as it relies on the number of units sold. Consequently, management accountants frequently utilize the idea of contributions. The contribution per unit stays the same regardless of changes in production and sales. The profit per unit changes with variations in produce and sales.

Total contribution = contribution per unit multiplied by number of sales.

Profit equals total contribution minus fixed overhead.

3. Absorption Costing

In absorption costing, the value of each stock item corresponds to its production cost. This includes an amount added to the price of each unit to account for the established manufacturing costs of that product, estimated at the start of the period.

The total cost of a product may be calculated by combining all of its direct costs and a portion of its manufacturing overhead costs. This may be accomplished by applying one or more overhead absorption rates. (More was discussed in the previous chapter.)

4. Impact of Absorption and Marginal Costing on Inventory Valuation and Profit Calculation

Absorption and marginal costing

With marginal costing, inventory is worth the whole variable cost of producing one unit of product. With absorption costing, the inventory is valued at the total cost of producing one unit of the output. As a result, inventory value will vary at the beginning and end of a period under both marginal and absorption conditions. This difference will affect the income statement. Hence, profits calculated using marginal costing will vary from those calculated using absorption costing.

4.1 Absorption Costing and Income Statement

Inventory valuation: Under absorption costing, open and closed inventory is valued at its full production cost.

Under- or over-absorbed overhead: In absorption cost income statements, you must adjust for under- or over-absorbed overhead.

4.2 Income Statement Using Marginal Costing

Inventory valuation: Open and closed inventory is valued at its marginal (variable) cost. To calculate the profit for the period, the actual fixed costs are deducted from the contribution generated.

5. Reconciling Profits Reported Under the Different Methods

Different methods give different profit levels as the inventory level rises and or falls.

When the inventory level goes up, the absorption method gives a higher profit. This is mainly because the fixed cost in the remaining inventory reduces the cost of goods sold. That remaining inventory (and the cost associated with it) is carried to the next accounting period instead of being written off in the current accounting period.

When the inventory level is down, the marginal costing gives higher profits. Under marginal costing, fixed overhead is expensed in the period incurred, so a decrease in inventory does not affect profit calculations (so it reports a higher profit than that of absorption costing).

When there is no change in inventory level, the profit remains the same under both methods.

6. Advantages and Disadvantages of Absorption and Marginal Costing

The positive and negative aspects of absorption and marginal costing

Absorption costing includes all costs associated with producing a product, encompassing both variable and fixed expenses. Marginal costing focuses solely on variable costs that change. Absorption costing is employed for external financial reporting in accordance with IFRS and GAAP. Marginal costing is primarily utilized for internal decision-making, such as determining pricing strategies and evaluating costs, sales, and profits.

6.1 Absorption Costing: Advantages

Adhering to IFRS and GAAP: Adheres to generally accepted accounting standards (GAAP) and IFRS, ensuring that information is accessible to external parties.

Accurate Profit and Loss Reporting: This approach aligns earnings with the reporting period by correlating all production costs to income.

Valuation: Provides an accurate assessment of goods by considering fixed costs.

Cost control identifies areas in the production process where costs are not being fully absorbed.

6.2 Absorption Costing: Disadvantages

Production level can be easily manipulated to influence reported profit

Dividing additional costs can be challenging when production rates fluctuate.

Fixed costs may not be relevant for short-term decision-making.

6.3 Marginal Costing: Advantages

The cost-volume-profit analysis simplifies the examination of costs, volume, and profit, aiding in the establishment of equitable pricing.

Helps in reducing costs by focusing on variable costs.

Profit varies with sales, allowing for a clearer assessment of the business's performance.

Decision Making: It provides essential insights for making swift decisions regarding price, production levels, and the choice between making or buying a product.

6.4 Marginal Costing: Disadvantages

This method is inadequate for external financial reporting as it does not follow IFRS and US GAAP.

Distinguishing between fixed and variable costs can be challenging.

Relying solely on variable costs for pricing may leave fixed costs uncovered.

Chapter 9: Job, batch and process costing

1. Costing Systems

Specific order costing is the costing system employed when an organization's work involves distinct, identifiable jobs or batches.

Continuous operation costing or process costing calculates the cost of goods or services produced in continuous or repetitive operations. It involves the average cost per unit, which is determined by dividing total production costs by the number of units produced during a specific time frame. This approach is especially beneficial for sectors with standardized production methods, like electricity generation or bottling.

2. Specific Order Costing Methods

2.1 Job Costing

Job costing or customer-requested task costing is a sort of customized order costing. Each work is priced differently. Job costing calculates and records order fulfillment expenses.

Cost sheets or work cards list the expenses of each task, which has a unique number.

Jobs' selling prices are decided by adding a profit margin to their cost. Costs of developing and building large, complex projects like airplanes or defense systems, event planning are some examples of job costing.

2.2 Batch Costing

Batch costing is a form of specific order costing. Batch costing is a method in cost accounting that involves tracking costs for a specific number of identical products produced in one run, referred to as a batch. This method is a form of job costing, treating each batch as a distinct cost unit, with a dedicated cost sheet for each one.

This method is common in footwear and clothing manufacturing, but it can also be used in pharmaceuticals, electronics, and bakery items. The selling price is calculated by adding profit to the cost of the batch.

3. Process Costing

3.1 Fundamentals

Process costing determines the expenses associated with goods or services generated through continuous or repetitive operations. The average cost per unit is calculated by dividing total production costs by the number of units produced within a given time period. This method is particularly advantageous for industries with uniform production processes, such as electricity generation or bottling.

A fundamental aspect of process costing is that all products in a process are uniform and indistinguishable from each other. A process account details costs and units, specifying materials, labor, and overhead inputs, along with the materials output at the end of the process. Therefore, a mean cost per unit is calculated for each process.

Expected output indicates the anticipated results of the process. One important feature of process costing is that the output from one process acts as the material input for the subsequent process.

The closing work-in-progress (WIP) at the end of a period serves as the opening WIP at the beginning of the subsequent period.

Average cost per unit = (Net cost of inputs/ Expected output)

3.2 Losses and Gains

3.2.1 Normal Losses

It is expeted loss in normal business activity. Normal loss is included in the production cost and distributed among the units produced. Sometimes, the total number of input units may differ from the total number of output units. Losses may occur due to the evaporation or wastage of materials, which may be an expected part of the process. Losses may sometimes be sold and generate revenue, generally referred to as scrap proceeds or scrap value. Normal loss is expected in a process and is often expressed as a percentage of the materials input to the process.

3.2.2 Scrap Value Handling

If the normal loss is sold as scrap, the revenue is used to reduce the input costs of the process.

If the normal loss is sold as scrap, then the formula for calculating the average cost of the unit's output does not change –the costs of inputs are reduced by the revenue received from the scrap that is sold, i.e., giving the net cost.

Average cost per unit = {(Total cost of inputs – Scrap)/ Expected output

If the normal loss has a scrap value, it is valued in the process account at this value. If the normal loss has no scrap value, it is valued in the process account as Nil.

3.2.3 Abnormal Losses and Gains

Abnormal loss is a loss that is not normally expected in usual business activity and is rare. Abnormal loss is more loss than expected. Abnormal loss is loss more than expected, while abnormal gain is less loss than expected. Abnormal losses and gains are not distributed into cost of goods sold.

3.2.4 Scrap Accounting

Losses and gains are transferred from the process account to the abnormal loss/gain account.

If there is no scrap value, the losses or gains are transferred to the Income statement at the value in the process account.

If there is a scrap value, then:

The abnormal loss is transferred from the abnormal loss/gain account to the scrap account at the scrap value. The cost of the loss transferred to the

Income statement is reduced by the scrap value of these loss units, and the same amount increases the cash received for scrap sales.

The abnormal gain is transferred from the abnormal loss/gain account to the scrap account at the scrap value. The savings associated with the gain are transferred to the income statement, reducing the cash received for the scrap sale.

3.3 Work-in-Progress Valuation

3.3.1 Equivalent Units Concept

At the end of the accounting period, some goods are partially completed. These items are called work in process (WIP). These items are called closing WIP. This closing WIP is the opening WIP for the next accounting period. The full cost of production cannot be allocated to these partially produced goods, so we use a concept of equivalent units (EUs).

The Equivalent units (EUs) idea is part-processed unit can be expressed as a proportion of a fully completed unit. For instance, a company with 100 units that are 60% complete regarding direct materials has 60 direct material equivalent units (100 * 60%).

3.3.2 Completion Stages

Equivalent units are determined individually for each cost component (direct materials, direct labor, and manufacturing overhead) due to their varying stages of completion. For example, materials may be introduced at the start of the process, whereas labor and overhead are incorporated over time.

3.3.3 Opening WIP Handling

Opening work in process (OWIP) inventory indicates the value of goods that are partially finished at the start of an accounting period. This reflects the expenses for materials, labor, and overhead that have been allocated to goods not completed by the end of the last period. It is the incomplete inventory that has been transferred from the previous period

WIP inventory = Beginning WIP inventory + Manufacturing costs - Cost of finished goods.

Partially completed units and completed units can be valued differently, like using weighted average and FIFO methods.

Opening inventory costs are added to current costs to provide an average cost per unit.

The FIFO method assumes that units in the OWIP must be completed prior to starting new units. The final output includes OWIP completed during the period and units produced from start to finish.

3.3.4 Mid-Production Losses/Gains

Losses or gains are recognized through a specific process. In this situation, EUs should be utilized to evaluate the degree of costs incurred at the time the loss or gain was recognized.

3.4 Joint and By-Products

3.4.1 Definitions

Sometimes, the process costing results in the production of multiple products. These extra products can be classified as joint products or by-products. Joint products are the primary outputs, while by-products are secondary and occur alongside the main products.

In other words, when two or more items of major value are made at the same time, they are called joint products. By-products, on the other hand, are secondary products that are made by accident while making the primary product and are not worth much in sales.

3.4.2 Product Examples

Wheat flour and bran are made when wheat is ground up in a grain processing plant. Gasoline, diesel, and kerosene come from the same refinery that refines crude oil.

Whey that comes from making cheese, glycerin that is left over from making biodiesel, and peanut shells that are left over from making peanut butter.

3.4.3 Cost Allocation Methods

Accounting treatment is different for joint products and by-products.

For joint products, the first step is to identify the split-off point.

The split-off point in manufacturing is when products made together become distinguishable.

Before this point, costs are considered as joint costs. After this point, the costs of further processing are specific for each product. Before split point the cost is distributed (proportioned) using one of following methods;

Physical units: The method employs a quantitative characteristic of the items, such as weight or volume, to determine their cost.

The Sales Value at Split-off: Method allocates expenses based on the value of each product at the split-off point.

The Net Realizable Value (NRV) Method allocates expenses by calculating the expected sales value and subtracting separable costs incurred after the split-off point.

3.4.4 By-Product Accounting

As by-products have an insignificant value, the accounting treatment is different.

1. The costs are allocated exclusively to the joint products. Like regular loss, the by-products absorb no costs.
2. The sales value of the by-product at the split-off point is viewed as a

cost reduction, again treated as a normal loss, rather than as income.

3. When a by-product has no value at the split-off point but increases in value after further processing, its net income is used to reduce the overall costs of the process.
   Net income, or net realizable value, is determined by deducting additional processing costs from the final sales price.

3.4.5 Process Accounting

Joint products ought to be regarded as normal output from a process. The handling of by-products in process accounts resembles that of normal loss.

The income from by-products is recorded as a credit in the process account and a debit in the by-product account.

To determine the number of units produced in a given period, by-product units, such as normal loss, decrease the total output of units.

Chapter 10: Service and operation costing

1. Service costing

Service costing is used by businesses in the business of services (instead of goods), like a law firm doing lawsuits for a company. The service provider businesses have outputs in the form of services (not goods) which are intangible, can be heterogeneous, and these services can be produced and provided at the same time. Moreover, these services cannot be saved (in contrast to goods).

2. Measurement of service costing

Measurement of service cost is complex. The business uses one or more methods to determine the cost of services. Working hours of staff who work to provide services can be used for costing services. If the service provided depends on more than one factor, the combined cost unit is used. For the hotel business, the cost of meals, laundry costs, and hotel staff working hours can be used to determine the cost of service. On the other hand, for the hospital business, the cost of medicine and other equipment, and the working hours of the doctors and nursing staff can be used.

3. Service unit cost

The whole cost of a service will include labor, supplies, fees, and overheads, which is the same as the prices of goods made in the manufacturing industry. In services, labor is usually used as a direct cost, and other costs like utilities and rents are considered as overhead. Costs can be classified as fixed, variable, or semi-variable. The semi-variable cost can be separated into determinable variable and fixed parts. To find the cost per service unit, you divide the total cost of giving the service by the number of service units used.

If companies in the same service business use the same service cost units, it is easy to see how the different companies stack up.

Chapter 11 Alternative Costing Principles

1. Modern Production Environment

Modern manufacturing varies from conventional production. The quantity of "direct" labor has decreased due to increased reliance on machines and computer-based processes in manufacturing, as well as lower batch sizes in response to customer needs and the usage of computers and automation. Increased indirect costs, including fees and taxes. Traditional cost-calculation methods, such as absorption and marginal costing, are becoming more unrealistic.

2. Modern Costing Methods

2.1 Activity-Based Costing (ABC)

Activity-based costing (ABC) monitors costs by analyzing a company's activities and assigning costs to those tasks. Ultimately, it allocates costs among items or services according to their usage. This method simplifies understanding the costs of a product or service by highlighting the specific actions that lead to those costs. For a manufacturing firm, cost drivers may include the number of machines used in production, while for a quality control firm, they may involve the number of inspectors. For instance, for a manufacturing firm, the cost drivers can be the number of machines involved in the production process, or for a quality control firm, the number of inspectors.

2.1.1 Advantages of ABC

Accuracy: ABC provides a clearer understanding of the costs associated with a product or service, aiding in precise pricing, profit analysis, and effective cost management.

Insight into Cost Drivers: ABC assists businesses in identifying activities that incur costs, enabling them to refine processes and reduce expenses.

Improved Choices: With accurate cost information, managers can make informed decisions regarding product creation, pricing, and resource allocation.

Better Performance Measurement: ABC can monitor the effectiveness of various tasks and identify areas for improvement.

2.1.2 Disadvantages of ABC

It can be difficult to implement and time-consuming in a business with diverse activities and products.

It requires more data to be collected, so the cost of implementation might be higher.

Employees might resist transitioning from the traditional method to the new one.

Cost determination for each activity can be a difficult task. Moreover, cost allòcation is also challenging.

2.2 Target Costing

Target costing is a price-based strategy in which management first decides at what price they can sell the product in the market and then targets a cost of making that product to get a desirable profit. It focuses on the market and customers in a competitive market. It is a more robust approach as traditional costing first determines the cost and then adds a margin to sell in the market.

Steps:

1. Estimate the competitive market price
2. Deduct the required profit margin to determine the allowable cost.
3. Engage the team to meet the cost target
4. Apply cost reduction tools.

2.3 Lifecycle Costing

Lifecycle costing takes into account all expenses related to a product, from acquisition to disposal or resale. I assist in making informed decisions by considering both initial and ongoing costs.

2.3.1 Benefits

- It provides a comprehensive Cost View.
- Lifecycle costing aids in forecasting future expenses, i.e, maintenance, repairs, and replacements, thereby helping to avoid unforeseen costs. This enables improved financial planning and reserve allocation for upcoming expenses.
- Lifecycle costing monitors and finds design or operational improvements that save money over time.

• It encourages the selection of energy-efficient and durable components, which results in reduced waste. This also offers investments in assets that provide better long-term benefits.

• Due to targeted maintenance strategies, the downtime can be significantly reduced, and the life of the asset can be extended.

• Lifecycle costing provides a rational basis for comparison of different options to choose the most efficient solutions.

• Lifecycle costing encourages sustainable investment decisions to reduce environmental impact.

• By considering the entire lifecycle, it helps optimize the value of the asset by using it more efficiently.

• It helps in making informed decisions about asset disposal, considering potential costs and environmental impacts.

3. Total Quality Management (TQM)

It is a management strategy that puts customer satisfaction first for long-term success. Management takes an active role in improving processes, goods, and services by collaborating with consumers, workers, and suppliers. It prioritizes customers, addresses problems, and makes data-driven solutions. This definition can be derived from the word Total Quality Management as total means everyone (i.e, consumers, workers, and suppliers) is involved, quality means meeting standards, and management means being actively managed (proactive approach).

3.1 Principles of TQM

(1) Stopping the problem before it happens costs less than fixing it afterwards. Therefore, TQM aims to achieve 100 percent satisfaction for the first time.

(2) TQM works continuously for improvement, as 100 percent accuracy the first time may not be possible.

(3) Pay attention to the customer`s demand and needs.

3.2 Quality-Related Costs

Not meeting customer expectations or making initial mistakes can result in businesses losing about 15% to 30% of their sales revenue. Quality-related costs are the expenses associated with ensuring product or service quality and the losses incurred when standards are not met. Costs are typically divided into four categories: prevention costs, appraisal costs, internal failure costs, and external failure costs. The prevention and appraisal costs are also called conformance costs, while internal failure and external failure costs are also called non-conformance costs.

3.2.1 Prevention Costs

Prevention costs are the cost of taking actions proactively to avoid defects and reduce the chances of quality problems arising in the first place. Firms that take actions for prevention can lower costly reworks, minimize returns, and increase long-term consumer satisfaction. The following are some examples to use prevention;

- Gathering customer feedback through surveys.
- Research on the needs of customers
- Training staff
- Evaluation of the supplier to ensure quality
- Applying precise production design to maintain product quality
- Implementing quality standards such as ISO 9001
- Encouraging a culture of continuous learning

3.2.2 Appraisal Costs

Cost of evaluating products, their components, and or processes to ensure quality. These costs are required to detect defects in the products before they reach customers. Appraisal cannot stop defects, but it detects them before the product reaches customers.

Common examples of appraisal costs can be:

- Purchasing inspection tools
- Conducting routine inspections and audits
- Monitoring process control
- Maintaining testing tools and maintaining them.

3.2.3 Internal Failure Costs

Internal failure cost arises when a defect is detected before reaching the market or customer. These costs are a result of not detecting the errors during the production process and often lead to wastage of time, material, and resources. Typical examples of internal failure costs are:

- Cost of repairing or reworking
- Loss of scrapped and unusable material
- Cost of disposing of defective items

- Downtime and production delays

3.2.4 External Failure Costs

External failure costs occur when the quality defect is detected after it reaches the customer or market. This can significantly damage the reputation of the company and customer satisfaction. Companies often contact customers directly in the event of an external failure. Common examples of external failure are:

- Investigating and resolving the complaints
- Handling customers' warranty and service claims
- Loss of future customers
- Cost of sales returns and replacements

4. Cost Control and Cost Reduction

4.1 Cost Control

Establishment of clear objectives for the cost centres and continuous tracking of their progress in accordance with those goals is a fundamental aspect of cost control practices. Crowningshield and Gorman have identified the following six requirements for designing an effective cost control system:

1. **Clear Allocation of Responsibilities**: For effective cost control, responsibilities regarding costs must be explicitly defined and allocated to accountable personnel. For this, proper authority and communication need to be established.

2. **Setting Realistic Goals**: Setting realistic goals and guiding managerial behavior is essential for cost control to work effectively. These goals must be aligned with broader organizational goals, and management must agree on them. Without proper goals and tasks, the management lacks a reference point for performance evaluation, resulting in inefficiencies and missed opportunities for cost improvement. Goals should be SMART- specific, measurable, achievable, relevant, and time-bound. These goals should be revised periodically.

3. **Motivation to Participate**: The cost control system must be collaborative. Individuals across departments can be motivated

when the goals are perceived as achievable and fair. The goals must be realistic and not overly lenient.

4. **Timely and Insightful Reporting**: Accurate and timely reporting is essential for cost control and identifying deviations from planned cost targets. Reports should include basic financials and other performance metrics highlighting cost-saving potential. Digital dashboards and ERP systems can enhance reporting efficiency.

5. **Implementation of Recommendations**: Critical recommendations must be translated into actions; otherwise, even well-crafted strategies may fail.

6. **Continuous Monitoring and Corrective Action**: Follow-up ensures corrective actions are implemented properly. Monitoring KPIs and post-implementation reviews encourage accountability and adaptability.

4.2 Cost Reduction

Cost-cutting involves lowering the cost per unit of product/service without lowering its quality or value. There is a misunderstanding about cost reduction. It is often associated with lowering quality and excessive frugality. However, effective cost reduction is all about identifying and avoiding unnecessary expenses while keeping the quality untouched or even improved. In some situations, profits can be improved without cutting costs, like increased investment in materials (bulk buying or acquiring the supplying source), a change in design, and greater customer support. One important point here is that if the company reduces the price, it should communicate effectively to its customers, as the customers can perceive it as a reduction in quality. A good cost reduction strategy also includes maintaining the perceived value of the product/service.

4.2.1 Value Analysis

One of the most effective and widely used methods for cost reduction is value analysis. Value analysis is a systematic method to examine the functions of a product/service to identify cost-saving potential. Its main objective is to achieve the desired level of output with minimized cost by optimizing resources and avoiding unnecessary expenditures.

Understanding Value:

◈ **Functional/Utility Value**: Practical value (e.g., fuel efficiency in a car).

◈ **Esteem Value**: Perceived value based on aesthetics/reputation.

Understanding this distinction is critical during value analysis. What may seem non-essential technically could hold high esteem value for certain customers. Value analysis must balance cost savings with consumer expectations.

4.2.2 Steps for Value Analysis

1. Determine exactly what the consumer wants.

2. Develop and compare approaches to meet client demands (specify costs for materials, labor, etc.).

3. Approve ideas by senior management.

4. Execute the plans.

5. Examine the substance of new ideas.

4.2.3 Value Engineering in Target Costing

Value engineering is a strategic approach essential for implementing target costing. This involves applying value analysis across organizational processes, starting from planning and product design. The main aim is to create products providing the highest customer value for the least cost. While value analysis lowers costs of existing products, value engineering is proactive—incorporated during development to ensure efficient design from the outset. After setting the target selling price, value engineering aligns design choices with financial objectives, ensuring competitiveness and economic feasibility.

Chapter 12: Forecasting techniques

1. Forecasts in Budgeting

Budgets are prepared for forecasted future events. Forecasting is primarily used to estimate predicted production, sales revenues, and expenses. In forecasting, the most reasonable assumptions are utilized to anticipate these outcomes, which are then used to plan. For example, a firm that has had a four percent increase in revenue over the last ten years may use the same growth percentage in the next year. Budget expenditures may also be projected using past or anticipated inflation rates.

2. Major Forecasting Techniques

Linear regression analysis
Time series analysis
Index numbers.

2.1 Linear Regression Analysis

The linear regression method is used to model the relationship between two or more variables (one is dependent, one or more are independent). This technique is widely used in forecasting and understanding relationships, particularly when the relationship is assumed to be linear.

For the time being, we are only interested in two variable relationships, one independent and one dependent.

In a linear equation, we can use many methods to find the relationship like

By drawing a scatter diagram and a line of best fit.

There are a variety of methods available for identifying the relationship: line of best fit, correlation, high-low method, and least squares.

2.1.1 Scatter Diagram

A scatter diagram or scatter plot is a graph used to display the relationship between two variables. A line of best fit (also called a trend line) is a straight line drawn through the scatter plot that represents the general trend of the data by minimizing the distance between the line and the data points.

The following method is used to draw scatter diagram and a line of best fit;

- Collect data sets and ensure you have the corresponding values of each variable for each point.
- Draw the x-axis and y-axis
- Plot the points in the graph corresponding to x and y values.
- Using a ruler, draw a straight line that best represents the overall trend of data points, aiming for roughly the same number of points on each side.
- Interpretation: the line best fit helps to understand the relationship between two variables, such as a positive slope, which means positive correlation. The closer the points are to the line, the stronger the correlation.

2.1.2 Least Squares Regression

In the least squares regression, we calculate the line of best fit mathematically. It's often represented by the equation $y = a + bx$, where "y" is the dependent variable, "x" is the independent variable, "a" is the intercept, and "b" is the slope of the line. Whereas

$$b = (n\sum xy - \sum x \sum y)/(n\sum x^2 - (\sum x)^2)$$

and "n" is the number of pairs of data or data points.

In budgeting, the linear regression analysis forecasts whenever a linear relationship is assumed between two variables, x and y.

2.1.3 Interpolation vs. Extrapolation

Interpolation estimates a value within known data points. Interpolation estimates the value of a missing data point between two known data points. If you have temperature data for 10:00 AM and 12:00 PM and want to predict 11:00 AM, you use interpolation.

Extrapolation is predicting a value outside known data. Extrapolation occurs when using morning temperature information to approximate 6:00 PM temperature. Interpolation prediction is considered safer than extrapolation.

2.1.4 Benefits of Simple Linear Regression

- It is simple to use and interpret the model's outcomes.
- It requires minimal computing power, allowing it to manage large numbers effectively.
- It can serve as a foundation for evaluating more complex regression models.
- Most computer spreadsheets allow the calculations for the linear regression.
- Forecasting is easy and simple.

2.1.5 Limitations of Simple Linear Regression

- Linear regression assumes a linear relationship, though it's not true all the time.
- Outliers can significantly reduce the accuracy of the result.
- It presumes that errors are independent, have constant variance, and follow a normal distribution. Breaking these assumptions can impact the model's reliability.
- Multicollinearity occurs when two or more independent variables are highly correlated, which can reduce the stability of the model.

◈ Limited Scope: It illustrates the relationship between two variables, yet many real-life scenarios involve multiple variables.

◈ Only interpolated predictions are reliable.

◈ Predictions are only reliable if the correlation between variables is strong.

2.2 Correlation

Regression analyzes the connection between two variables, consisting of one independent and one dependent variable.

Correlation quantifies the strength and direction of a linear relationship between two variables. The correlation coefficient (r) ranges from -1 to +1.

2.2.1 The Correlation Coefficient

The degree of correlation can be measured by Pearson's correlation coefficient, r. The correlation coefficient (r) ranges from -1 to +1.

+1 indicates a perfect positive linear relationship.

Zero: no linear correlation

-1 indicates a perfect negative linear relationship.

Values between +1 and -1 are called partial correlation.

The degree of correlation can be measured by Pearson's correlation coefficient, r (the product-moment correlation coefficient).

r must always be between –1 and +1.

If r = 1, there is a perfect positive correlation.

2.2.2 Formula for Correlation Coefficient "r"

$r = (n * \Sigma XY - (\Sigma X * \Sigma Y)) / \sqrt{[(n * \Sigma X^2 - (\Sigma X)^2) * (n * \Sigma Y^2 - (\Sigma Y)^2)]}$.

Here's a breakdown of the formula:

n: The number of data points.

ΣXY: The sum of the products of each pair of x and y values.

ΣX: The sum of all x values.

ΣY: The sum of all y values.

2.3 Time Series Analysis

Regression analysis looks at the connection between variables, not the order in which they happened, to see how changes in one variable might affect changes in another.

Time series analysis looks at data points that were collected over time and models the connections and trends that can be found in that order. This is usually done to make predictions. It is a sequence of data points collected or recorded at regular time intervals—e.g., monthly sales, daily temperatures, or annual GDP figures.

2.3.1 Purpose of Time Series Analysis

- Identify historical trends
- Forecast future values based on historical patterns
- Detect seasonal variations
- Adjust forecasts using seasonal effects

2.3.2 Components of Time Series

There are four components of time series analysis:

Trend (T):

A long-term movement or direction in data (upward, downward, or flat). A Trend is estimation by any of the following methods:

- Graph
- Least squares regression
- Moving average

Seasonal Variation:

Seasonal variation means repeating short-term trends based on time of year, day, month, etc. For instance, more grocery demands increase over weekends.

Two methods to measure seasonal variations are the additive model and the multiplicative model.

Additive model:

In a seasonal model, an absolute value is added to the trend to forecast the future. For instance, coffee sales in winter will be over 10000 above the trend.

Prediction = trend + seasonal variation.

Multiplicative model:

In this model, the seasonal variation is expressed in ratio/proportion or in percentage form.

Prediction = trend x seasonal variation. For example, the coffee sales would be 1.5 times the trend in summer.

Cyclical Variation (C):

The variations in sales (or any other amount) due to business cycle fluctuations (good business times, bad business times, in other words, boom, recession, depression, peak). This forecasting is one of the hardest, as the fluctuations are always unpredictable and their magnitude and duration cannot be predicted.

Residual/Random Variation:

Unpredictable fluctuations in business revenues/sales, expenses, etc, due to natural disaster, sudden political unrest, unexpected market shocks, and other anomalies and noise.

Note: the forecaster mostly focuses on trends and seasonal variations to forecast, as the other two are very hard to estimate.

2.3.3 Moving Averages

A moving average is a statistical method that helps to reduce short-term variability and reveal the main trends in time series data. Calculating the average of a set of consecutive observations helps analysts grasp long-term trends and reduce the impact of irregular fluctuations in the data.

Choosing the right number of periods for calculating moving averages is essential when estimating trend lines. The ideal period length is typically determined by the characteristics and frequency of cyclical patterns present in the data, although there is no single correct value. For example: A seven-day moving average is often utilized in daily observations to address weekly cycles. A four-quarter moving average is typically used when analyzing quarterly data to reflect the complete annual cycle. A 12-month moving average for monthly datasets offers a comprehensive perspective on annual trends, while shorter periods may better reflect recent shifts.

2.3.4 Advantages of Time Series Forecasting

Transparent and Logical Assumptions make it easy to interpret.

With the availability of new data, trend lines and patterns can be updated regularly. This enables organizations to evaluate the precision of past forecasts and implement prompt adjustments, enhancing reliability progressively.

As analysts become more experienced, their ability to interpret patterns, identify anomalies, and refine models based on past performance improves.

2.3.5 Limitations and Challenges

An essential premise is that historical trends will persist moving forward. This may not always be the case, particularly in times of major change.

Assumption of Linear Trends: Many models assume the presence of a consistent, straight-line trend, which may oversimplify real-world dynamics.

Fixed Seasonal Patterns: Time series models typically assume that seasonal variations are stable over time, either as fixed values in the additive model or as consistent proportions of the trend in the multiplicative model. Seasonality can change based on consumer behavior, external events, or economic shifts.

3. The Product Life Cycle and Its Role in Forecasting

Product life cycle describes the stages a product passes through in the market to get insights about its sales forecasting. Understanding the life cycle stage of the product helps to estimate future sales and other important indicators with more precision.

3.1 Sales Forecasting at Different Life Cycle Stages

Development Stage: At this stage, the product is in its development phase and not yet introduced to the market. The main focus is on development, research, and testing.

Introduction Stage: Introduction is the launching stage of the product, and sales have started at a lower level. Significant marketing efforts are being utilized to promote the product. Forecasting expectations in this stage should be modest.

Growth Stage: as the market accepts, sales start to improve and rise rapidly. There is an increase in sales, interests, and distribution channels. The profits start to rise. Forecasting at this stage can be substantial with a caution of overestimation.

Maturity Stage: At this stage, sales peak and begin to stabilize. Market saturation often occurs and competition intensifies. Total sales are still high but the sales growth slows down. Forecasting in this stage should be on maintaining the existing level rather than expansions.

Decline Stage: Eventually, sometimes the product faces a drop in demand due to technological change, market shift, or any other factor. Forecasting should be conservative at this stage.

3.2 Uses of the Product Life Cycle in Forecasting

The product life cycle offers several benefits for managerial planning, including:

- Coordinating marketing and investment approaches with anticipated sales patterns.
- Forecasting inventory and production requirements
- Assisting with budget planning and financial forecasts

3.3 Limitations

◈ The PLC model suggests a uniform sequence of stages; however, not every product adheres to a clear or consistent path.

◈ Determining the exact stage of a product in its life cycle can be difficult, particularly when market signals are unclear or conflicting.

◈ External factors like technological disruption, regulatory changes, and consumer trends can change the anticipated trajectory of the life cycle.

4. Index Numbers

4.1 Introduction

In financial analysis, data over various periods—like revenues or costs—often shows trends. For instance, a shoe manufacturer experience an increase in revenue, could indicate growth via expansion. However, these increases may merely stem from rising prices caused by inflation, not from heightened activity. Analysts use index numbers to adjust for price-level changes, allowing them to distinguish between nominal and real growth and evaluate actual performance over time.

An index number is a statistical measure used to track changes in a particular variable (such as prices, quantities, or revenues) over time, relative to a selected base year (serves as the benchmark, usually assigned a value of 100). It expresses each year's data as a percentage of the base year value, facilitating meaningful comparisons across different time periods. The base year should be selected carefully. Ideally, it should represent a "normal year". A normal year is free from any major economic fluctuation. Base year can be changed and adjusted periodically.

4.2 Practical Application

The shop made $500,00 in sales in 2020. The income went up to $650,00 in 2024. Prices, on the other hand, also went up at this time.

The selling price index (base year 2020 = 100) for 2024 is 130.

To adjust 2020 revenue to 2024 prices:

Adjusted Revenue=500,00× (130/100) =650,00

The increase in income is attributed not to higher sales but to rising prices. The index figure indicated that sales volume remained stable, with only pricing experiencing an increase.

4.3 Types of Index Numbers

The use of index number is diverse so they can be divided into several types according to their usage. Following are some most common used index number types. These index number can be modified for specific need.

- Simple indices
- Chain-based indices
- Multi-item (or weighted) indices.

4.3.1 Simple Indices

A simple index measures a single item's price or quantity changes. In the first example of index number we used simple index. There are two type of simple indices; Price index, Quantity index.

When we calculate simple index using prices it is price index and when we use it with any quantity it is quantity index.

Formula for price index = (price of goods in current period / price of goods in base period) * 100.

While current prices are symbolized as p1 and p0 as previous /base year price.

So Pi = (P1 / P0) * 100.

Same formula can be used for quantity index as Qi = (q1 / q0) * 100

4.3.2 Chain Base Index Numbers

Chain basis index numbers allow for the calculation of index numbers by comparing the index of one period to that of the preceding period, instead of relying on a fixed base year.

It assesses changes from one year to the next.

Index values rise with an increasing variable, remain steady during stabilization, and fall when the trend declines. The chain base technique is useful for managing frequently changing index item weights. The chain base index is better suited for long-term analysis than the fixed-base method, which often needs full adjustments for weight changes.

It's calculated by dividing the current period's index number by the previous period's index number and then multiplying by 100 to express it as a percentage.

Chain Base Index (for a period t) = (Value in period t / Value in period t-1) * 100

4.3.3 Multi-Item (Weighted) Indices

Index changes can be monitored by using the "weight" of each item to observe variations in the overall price or quantity of several items. Businesses offering various products can utilize this to analyze changes in prices or quantities from a reference year.

A store with three products might consider developing a pricing index to examine the impact of price changes on the total cost. Each factor may influence sales or revenue in distinct ways, so assign appropriate weight to highlight its significance.

Steps to Construct a Weighted Price Index:

1. Calculate the Price Relative for Each Item:

Price Relative= (Current Price/Base Year Price) $\times$100

2. Apply Weights to Each Price Relative:

Multiply each price relative by its corresponding weight (e.g., quantity sold, revenue contribution).

3. Calculate the Weighted Average:

Overall price index = (Sum of weighted price relatives) / (Sum of weights)

Weighted indices more accurately represent reality because they prioritize factors that significantly impact value, like sales volume or revenue share. They are essential in business, economics, and cost analysis.

Same way we can calculate weighted index for the quantity.

4.3.4 Laspeyre and Paasche Indices

Laspeyre Price Index: it is a special case of a weighted index. In a weighted index, the weight can be assigned on any basis, like current year prices/ quantities, base year quantities, or price. In the Laspeyre index, the weights are only assigned on a base year basis.

Laspeyre Price Index = [Σ (Current year price × Base year quantity) / Σ (Base year price × Base year quantity)] x 100

Quantity index = [Σ (Current year quantity × Base year price)/Σ (Base year quantity × Base year price)] x 100

Advantages of Laspeyres Indices:

◈ Relies on quantities from a base year, eliminating the need for annual data updates.

◈ Denominator remains constant, simplifying index calculations.

◈ Effective for long-term comparisons.

Drawbacks:

◈ Employs fixed base-year quantities that may not reflect actual behavior.

◈ Exaggerates effects of price hikes by ignoring consumer substitutions.

Paasche Index:

Paasche index numbers are also a special case of weighted index. In this index current prices or current year quantity is used to weight the index.

Paasche Price index = [Σ (Current year price × Current year quantity)/Σ (Base year price × Current year quantity)] *100

Quantity index = [Σ (Base year quantity × Current year price)/Σ (Base year quantity × Current year price)]*100

Benefits:

◈ Accurately represents current behavior using current-year weights.

Drawbacks:

◈ Requires annual updates, increasing effort.

◈ Underestimates inflation by minimizing effects of price rises.

4.4 Benefits of Index Numbers

◈ Enhanced Managerial Insight: Clarifies complex information to identify trends.

◈ Time-Based Percentage Comparison: Facilitates evaluation of pricing/cost changes.

◈ Standardized Comparisons: Simplifies interpretation via base-100 standardization.

◈ Impact Assessment: Distinguishes price-driven vs. volume-driven changes.

4.5 Issues

◈ Construction Complexity: Requires methodological scrutiny for accurate interpretation.

◈ Limited Applicability: Only valid for original data groups.

◈ Inflation Adjustment: Predictions must incorporate inflation for accuracy.

4.6 Numerical Data Applications

Utilize past and projected data to make estimates, considering inflation factors. Basic revenue or cost figures, when not adjusted for inflation, may not effectively indicate success, but rather reflect a change in price.

Future predictions should incorporate inflation to maintain accuracy.

Chapter 13: Budgeting

1. The Purpose of Budgeting

1.1 The Budget Theory

A budget is a list of numbers that shows how you plan to spend your money over a certain length of time. It lists projected income and expenses and acts as a financial road map to help the group reach its goals. Most companies make a master budget for the whole company, but also make smaller, more specific budgets to go with it.

Organizations may also be involved in many different types of budgeting;

Departmental budgets: Marketing, HR, and production, so there is more control and responsibility at the smaller level.

Budgets for cash flow: These show how much money is expected to come in and go out. This helps them keep track of their cash flow and make sure they have enough to pay their bills.

Functional budget: Budgets help keep an eye on and run each business function smoothly by focusing on certain operating areas like sales, production, or purchasing.

Forecasted Statements of Financial: These include statements of predicted income and statements of financial situation, which show how profitable and healthy the business is expected to be.

1.2 Primary Functions of Budgeting

1. **Planning Strategies and Achieving Goals**:

   Budgets direct future activities in alignment with the company's long-term goals.

2. **Cost Control and Performance Monitoring**:

One primary objective of budgeting is to manage costs. Analyze the actual outcomes against the budgeted figures and examine significant discrepancies.

3. **Coordination**:

Budgets connect departmental strategies and activities with the goals of the organization. Budgeting brings together operations, sales, and finance under a unified strategy, fostering integration and collaboration.

4. **Stating Goals**:

The organization conveys its strategic and financial objectives through a budget.

5. **Motivation and Incentives**:

Budgets can inspire by establishing challenging yet achievable performance objectives. Numerous organizations provide performance-based incentives to managers and employees who surpass budget expectations.

6. **Assessment of Performance**:

Budgetary performance is a common measure of managerial efficiency. Budgets play a crucial role in accountability and assessment as performance evaluations typically measure how well a department or individual adhered to budget constraints.

7. **Approved Spending**:

Budgets limit spending, managing it effectively.

2. Steps for Budgeting

- Organizations develop and establish a budget that connects long-term financial goals and short-term objectives. Typical budgeting steps include;

1. **Establishing strategic goals**:

The organization should establish long-term goals prior to budgeting and outline spending needs.

2. **Formation of the Budget Committee**:

A budget committee manages and organizes the planning process. Budget committee can include the Chief Executive Officer, the budget manager, and a senior representative from sales, purchasing, and production.

3. **Creating the budget guide**:

Budget guides outline the process for creating, submitting, and tracking budgets. Contents: Processes and timelines, reporting structures and responsibilities.

4. **Identify the primary budget element**:

Identifying the limiting factor, or key spending element, is a critical phase. The amount of labor performed is constrained, influencing expenses. Typically, sales demand is a limiting factor. The restricted factor budget should be prepared first, as it influences the scale and feasibility of the other budgets.

5. **Creating an effective budget**:

Once the limiting factor budget is established, managers in production, marketing, and HR begin to budget for their respective departments or functions. The individual restrictions should align with the previously stated limits.

6. **Distributing and evaluating initial budgets**:

Drafts of functional budgets are submitted to the budget group. Managers might deliberately lower revenues or overstate expenses to generate "budgetary slack" for achieving targets. The committee assesses the proposals, formulates a budget, and verifies alignment with the objectives.

7. **Approval and creation of the master budget**:

Upon examination and modification: All finalized budgets create a master budget. The master budget typically comprises: An anticipated income statement, a planned balance sheet report for the company, and a cash flow estimate. The master budget is submitted to upper management for final approval.

8. **Ongoing Variance Observation and Evaluation**:

Budgets undergo regular reviews following their implementation. Actual outcomes are assessed against projected figures, and significant discrepancies are examined to understand the reasons behind them. This encourages accountability and advancement.

3. Behavioral Aspects of Budgets

3.1 Behavioral Aspect of Budgeting

The Human Factor in Budgeting and the Role of Motivation:

For a budgeting system to be truly effective, it must go beyond technical accuracy—it must also account for human behavior, organizational dynamics, and individual motivation. The success or failure of a budgeting system is often less about the system itself and more about how it is implemented, perceived, and used by people within the organization.

A major strength of budgeting lies in its comprehensiveness—it influences all aspects of the organization. However, this strength can become a weakness if the process lacks credibility, transparency, or trust. When employees and managers feel disconnected from budget goals or processes, the risk of non-compliance, low morale, or passive resistance increases. While senior management plays a key role in setting strategic direction, lower-level management is essential for budgets to translate into action.

Influencing Behavior through Budget Responsibility:

Assigning budgetary responsibility is one of the most direct ways to influence managerial behavior. Every decision made by a manager has financial implications, and these are reflected in budget comparisons—planned versus actual results. As such, budgeting becomes a mechanism for accountability, but also a tool for guiding decisions and actions. In a budgeting context, motivation is crucial—without it, even the best-formulated plans can fail to produce results.

3.2 Motivation and Budgeting

In management accounting, budgeting aids in financial preparation and encourages employee motivation through behavioral adjustments. Planning systems should function with programs that incentivize managers, involve workers, and maintain technical accuracy. The motivation of managers and workers is influenced by the allocation, monitoring, and management of resources.

"Identifying the Suitable Financial Barrier":

Select the appropriate combination of spending targets for motivation: When objectives are overly simplistic, employees may engage in unproductive tasks due to a lack of challenge. Aiming for high objectives can negatively impact employee engagement, motivation, and retention. Establishing clear and realistic goals can motivate managers and individuals to pursue continuous improvement. Keep in mind that different amounts of hardship impact individuals in various ways. Some managers excel in high-pressure situations, whereas others thrive when faced with minor challenges.

Five methods to inspire financial planners:

Even when money doesn't motivate people, real rewards and consequences can drive them to take action. Managers tend to use finances more responsibly when they perceive their goals as important. All employees, irrespective of their position, must be considered for performance evaluations and recognition. This promotes responsibility, equity, and collaboration for success. Effective reward systems typically consist of the following elements: Equity: A just reward should correspond to the effort put into corporate growth. Award requirements must be clear and straightforward. The system should motivate employees to help the company reach its long-term goals. When possible, use the same system for similar tasks. Regardless of feasibility, it is essential for everyone to understand the norms and expectations. Evaluations must prioritize measurable success indicators over personal opinions or dishonesty.

3.3 Participative Budgeting: A Bottom-Up Approach

The bottom-up approach involves middle and lower officials in the budget creation process. This approach enables managers to establish realistic and achievable spending goals based on their daily observations and activities.

Advantages of the Bottom-Up Approach: It encourages individuals to take responsibility and be accountable for their actions. Budgets are accurate and logical, reflecting the true operations of the business. Enhances motivation and engagement, resulting in improved outcomes.

Cons: It may lead to financial slack, where managers deliberately underreport income or overstate expenses to simplify goal attainment. Creating various budget plans requires time and careful organization. To reduce economic bias, it is essential to implement robust controls and an annual review process.

3.4 Process for Integrated Budgeting

Many businesses in practice utilize a plan that merges the strategic guidance of top-down spending with the practical insights from bottom-up feedback. Combining practical perspectives with long-term objectives ensures balance.

3.5 Rolling Budgets

Incorporating a new financial period, whether a month or a quarter, as the previous one concludes ensures that the budget remains current. A rolling 12-month budget consistently projects one year into the future.

Benefits: It maintains an updated and adaptable budget. Facilitates the regular reassessment of beliefs. Assists individuals in organizing their plans for the entire year.

4. Effective Budgets

Functional budgets are distinct plans tailored for various operational areas. Examples include:

Sales Budget: A projection of anticipated revenue from sales activities.

The production budget indicates the quantity of items to be produced.

Materials Budget: Estimates the quantity and cost of required items.

Estimates the required workforce and associated costs.

Overhead Budget: This budget forecasts fixed and variable operating expenses.

Creating a budget for sales and production:

Step 1: Develop a sales forecast. Estimate potential sales by analyzing market trends, previous performance, and marketing strategies.

Step 2: Allocate funds for production

Step 3: Allocate funds for materials: Determine your requirements: Numerical theory: Required materials = Number of units × Material required per unit. Next, determine the quantity to purchase by considering variations in supplies.

An effective spending method serves as a tool for financial planning, enhances communication, motivates individuals, and assesses performance. The choice of method—top-down, bottom-up, or a combination—depends on the company's goals, structure, and culture.

5. Budgeting for Cash Flow

5.1 Cash Flow Budgeting

A cash budget is a financial planning tool that projects the inflow and outflow of cash over a specific time frame. Companies must monitor their cash flow, address any cash shortages or surpluses, and ensure that daily operations align with strategic objectives.

Businesses can utilize a cash budget to: Prepare for potential cash flow issues or excesses and make informed choices regarding your business financing. Monitor cash flow timing according to scheduled tasks. Assess the difference between your expected cash and your actual cash requirements. Plan carefully for significant purchases, such as acquiring assets. Verify whether the company can fulfill its financial commitments, such as timely payments to employees and customers.

5.2 Components of a Cash Budget

Revenue Inflow: Receipts from cash sales or credit sales. Loans, interest income, or asset sales.

Cash expenditure: Purchases made on credit involve payments to sellers. Compensation and earnings. Certain expenses remain constant, such as rent and depreciation. Fluctuating production costs (such as materials and labor). Expenditure on capital goods and other infrequent expenses. Repaying a loan along with interest.

5.3 Considerations for Cash Flow Timing

Receiving cash from credit sales in a credit sale, cash flow remains unrecorded. Payment is recorded upon receipt. Consider the following points: Sales are received as a percentage each month, with 80% in the month following the sale and 20% in the month of the sale. Receivables are being established that will convert to cash during the budget period. Similarly, expenses from credit purchases are recorded at the time of payment, rather than at the time of the transaction. Key points: Payments made a month after the purchase of an item are considered late. Outstanding payables for the budget period are identified. Net Cash Flow is calculated by subtracting Total Cash Going Out from Total Cash Coming In. Determine the bank's closing balance: Opening Balance plus Net Cash Flow equals Closing Balance.

6. Master Budget

6.1 Putting Budgets Together

Company budgets consist of various smaller budgets merged into a single comprehensive budget that is the master budget. The master budget serves as a comprehensive planning instrument. The master budget directs an organization's financial decisions for the fiscal year. It is used in management accounting and financial planning. The master budget facilitates planning and control, enabling managers to align departmental activities, optimize resources, and assess performance against goals.

The Purpose of the Master Budget: Align regional initiatives to achieve the organization's objectives. Forecast the company's revenue, expenses, cash flow, and overall condition. Communicate the strategic goals with the organization. Help financial planning and support decision-making.

6.2 Components of Master Budget

The master budget consists of two primary components: Operating Budget and financial budget.

The operating budget outlines the organization's expected earnings and expenditures for its main activities. Typically, operating budget include: The sales budget, a key component of the master budget, predicts sales and revenue. This is the sole budget based on sales. Production Budget: This budget calculates the number of units required to meet sales and inventory needs. The Direct Materials Budget outlines the quantity of each raw material needed for acquisition and inventory for production purposes. The Direct Labor Budget calculates the hours and expenses required to achieve output goals. The Manufacturing Overhead Budget estimates all manufacturing costs, excluding materials and labor. It encompasses depreciation, utilities, and additional labor. The Selling and Administrative Expense Budget includes costs for rent, office supplies, wages, and advertising. Budgeted Revenue Statement: This outlines expected revenue and expenses to determine net profit or loss.

2. Financial budget: The financial budget emphasizes cash flow and financial resources. Include: The capital expenditure budget includes long-term

assets such as buildings, machinery, and technology. Cash Budget: This plan predicts cash flow, enabling the firm to meet its obligations and avoid cash flow problems. The study analyzes credit conditions, loan returns, and payment and receipt dates. The Budgeted Balance Sheet shows the assets, liabilities, and equity at the end of the budget period, reflecting information from previous budgets.

6.3 Steps for Master Budgeting

Set company goals. This process include; The market and historical trends, and forecasted sales to set the sales budget. Identify production budgets and related costs such as direct supplies, labor, and fees. Allocate funds for company operations, encompassing sales and management activities. Finalize the projected income statement. Develop a cash budget that outlines sales revenue alongside expenses for bills and investments. Create a Capital Expenditure Budget if needed. Finalize the Budgeted Balance Sheet. The master budget is reviewed and approved by top management to confirm its alignment with the plan and its feasibility.

7. What-If Analysis and Scenario Planning

7.1 Budgeting, "What-If" Analysis, and Scenario Planning

Effective budgeting requires prediction, assessment, and adaptation to uncertainty through strategic choices. Achieving success in these situations necessitates conducting what-if analyses and preparing scenarios. These tools for advice and budget management assist businesses in remaining adaptable and resilient.

What-If Analysis: Impact of Changes: Conducting a "what-if" analysis can reveal how key factors influence results before making a decision. What-if research examines the impact of sales volume, material costs, and work hours on total revenue, cost structure, and net profit. Unexpected circumstances have caused outcomes to differ from predictions. Budgets are often created in uncertain environments. This approach is effective for: Evaluating risks and uncertainties, recognizing essential elements, replicating backup strategies. A corporation can quickly assess the impact of a 10% sales decline on revenue and expense coverage through "what-if" research. Using spreadsheet tools such as Excel to automate recalculations can simplify this analysis.

Preparing for events: readiness for uncertainty: What-if analysis develops future scenarios based on assumptions regarding external factors such as the economy, market demand, and regulatory changes. Planning for the future involves evaluating multiple possibilities. This benefits businesses by: Consider the possibilities. Formulate responses that can accommodate disruptions. Scenario planning encompasses more than just numerical data. The context is analyzed in greater detail. This differs from what-if analysis, which emphasizes minor changes. A firm may create sales and cost budgets in response to an economic rebound, prolonged recession, or regulatory changes.

Steps to do scenario planning: Budgetary control cycle: Control is defined by management as the process through which an organization's leadership guarantees the direct and efficient achievement of its stated goals. This role involves setting goals, tracking progress, and adapting to new situations. Creating a mission statement—a brief description of the organization's purpose—is the initial step in this process. Next, we need to set long-term goals. The company aims to achieve specific, measurable, and time-bound objectives. Once the organization's purpose and objectives are established, leadership develops a strategy that acts as a guide for achieving those goals. Creating a budget transforms a plan into numerical form, bridging strategy and finances. The budget allows for monitoring the company's progress and pinpointing areas needing improvement. Management can identify discrepancies by comparing actual outcomes with expected statistics, determining their causes, and implementing solutions. If the organization strays from its planned path, the budget offers a clear framework to reevaluate goals, redistribute resources, and adjust operations.

1. Addressed feedback: Therefore, challenges should be assessed following the financial period. This enables the company to accomplish the following: Assess performance, determine the issue, prevent it from occurring again. Reflexive feedback control presents challenges. Results cannot be altered after the deadline. Utilize feedforward control. Managers can anticipate issues and adjust plans

through feedforward control. A cash budget enables managers to predict cash flow challenges by forecasting future cash flows, which helps them delay expenditures or seek alternative funding sources.

Techniques for Tracking Budgets: Financial management loops are ongoing yet efficient. Formulate a clear strategy and outline the primary objectives of the organization. Master budget: Utilize it to convert your objectives into financial resources. Allocate the funds to finalize projects. Monitor outcomes throughout the deadline period. Analyze the differences between actual and budgeted expenses. Adjust plans based on feedback or indicators of future success. This loop connects strategic goals to their outcomes.

8. Fixed and Flexible Budgets

A fixed budget is prepared according to anticipated activities. It assumes consistent work or output during the spending period. However, this is not always the case in situations where labor volume fluctuates significantly. Flexible budgeting is beneficial in this context. Implement a flexible budget that adjusts according to work volume to enhance performance management and evaluation.

Function of a flexible budget: The flexible budget modifies expected costs and revenues to align with production, allowing for more precise comparisons. This allows superiors to: Assess actual expenses against forecasts to inform decisions. Assess whether the issues stem from quantity or efficiency differences. It focuses on variance analysis. This aids managers in identifying and resolving issues by pinpointing the areas and reasons for performance discrepancies. For instance: The flexible budget will indicate if the increased labor cost was justified by enhanced output or if the workforce was not performing adequately. If output decreased while prices remained elevated, the variable budget will reveal inefficiencies or elevated fixed costs. A fixed budget relies on anticipated production, whereas in a variable budget, workload is taken into account. Flexible budgets enable managers to maintain control and adjust to actual changes in the environment. Understanding that changes in spending are frequently linked to activity levels and do not necessarily reflect poor performance which helps individuals in maintaining accountability.

9. Responsibility Accounting

Many individuals share certain aspects of budgeting and money management. Every manager should understand their role and make informed decisions within their domain to ensure the firm's success. Authority should be clearly defined, leaving no room for ambiguity.

Organizations often allocate tasks into responsibility areas according to the authority of supervisors. Cost Center—In manufacturing sector, the manager solely oversees expenditures. Profit Center: The manager oversees income and costs to enhance profitability. The Investment Center is responsible for determining revenue, expenses, and financial investments for various departments or enterprises. The budget must outline these areas clearly.

Despite having a clear structure, it can be challenging to assign responsibilities. For instance: Marketing managers can create agreements (crash production) that increase product prices. Who is to be held accountable? Which team should we focus on: the work team or the marketing team? When responsibilities are shared, accountability becomes challenging. Costs can be confusing due to the sharing of supplies and salaries across sectors. What is the solution? Clearly specify who holds authority in the planning and reporting tools. Some expenses are not related to production. For example conducting research and development. These costs are considerable, yet they are independent of production. Various assessments may be employed to assess them: i.e Cost associated with each sale or charges for each delivery.

9.1 Controllable vs. Uncontrollable Costs

Controllable costs refer to expenses that a manager can modify through their decisions, whereas uncontrollable costs are expenses that remain largely fixed and cannot be significantly changed by the manager. Controllable costs can be changed in the short run while uncontrollable costs can only be adjusted (may not be entirely) in the long run.

Examples of controllable costs are: Marketing expenses, direct materials and labor costs, training and development costs, maintenance expenses. Managers can oversee labor hours, manage supplies, and regulate advertisements.

Uncontrollable cost: Persistent expenses such as rent, taxes, and depreciation. Costs that seem "uncontrollable" can change over time. Upper management decides whether to renegotiate rent or relocate the firm. Therefore, it is important to identify who has the authority to alter this cost.

Chapter 14: Capital budgeting

1. Capital Budgeting

Capital budgeting: It is a process or method used by companies to evaluate capital projects. Capital budgeting helps in decision making of which project to choose and which project to leave, based on cost–benefit analysis. Capital project means a project whose lifespan is more than one year.

Capital budgeting is very important, and the finance manager should take good care in the process. Capital projects can include the purchase of costly machinery, the installation of new plant, etc. Buying long-term assets is called capital investment.

2. Difference Between Capital and Revenue Expenditure

Recognizing the distinction between capital expenditure and revenue expenditure is crucial, as they are reported differently in financial statements.

2.1 Capital Expenditure

Capital expenditure is the money used to acquire or enhance long-term assets that will provide benefits to the business over multiple accounting periods.

This encompasses:

machinery, land, buildings, or vehicles intended for business use rather than resale.

Enhancing or refining assets to boost their capacity, efficiency, or longevity.

Method of recording: Capital expenditure appears initially on the Statement of Financial Position as a non-current asset.

Over time, the cost is systematically allocated to the Income Statement via depreciation.

2.2 Revenue Expenditure

Revenue expenditure is the money allocated for the daily operations of a business. These costs support the business's capacity to earn income during the present period.

This encompasses:

Acquiring raw materials for resale or production purposes, Expenses like salaries, rent, utilities, and administrative costs, regular repairs and maintenance ensure assets function properly without substantial enhancements.

Method of recording: Revenue expenditure is recorded in the Income Statement during the period it occurs.

Determining if an expense is capital or revenue can be challenging. For instance: Upgrading an outdated heating system to a newer, more efficient model can be viewed as an enhancement. However, if the goal is merely to uphold the existing level of comfort, it could be viewed as revenue expenditure.

3. Investment Appraisal

Investment appraisal is a key part of the capital budgeting process. It involves assessing potential projects to determine whether they are worth investing in.

3.1 Steps in Investment Appraisal

1. **Idea generating**: Generating good ideas is the first and important step.

2. **Analyze individual proposals**: Gather maximum information about each idea. Evaluate and forecast the cash inflows and outflows and their timings and profitability.

3. **Plan capital budget**: Prioritize and organize all those projects that are within the firm's strategies.

4. **Assessing, monitoring, and post auditing**: Examining how the project is performing, related to forecasts.

3.2 Stages of the Capital Budgeting Process

Capital Expenditure Committee:

This committee typically oversees the capital budgeting process. Its main responsibilities are:

Coordinating overall capital expenditure policy.

Appraising and authorizing spending on specific projects.

Reviewing actual project costs and comparing them to budgeted amounts.

Many organizations set up special teams to investigate each proposal in detail and report findings to top management.

A project team may include:

Project engineer – for technical feasibility, Production engineer – to assess how the project affects operations, Management accountant – to evaluate financial impacts, Specialists as needed like Personnel officer for employee-related projects (e.g., staff facilities), Health and safety officer for compliance matters, Economist for broader economic evaluation.

4. Cash Flows in Investment Appraisal

Decisions on capital budgeting are based on cash flows and not only accounting concepts like net income. Moreover, intangible assets (patent rights, goodwill, etc.) are only considered when they cause a cash flow.

Timings of cash flows: Timings of cash flows are very important. The managers should take good care to forecast the timings of each cash flow. It is mainly because early inflows and delayed outflows are better than early outflows and delayed inflows due to the time value of money.

Cash flows are based on opportunity costs: Opportunity costs are those incomes that will be lost if we undertake a project.

Cash flows should be considered after deduction of taxes.

Financing cost is ignored in capital budgeting because it is already being reflected in the required rate of return (RRR or discount rate).

Cash flows are not considered as net income because net income means revenues minus all costs, but here, costs are not deducted from cash inflows.

4.1 Key Concepts

◈ **Sunk cost**: It is the cost which is already been incurred and cannot be recovered. Sometimes it is incurred before even starting a project, like consultation costs.

◈ **Incremental cash flows**: The cash flows if we have undertaken a project.

Incremental cash flows = cash flows after the decision about a project has been undertaken minus the cash flows before that decision.

◈ **Externalities**: The effect of investment on the cash flows of other projects of the same firm. When a new project decision has a negative impact on another ongoing project, it is called cannibalism. For example, a company introduces a new car and existing customers of the old model move towards the new car. In capital budgeting, these externalities must be considered.

◈ **Conventional cash flows**: It is the series of cash flows in which there is an initial cash outflow and then there are cash inflows.

◈ **Unconventional cash flows**: These cash flows do not follow the patterns of conventional cash flows. There might be an initial inflow and then an outflow. The direction of cash flows can change over time.

5. Time Value of Money

When evaluating capital investment of a project, one important concept is time value of money is used. Time value of money concept tells us that a dollar received today is worth more than a dollar received in the future.

As the cash flows of capital investments usually spread over a longer period, the timing of cash flows is very important. The managers should take good care to forecast the timings of each cash flow. It is mainly because early inflows and delayed outflows are better than early outflows and delayed inflows due to the time value of money.

5.1 Causes of Time Value

Three primary reasons exist:

1. **Potential for Earning Interest** - Funds received today can be promptly invested to generate interest or returns. Delayed funds result in missed investment chances.

2. **Inflation**: Prices rise over time as a result of inflation. This indicates that money in the future will have less purchasing power than it does today.

3. **Risk and Uncertainty**: Future payments may not always be guaranteed. Immediate cash is guaranteed, whereas future cash involves uncertainty.

5.2 Handling Time Value in Decisions

To account for the Time Value of Money, we use Discounted Cash Flow (DCF) techniques when appraising investments.

Discounted cash flow method: In this model, all the future expected cash flows are discounted to get the present value of a project. These cash flows can include all cash in and outflows. If the present value is positive or higher than any other available project, it means the project is viable.

6. Interest Concepts

6.1 Simple Interest

Simple interest is calculated only on the original amount (also called the principal) that is invested or borrowed. It does not include any interest that was earned in earlier periods.

Simple interest is used for a single investment for a short period.

Formula:

I = Prt, where:

- **I**: is the interest earned.
- **P**: is the principal amount.
- **r**: is the annual interest rate (as a decimal).
- **t**: is the time the money is invested or borrowed for, in years.

6.2 Compound Interest

Compound interest allows you to earn interest on both the original amount and any interest that has been earned before. It's used when investments or loans are held for longer periods and interest is added at regular intervals (e.g., yearly).

Formula:

A = P (1 + r/n)^(nt)

- **A** = Final Amount, which is the total you will possess after interest has been compounded over the specified duration.

- **P** = Principal: This refers to the original sum of money that is either invested or borrowed.

- **r** = Annual Interest Rate in percentage. This represents the percentage of the principal amount that is accrued as interest annually.

- **n** = Number of Times Interest is compounded per Year: This shows the frequency at which interest is calculated and added to the principal amount. For instance, when interest is compounded annually, n equals 1; when compounded semi-annually, n equals 2; and when compounded monthly, n equals 12.

- **t** = This represents the entire duration in years for which interest is compounded.

6.3 Nominal vs. Effective Interest Rate

Nominal Interest Rate:

The nominal interest rate refers to the declared interest rate for a specific time frame, like monthly or yearly. It does not independently consider compounding.

A bank's advertised annual interest rate of 9% is referred to as the nominal rate. When interest is compounded more frequently, such as monthly, the actual return exceeds 6% due to the effects of compounding.

Effective Interest Rate:

The effective interest rate is the true rate of return on investment (or true cost of capital) when compounding is taken into consideration. This is in contrast to the nominal rate. The effective interest rate is the actual percentage return on the investment. The nominal rate is the stated rate without the compounding effect.

Effective Rate Formula:

r = [(1 + i/n)^n] – 1

Where:

- **r** = Effective interest rate
- **i** = Nominal interest rate
- **n** = Number of Time periods. Common compounding periods include monthly (n=12), quarterly (n=4), or semi-annually (n=2).

It allows for an equitable assessment of financial products that compound at varying frequencies. Therefore, the actual rate of return helps in decision making and long-term planning.

7. Discounting and Present Value

Discounting contrasts with compounding. Compounding indicates the future value of a current investment. Discounting indicates the present value of a future sum of money (PV).

The Importance of Present Value in Investment Choices:

When a business assesses a potential project, it must grasp the present value of future cash inflows, such as profits or savings. Future cash flows hold less value than present cash flows, so we apply discounting to modify those future sums.

7.1 Fundamental Assumptions

- **Timing of Cash Flows**: To keep it simple we assume all cash inflows and outflows occur at the beginning or end of a year.

- **Investment Timing**: Most investment projects necessitate initial expenditure at the outset, referred to as T0. The project begins to generate returns after one year, referred to as T1.

7.2 Discount Rate and Discount Factor

To convert future amounts into present values, we apply a discount rate that considers: The cost of capital (the expense incurred by the business to obtain funds), the investment's risk, and the return expected by investors or the business.

This rate is often referred to as the required return, the discount rate, or the cost of capital.

We use a discount factor on future cash flows to determine their present value. Discount factors are usually calculated using formulas or financial tables.

8. Capital Investment Appraisal Methods

Investment Appraisal Methods:

There are many techniques used which help in decision-making of capital investment, which are as follows:

- Payback Period (discounted and non-discounted)
- Net Present Value (NPV)
- Internal Rate of Return (IRR).

8.1 Payback Period

It measures how much time it will take to return our original investment. We use the negative signs with outflows (and initial investment) and positive signs with inflows and take a sum until we reach zero.

Example

year	0	1	2	3
Cash flow	-500	100	400	300
Cumulative cash flow	-500	400	0	300

As we see in this example, the cumulative cash flows become zero in year 2, so the payback period is two years. In the payback period, the years 3 and following are ignored.

If we have a project with the following cash flows in which the payback is not a whole year, then we use the following formula;

year	0	1	2	3
Cash flow	-500	100	450	300
Cumulative cash flow	-500	400	50	350

Payback period=

$$\text{Full years until recovery year} + \frac{\text{un-recovered cost at the begining of recovered year}}{\text{Cash flow during recoverd year}}$$

$$\text{Payback period} = 1 + \frac{100}{450} = 1.223 \text{ years}$$

Decision: Choose the project with the shortest payback period, as it recoups the original investment the fastest.

8.2 Discounted Payback Period

This method is the same as the simple payback period, but here we use discounted cash flows.

We first discount each cash flow with the cost of capital (the discounting concept will be discussed later) and then add them up to get our payback period, just like the payback period.

A project with a shorter payback period is better. The payback and discounted payback period methods measure the liquidity. But the decisions cannot be made solely on these two measures. These methods ignore the salvage value (sale value of the asset after its useful life) and the cash flows beyond the payback period. The payback period method is easy to understand, simpler calculation of risk uses cash flow instead of accounting profit (which is a more tangible way).

8.3 Net Present Value (NPV)

Net present value: Net present value is the present value of all future cash flows minus the initial investment.

The discount rate is the cost of capital adjusted for the risk.

Formula:

NPV = Initial investment + [Cash $flow_1$ / $(1+r)^1$] + [Cash $flow_2$ / $(1+r)^2$] + ... + [Cash $flow_n$ / $(1+r)^n$]

[Initial investment is used with a negative sign]

or

NPV = Σ [CF_t / $(1+r)^t$] for t=0 to n

[Remember, initial investment is used with a negative sign and is included here]

Where:

- **t** is the time of the project or the point of time of each cash flow
- **CF** is the cash flow (after tax)
- **r** is the required rate of return or cost of capital.

Decision for independent projects:

- Projects with **NPV > 0** can be accepted because this project will increase the shareholders' wealth.
- Projects with **NPV < 0** can be rejected because this project will decrease the shareholders' wealth.

◈ Projects with **NPV = 0** can be accepted or rejected because this project will not have any impact on shareholders' wealth.

8.4 Internal Rate of Return (IRR)

IRR is the discount rate that makes the net present value of all the cash flows equal to zero.

Formula:

NPV = [Cash $flow_1$ / $(1+IRR)^1$] + [Cash $flow_2$ / $(1+IRR)^2$] + ... + [Cash $flow_n$ / $(1+IRR)^n$] = 0

or

NPV = Σ [CF_t / $(1+IRR)^t$] = 0 for t=0 to n

Solve for **IRR.**

Decision for independent projects:

◈ Projects with **IRR > r** can be accepted because this project will increase the shareholders' wealth.

◈ Projects with **IRR < r** can be rejected because this project will decrease the shareholders' wealth.

◈ Projects with **IRR = r** can be accepted or rejected because this project will not have any impact on shareholders' wealth. It will generate a return just equal to the cost of capital (cost of borrowing).

r is the cost of capital.

Limitations of NPV and IRR: These methods cannot be used when future cash flows are uncertain. These measures are also very sensitive to inflows and outflows of cash (timings and amounts).

9. Annuities and Perpetuities

9.1 Annuities

Annuity Definition:

An annuity is a series of equal payments (cash inflows or outflows) made at regular intervals over a period of time — for example, $1000 every year for 3 years.

NPV of Annuities:

It is the present value of future cash flows minus the initial investment.

NPV = Initial investment + [Cash $flow_1$ / $(1+r)^1$] + [Cash $flow_2$ / $(1+r)^2$] + ... + [Cash $flow_n$ / $(1+r)^n$]

NPV = PV - Initial Investment

As all the future cash flows are same, the formula can be reduced to:

$PV = \text{Cash flow} \times [1 - (1 + r)^{-n}] / r$

- **PV** is the present value of the annuity.
- **Cash flow** is the periodic payment amount.
- **r** is the discount rate per period (interest rate).
- **n** is the number of periods.

On the other hand, the PV of an annuity can be calculated from a financial table called the annuity factor.

IRR of Annuities:

The internal rate of return (IRR) for an annuity is the discount rate that makes the net present value (NPV) of its cash flows equal to zero.

$NPV = \Sigma [CF_t / (1+r)^t] = 0$ for t=0 to n

Here **r** is IRR and can be solved with hit and trial method or using financial table.

9.2 Perpetuities

A perpetuity refers to an endless sequence of equal annual cash flows, such as a pension or a guaranteed annuity that continues indefinitely.

NPV of a Perpetuity:

NPV = (Fixed cash flow / r) – I

- **r** is interest rate.
- **I** is initial investment.

IRR of a Perpetuity:

The internal rate of return (IRR) for Perpetuity is the discount rate that makes the net present value (NPV) of its cash flows equal to zero.

IRR = Annual Cash Flow / Investment Cost

Chapter 15: Standard costing

1. The Purposes of Standard Costing

1.1 Standard Costing

A standard cost is the predetermined or estimated cost of production of a product or a unit of service. It represents what the cost should be under efficient operating conditions. Because of this, standard costs are often referred to as "target costs". These standard costs are essential in planning, Control, and Motivation.

1.2 Types of Cost Standards

There are four main types of cost standards.

- Basic standards.
- Ideal standards.
- Attainable standards.
- Current standards.

Basic Standards are long-term estimates of costs that don't change over time. It's major goal to keep an eye on long-term trends, like changes in prices for materials, wages, and how well workers do their jobs.

In modern practice, basic standards are rarely used, even though they can help you see long-term trends or the results of different approaches. This is because they quickly become out-of-date and useless in changing business settings, making them the least useful type of standard cost for making decisions right now.

Ideal standards are theoretical cost targets that assume perfect operating conditions, which seldom occur in reality. These standards presume a perfect and continuous production process. They act as a goal to strive for; although seldom reached, they assist in recognizing the highest possible efficiency.

Ideal standards can inspire ambition, but they may also harm employee motivation if perceived as unrealistic.

Attainable standards are realistic goals for costs or performance, assuming efficient, though not flawless, operating conditions. They indicate the anticipated performance level when operations function effectively, though not perfectly.

These standards account for typical inefficiencies, including expected material losses, employee fatigue and rest periods, minor machine breakdowns and maintenance delays, and routine inefficiencies encountered in daily operations. They expect capable performance, not flawless execution.

Current standards reflect the existing efficiency and performance levels in an organization.

They illustrate the current methods in use, including:

The usual amount of material waste

Equipment failures

Work efficiency

Existing delays or inefficiencies in the system

They reflect the current state of operations without anticipating any enhancement or alteration. For instance, if 3% of materials are wasted in production, the current standard reflects this 3% wastage.

These are commonly utilized when a company aims to assess its performance in relation to the standard.

2. Standard Costs per Unit

To develop a standard cost card for a product, decompose all anticipated (standard) costs into their components. Standard cost may fall under either marginal costing or absorption costing, as previously discussed.

Prime cost

This includes direct labor and direct materials. Multiply the standard time for each department by the hourly rate to get the labor cost. Add in the cost of materials (if provided) to get the total prime cost.

Marginal cost

This includes the prime cost plus variable production overheads. Variable overheads are the running costs that change with how many units you produce (e.g., electricity, indirect labor). You calculate these overheads based on the number of labor hours used — more hours mean more cost.

So, marginal cost = prime cost + all variable overheads.

Total absorption cost

This includes marginal cost + fixed production overheads. Fixed overheads don't change with production level (e.g., rent, equipment). These costs are "absorbed" by each unit by dividing the total fixed cost by the number of units produced. This tells you what each unit "owes" in terms of fixed cost.

Total standard cost

- This is the complete cost per unit, including:
- Direct labor
- Direct materials
- Variable production overheads
- Fixed production overheads
- Selling and admin costs (if included)

3. Variance Analysis

Standard costing is closely linked to variance analysis.

Standard costs represent established benchmarks for expected expenses under typical circumstances. When actual results are available, variances represent the differences between our expectations (standard) and the actual outcomes.

Flexible Budget Compared to Actual Outcomes

- A flexed budget modifies the initial budget according to the actual activity level (for instance, if production was 900 units instead of 1,000).
- This ensures a more equitable comparison with actual results.

Variance analysis begins with a comparison of the flexed budget to actual results.

Variance Analysis in Detail: Exploring Further

After identifying a difference, we seek to understand the reasons behind it. Detailed variances play a crucial role here. Let us analyze this step by step:

The variances that will be looked at are:

- Sales variances
- Raw material variances
- Labor variances
- Variable overhead variances

• Fixed overhead variances

3.1 Sales Variances

Sales variance describes discrepancies between actual and predicted sales, and whether volume or pricing is the source.

◈ **1. Sales Volume Variance**: Shows whether we sold more or less units than projected.

• More units sold often increase revenue and profit (assuming reasonable price reduction).

• A decrease in sales leads to lost revenue and profit.

How we value:

It depends on the costing approach employed.

In marginal costing, usage contribution per unit measures how much each sale covers fixed expenses and generates profit.

Absorption costing: utilizes profit per unit (after covering variable and fixed manufacturing expenses).

Interpretation:

• Higher sales than projected result in positive variance (greater profit).

• Lower real sales result in negative variance (loss of revenue).

◈ **2. Sales Price Variance**: It shows if we sold for more or less than planned.

Prices impact revenue and profit, even if we sell the proper number of units.

Selling at a discount may lower earnings, whereas selling at a premium improves it.

The calculation involves comparing the actual selling price to the budgeted price, multiplied by the number of units sold.

Interpretation:

• If the real price exceeds the projected price, we make more per transaction.

• Adverse variance (less revenue per sale) if actual price < anticipated price.

Possible causes of sales variances

Causes of sales variances include the following:

• unplanned price increases (sales price variance)

• unplanned price reduction, to attract additional business (sales price variance)

• unexpected fall in demand due to recession (sales volume variance)

• additional demand attracted by reduced price (sales volume variance)

• failure to satisfy demand due to production difficulties (sales volume variance).

3.2 Material Cost Variances

A business determines the quantity of materials required for production and estimates their costs. In practice, events seldom unfold as intended. Variances arise from the differences between planned and actual outcomes.

Two primary factors may cause material costs to deviate from the budget:

The cost per unit of material varied.

The amount of material utilized varied.

Material cost variance is divided into:

1. Variance in Material Costs

Did we spend more or less per unit of material than anticipated?

• This indicates if the cost per unit of raw material exceeded or fell below the budgeted amount.

• It centers exclusively on the purchasing choice, rather than the quantity utilized.

Possible causes include: • Variations in supplier pricing.

• Purchasing in varying amounts (which could influence discounts).

• Changes in prices across the market.

• Employing varied materials (distinct quality or grade).

For instance, if you planned to purchase high-quality steel but opted for a less expensive alternative, you might notice a positive price variance; however, this choice could lead to negative outcomes, such as increased waste.

2. Materials Usage Variance

Did we utilize more or less material than necessary for the quantity produced?

• This indicates if the actual material used was more or less than anticipated for the given output level.

• Emphasizes usage efficiency rather than cost.

Possible causes include: • Inadequate handling or storage leading to spoilage.

• Defective machines resulting in increased waste.

• Skilled labor versus unskilled labor (some may utilize materials with greater care).

• Adjustments in design that necessitate varying amounts of material.

For instance, if employees lack experience or are inattentive, they may use more fabric than anticipated during garment cutting, leading to a negative usage variance.

Overall Variance in Materials

This represents the difference between your expected material cost for the achieved output and the actual cost incurred.

Consider it as the total of:

• Price variance (Did we incur a higher or lower cost per unit?)

• Usage variance (Did our usage exceed or fall short of expectations?)

3.3 Labor Cost Variances

Labor cost variances occur when there is a discrepancy between the expected labor costs, as outlined in the budget, and the actual labor expenses incurred. This difference can be attributed to two primary factors: labor rate variance and labor efficiency variance.

1. Labor Rate Variance

Did we pay a wage rate that was higher or lower than our plan? This variance indicates whether the hourly wage paid to workers differed from expectations.

Possible causes:

• Unexpected salary hikes resulting from market dynamics or legislative updates (e.g., revised minimum wage).

• Compensating for overtime, bonuses, or allowances that are outside the budget.

• Employing a workforce with greater skills than anticipated, resulting in higher costs.

• Labor unions are seeking a higher rate following the establishment of the budget.

When is this favorable?

• If the company pays less per hour than planned, without compromising quality or efficiency.

2. Labor Efficiency Variance

Did workers spend more or fewer hours than anticipated to complete the output?

This variance examines the efficiency of the workers. The focus is on the length of time invested, rather than the hourly wage.

Potential factors include:

• Improved or diminished supervision of personnel.

• Employment of workers with varying levels of experience (impacting efficiency).

• The adoption of new technology or improved tools accelerates work efficiency.

• Fatigue, low motivation, or insufficient training is hindering progress.

• Replacing a highly skilled worker with a lower-skilled one.

When is this favorable?

• When employees achieve the same level of productivity in a shorter time than anticipated.

Labor Total Variance

This represents the overall discrepancy between the actual labor costs and the expected costs based on the level of production achieved (the "flexed budget").

It's made up of:

• Rate variance: Was the hourly rate increased or decreased?

• Efficiency variance: Were the hours worked greater or less?

3.4 Variable Overhead Variances

Variable overheads are indirect costs that fluctuate with activity levels, similar to direct materials and labor. Examples are: • Indirect materials Maintenance

• Indirect labor.

Producing more units or working additional hours will likely lead to an increase in variable overhead costs. If not, we must explore the reasons, and this is where variance analysis is useful.

Elements of Variable Overhead Variance

1. Spending Difference

Did the actual cost per hour of variable overhead exceed or fall short of expectations?

This evaluates if our expenditure per unit of activity, typically per labor hour, was above or below the budgeted amount.

Potential causes include: • Higher power rates than anticipated • Unscheduled maintenance • Increased costs of indirect materials (such as lubricants and cleaning supplies) • Inaccurate or outdated budgeting. An actual cost per hour that exceeds expectations indicates an unfavorable variance. If it is less, it is favorable.

2. Efficiency Variance

Did the hours worked align with the expected output? This evaluates the hours utilized versus the hours that should have been used for the actual production level. It is based on the premise that overhead costs are allocated according to labor hours.

Possible causes:

• Improved or diminished staff performance • Effects of the learning curve (progress over time) • Downtime due to breakdowns or inadequate planning • Changes in staff motivation, training, or supervision

A favorable efficiency variance occurs when fewer hours are used than anticipated for the same output.

3.5 Fixed Overhead Variances

Fixed overheads, such as rent and insurance, remain constant regardless of activity levels in the short term. These costs are based on time rather than volume. When we include them in product costs through absorption costing, variances may still occur because of discrepancies between budgeted, incurred, and absorbed amounts.

In marginal costing, only one variance is pertinent: **Variance in Fixed Overhead Expenditure**

This indicates if our spending exceeded or fell short of the budget.

Formula: Actual Fixed Overheads minus Budgeted Fixed Overheads

- When actual exceeds budgeted, it results in an adverse variance.
- If actual is less than budgeted, it results in a favorable variance.

What is the reason for selecting this variance?

Under marginal costing, fixed overheads are not allocated per unit; instead, they are considered a period expense. No impact on volume is observed.

In Absorption Costing, Variances increase due to the allocation of fixed overheads to units based on a predetermined rate, known as the Overhead Absorption Rate (OAR).

1. Fixed Overhead Expenditure Variance (Identical to marginal costing)

- Analyzes the differences between actual and budgeted fixed overhead expenditures

2. Fixed Overhead Volume Variance

This illustrates the effects of producing more or fewer units than anticipated.

Formula:

Actual output overheads absorbed - budgeted overheads

Fixed overheads remain constant regardless of volume; however, absorption costing distributes them according to volume levels. Thus, insufficient or excessive production results in inadequate or excessive absorption.

Breakdown of Volume Variance (applicable only if OAR is hour-based):

a. Capacity Variance

Did workers log more or fewer hours than anticipated?

- Comparison of actual hours to budgeted hours • Assessment of idle time, sick leave, overtime, and more.

b. Efficiency Variance

Was the time taken per unit for production more or less than anticipated?

- Standard hours for actual output compared to actual hours • Assesses productivity or inefficiency

Efficiency and capacity variances together account for the differences between actual production volume and the budgeted amount.

Total Variance of Fixed Overhead

The total consists of: • Expenditure variance • Volume variance

It indicates the overall difference between actual and planned fixed overhead absorption.

Common Causes of Variances

Expenditure Variance

• Unforeseen rent hikes • Additional depreciation expenses • Variations in utility or insurance costs

• Errors in budgeting (e.g., neglecting seasonal impacts)

Variance in volume

• Variations in demand • Equipment failures or labor disputes • Improvements in efficiency (e.g., automation) • Employee absenteeism, overtime, or downtime • Adjustments in inventory policies (increasing production to stock or reducing output to sell from inventory)

4. Relationships Among Variances

Variances are interconnected when the cause of one variance influences another, whether in a positive or negative manner. Variances should not be interpreted in isolation. A positive variance in one area may lead to or result from a negative variance in another.

For example

1. Inexpensive Material Acquisition → Consequential Impact

• Materials Price Variance: Favorable (less expensive material)

• Materials Usage Variance: Adverse (lower cost leads to reduced quality and increased waste)

• Fixed Overhead Volume Variance: Unfavorable (production decreases due to material problems)

• Sales Volume Variance: Adverse (failure to meet customer demand resulting in lost sales)

A positive material price variance might negatively impact the business as a whole. The buying choice resulted in several concealed expenses.

2. New Costly Equipment

• Fixed Overhead Expenditure Variance: Unfavorable (increased depreciation cost)

• Labor Efficiency Variance: Favorable (the machine operates more quickly, resulting in fewer labor hours per unit)

• Fixed Overhead Volume Variance: Favorable (increased production leads to greater overhead absorption)

Interpretation: While the machine raised fixed costs, the improvements in efficiency could warrant the investment. Management should not be penalized for an unfavorable variance resulting from a strategic investment.

3. Labor Productivity Enhancement

• Labor Efficiency Variance: Positive (increased speed of work)

• Materials Usage Variance: Negative (hasty or negligent handling leads to increased waste)

Interpretation: Striving for labor efficiency may negatively impact material quality. Excessive rewards in one area may lead to issues in another.

Management Implications

Do not indiscriminately reward short-term gains.

When buyers or production managers focus solely on cost savings or efficiency, they might compromise quality, resulting in losses later on.

b) Examine Net Impact

To evaluate performance, merge related variances to grasp the underlying cause and overall impact.

For instance, when a buyer opts for less expensive materials, it is useful to combine price and usage variances to evaluate the overall material variance and determine the wisdom of that choice.

Systemic thinking is essential.

Cost control involves optimizing the whole system rather than just achieving individual targets.

5. Operating Statements

Operating statements—a key managerial accounting tool for reconciling budgeted profit with actual profit through the use of variances.

Operating Statement Logic

You're reconciling from Budgeted Profit to Actual Profit. Here's how:

Add/Subtract the Variances:

- Add: Any Favorable (F) variance (increases profit)
- Subtract: Any Adverse (A) variance (reduces profit)

Note:

- Variances must be calculated first based on production and budget info.
- Then, plug them into the statement.
- Net out favorable and adverse totals to see the overall impact on profit.
- The operating statement gives a detailed explanation of how and why actual profit differs from budgeted profit.
- It's a key managerial tool for performance evaluation and control.
- Use this logic every time you're given a set of variances and asked to prepare the reconciliation.

Working Backwards in Variance Analysis

In variance analysis, particularly within exam contexts, learners may be required to work backwards from variances to determine unknown figures. Instead of performing straightforward variance calculations, this method challenges understanding by requiring the reconstruction of:

- Actual figures using known variances and standard data
- Standard figures using known variances and actual results

This approach reinforces conceptual understanding and the interrelationships among various cost elements.

Fixed Overhead Variances

When analyzing fixed overhead variances, standard costing often provides a per-unit allocation of fixed costs. If variances are known, one can derive either:

- The actual fixed overheads incurred, using the expenditure variance
- The actual production volume, using the volume variance

These calculations help to evaluate performance by comparing actual outcomes with budgeted expectations.

Contribution Analysis

Under marginal costing, variances such as sales price, variable costs, and sales volume contribute to changes in the actual contribution. Given standard contribution figures, these variances can be used to deduce the actual contribution achieved in the period.

Working Backwards from Variances

A series of standard costing variances, such as price and efficiency variances, can be used to determine:

1. Actual output levels based on efficiency or usage variances

2. Actual input prices from price variance formulas

3. Material usage variances, reflecting efficiency in resource use

4. Standard labor rates, which assist in interpreting wage-related variances

5. Labor rate variances, indicating whether actual wages differed from expectations

6. Fixed overhead expenditure variance, reflecting differences in spending versus the budget

7. Absorption rates, showing how fixed overheads are allocated

8. Capacity and efficiency variances, which explain deviations in labour or machine usage

9. Volume variance, summarizing the total production variance due to output differences

These reverse calculations require a strong command of standard costing formulas and the logic underlying each variance type.

By practicing both direct and reverse variance calculations, students develop a more holistic grasp of performance measurement and cost control in managerial accounting.

6. Reporting of Variances in Management Accounting

1. Responsibility Accounting

Variance reports must adhere to the principle of responsibility accounting. Reports must only reflect variances that a manager can influence. Additional data may be provided as "for information only" to assist the manager in grasping the wider business context.

2. Deciding Whether to Investigate a Variance

Not every variance requires investigation. Minor, intangible, or unmanageable differences may not warrant the expense and effort of examination. Prior to examining a variance, management must assess:

- Can the variance be influenced by the manager?
- Will the benefit of corrective action exceed the cost?
- Is it likely that the corrective action will be effective?
- Is the variance large or significant?
- Is the variance worsening over time?

3. Cost vs. Benefit

Investigating and correcting variances involves expenses. A variance should be considered only if the anticipated benefit, adjusted for the likelihood of success, surpasses the cost of the corrective measure. This includes analyzing expected value, particularly in situations with uncertain outcomes.

4. Management by Exception

This principle indicates that only significant variances should be emphasized and communicated to management. It minimizes information overload by directing focus on exceptions instead of routine, minor discrepancies.

Designing Effective Control Reports

To ensure variance and control reports are useful, they should meet the following criteria:

Criterion	Explanation
Relevance	Include only information related to the manager's decisions and responsibilities.
Responsibility-linked	Reports should reflect areas the manager can control.
Timeliness	Reports must be delivered before decisions are made, not afterward.
Reliability	Information should be trustworthy, even if not perfectly precise.
Effective communication	Use clear language, avoid jargon, and consider graphs/charts for clarity.
Cost-effectiveness	The benefits of the report should outweigh the cost of producing it.

Chapter 16: Performance measurement techniques

1. Performance Measurement

Performance measurement shows the effectiveness of the firm and its employees by comparing actual results to set budgets or objectives. Performance can be assessed through long-term objectives, such as reducing expenses, or short-term goals, like enhancing customer satisfaction.

2. Different Types of Companies Have Different Goals

The primary objective of a for-profit business is to maximize profits for its shareholders. This is typically accomplished by:

Enhancing profits through increased sales and reduced expenses.

Enhancing market share by outperforming competitors in the industry. Key performance indicators (KPIs) consist of gross profit margin, net profit margin, return on equity (ROE), return on assets.

A primary objective of a government organization could be to deliver high-quality services efficiently and promptly. The key idea is to maximize the value of your money by ensuring effective use of tax funds. Minimize costs while maintaining service quality.

All organizations generally share a common structure: they establish long-term goals alongside tactical and operational targets.

3. Goals for the Future

This outlines the organization's long-term direction. Long-term objectives typically span three to five years or even longer.

Operations and tactics are essential components of long-term objectives.

Tactical objectives are short-term goals that demonstrate how the plan will be executed.

Operational objectives are the daily tasks that facilitate smooth operations and help achieve tactical goals.

4. The Mission Statement

Utilizing the Mission Statement to Direct Performance Evaluation

A mission statement defines the long-term goals of an organization. It acts as both a strategic base and a guide for creating performance measures. The components of the mission statement:

1. **Purpose**: This outlines the main objectives of the organization. Performance measures must evaluate if the organization is meeting its main goals, which include maintaining high customer satisfaction and providing innovative, valuable products or services.

2. **Strategy**: A strategy describes the organization's approach to fulfilling its objectives. Performance indicators may include if the organization is providing the intended products or services and if these offerings align with the envisioned strategy.

3. **Policies and Culture**: This pertains to internal conduct and criteria. Performance can be assessed by examining if employees align with organizational expectations and the quality and consistency of customer service.

4. **Values Core values**: Represent the ethical standards and internal culture of the organization. Possible measures include how well the organization's principles are practiced, levels of staff morale and satisfaction, and employee retention rates, such as staff turnover as an indicator of workplace culture.

5. Planning

To achieve their objectives, organizations must plan by defining goals and developing strategies. A solid foundation for future planning is built on understanding the past. This allows for informed and achievable decisions. For instance, a sales manager relies on past sales data to accurately forecast future performance. Planning can be approached strategically, focusing on long-term vision, or tactically, addressing mediate needs.

1. **Strategic (Corporate) Planning**

Strategic planning covers three to five years or more of the organization's long-term orientation. It entails establishing ambitious growth, competitiveness, innovation, and sustainability goals.

This level measures success using broad financial and strategic factors like:

- Overall profitability
- Return on investment (ROI)
- Market share growth
- Long-term value creation for stakeholders

2. **Tactical Planning**

Tactical planning converts the strategic vision into medium-term goals for particular departments, business units, or functions. It guarantees that every section of the organization aligns with the overall strategy by establishing clear goals.

Performance at this level is typically assessed by:

- Comparing actual departmental costs and revenues to budgeted figures
- Evaluating the efficiency of resource allocation
- Monitoring the achievement of functional targets.

3. **Operational Planning**

Operational planning emphasizes the daily activities that align with tactical and strategic objectives. This involves establishing clear tasks, timelines, and performance standards for staff.

Performance measures at the operational level are more detailed and immediate, such as:

- Meeting daily or weekly production targets
- Achieving sales or customer service goals
- Minimizing errors, defects, or waste

Effective performance measures need to be thoughtfully chosen at every level to guarantee that operational and tactical efforts align with overarching strategic goals. This alignment aids in maintaining focus, boosting accountability, and enhancing overall organizational performance.

6. Critical Success Factors (CSFs) and Their Role in Organizational Success

Critical Success Factors (CSFs) are the essential activities that must be performed well for an organization to fulfill its mission, objectives, and strategic goals. They act as a key reference for evaluating organizational success and coordinating efforts throughout the business.

Focusing on critical success factors allows teams to prioritize tasks that directly influence the organization's success, enhancing coordination and overall performance.

Critical Success Factors connect strategic goals with daily operations, ensuring that routine tasks align with larger objectives.

Measuring CSFs with Key Performance Indicators (KPIs)

KPIs are quantifiable metrics that monitor success in relation to CSFs and can be:

- Financial, such as profit margins, return on investment, or cost efficiency

• Non-financial, such as customer satisfaction, staff turnover, or product quality

By developing appropriate KPIs, businesses can track progress, identify gaps, and make informed decisions to stay on course toward achieving their strategic objectives.

7. Financial Performance Measures

Financial performance measures are key tools used to monitor the financial health of a business. They focus on the inflows (revenues) and outflows (costs) associated with business activities and help assess how effectively financial resources are being managed. These measures are primarily derived from the Income Statement (Profit and Loss Account) and the Statement of Financial Position (Balance Sheet). An organization can use these financial performance indicators for CFS, overall performance, or any department, but they should be applied consistently to ensure reliable comparison.

Measuring Profitability

A company's main goal is to increase profitability. Profitability ratios help track the success of this goal. Following some major profitability ratios.

Return on capital employed = (EBIT/capital employed) *100

Operating profit (EBIT) = earnings before interest and taxes

Capital employed = Total assets – current liabilities.

In this ratio, we measure the return on each dollar of capital invested. A very low ratio from industry norms should alarm the analyst.

Gross profit margin = gross profit/revenues.

Gross profit margin indicates the amount of sales left over after accounting for the cost of goods sold. It is a comparison of Gross profit with sales. A higher gross profit margin indicates a company's ability to charge a higher price for a product that it can manufacture for a lower cost and vice versa. Gross profit margin also helps the management in cost control.

Profit for the period margin

This is the profit (revenue less all expenses) as a percentage of revenue.

Profit from operations

Also known as operating profit margin or EBIT margin.

EBIT margin = (EBIT/sales revenue) *100

A higher ratio is desirable.

Asset turnover

Asset turnover (Sales / Average Total Assets) *100

It tells us how efficiently the company is generating revenue from its assets.

Interpretation: A higher figure indicates that the company is effectively or efficiently utilizing its assets to generate revenue. A lower figure would indicate inefficiencies or that the firm is in a very capital-intensive business.

Measuring Liquidity

The liquidity of a company is measured through liquidity ratios. Liquidity ratios measure a company's ability to meet its short-term obligations.

We have 3 major liquidity ratios: the current ratio, the quick ratio, and the cash ratio.

Current ratio = Current assets /current liabilities.

Quick ratio = Liquid assets / current liabilities. Where, Liquid assets = cash+ marketable sec. + receivables

Cash ratio = (cash + marketable securities) / current liabilities.

Interpretations

A current ratio of one indicates that the company's current assets are equal to the dollar value of its current liabilities. So, the short-term obligations are just covered. A ratio less than one means that the company is relying on operating profit to meet short-term obligations because current assets are not enough.

Quick ratio is a more realistic approach to our ability to convert certain current assets into cash. Pre-payments, for example, might be included in the current assets of a company but would be very difficult to turn into cash. The same is the case with inventory. So, we exclude these two from the quick ratio to have more meaningful results.

With the cash ratio, we are more conservative about the asset`s ability to meet short-term obligations. We only include the most liquid assets. We only include cash and marketable securities that the company has right now to pay its short-term obligations.

Other Liquidity Ratios

Days inventory in hand = 365/ inventory turnover

Or

Days inventory in hand = (inventory/cost of sales) * 365

It tells us how many days a firm takes to process its inventory. Again, these (Inventory turnover and Days inventory in hand) should be close to industry norms. A higher inventory turnover ratio means fewer days of inventory on hand. It might indicate a highly effective inventory management, or the company is not holding enough stock and is potentially on the verge of shortages and falling sales revenue. Analysts must see revenue growth to assess the explanation. A higher (or same as industry) growth with high turnover means effective inventory management and vice versa. A lower inventory turnover means a higher number of days inventory on hand, which may indicate that too much capital is tied up and there is a high processing time. It means inventory could be getting obsolete. The cost of goods sold may not be according to current circumstances.

Receivables collection period (in days)

Also known as the number of days' sales outstanding. This represents the typical duration for a company to collect payments on its receivables.

Receivables collection period (in days) = (Receivables/Revenue) *100

or

Number of days sales outstanding = 365/ receivable turnover

This ratio should be close to industry norms. If it is too high, it means the firm is not collecting cash easily (inefficiency). A ratio that is too low shows a very strict credit policy, which might be affecting sales, or the firm is collecting cash very efficiently.

Payables period

Payable turnover ratio = purchases/ average payables. It means how many times the company pays its payables completely (theoretically).

Number of days of payables = 365/ payable turnover ratio

This is the average period it takes for a company to pay for its purchases.

These two should be close to industry norms. If the company has a relatively higher payables turnover (which would mean a relatively lower number of days payables are outstanding), the company might not be effectively taking advantage of credit facilities made available to them, or they might be taking advantage of early payment discounts. We must look at the liquidity ratios to get a proper understanding. If a company has better liquidity ratios but higher days payable (lower payable turnover), it means they are taking advantage of available credit facilities. If the liquidity position is bad, with lower payable turnover, they might have trouble with cash generation.

Measuring Risk

In addition to profitability and liquidity, it is important to manage the risks attached to the company. The following are major ratios that can be used to calculate risks.

Financial gearing or debt-to-equity ratio

Debt to equity = (Total debt / total equity) * 100

And

Total equity = debt + equity

This ratio compares the debt side of the capital structure to the equity side. It shows how much debt a company is using to finance its assets in comparison to equity. A higher figure would indicate a less solvent company.

Interest coverage ratio= EBI/interest payment

EBI is earnings before interest. It measures how many times a company's earnings before interest cover its interest obligations.

A higher number is desirable here because it indicates that the earnings are quite larger than the interest payment. A lower value of this ratio means they have difficulty paying interest.

Dividend payment ratio = CFO /dividends paid. It measures the company's ability to pay dividends out of operating cash.

CFO is the cash flow from operations. Sometimes, net profit is also used instead of CFO.

8. Problems with Using Only Financial Performance Indicators

Ratio analysis benefits: Ratio analysis is used for

- Internal and external comparison.
- To project future earnings and cash flow.
- To evaluate a company's financial flexibility (ability to obtain cash) to meet its obligations and to grow even in the case of difficult financial circumstances.
- To measure the performance of a company's management.
- To look at how the company or the industry is changing over time.

• To compare the company with its peer companies or relevant industry benchmarks.

Limitations of ratios: 1. They are not useful in isolation. They are only useful when they are combined with an overall understanding of the company, the company's industry, and the macroeconomic environment.

1. Ratio analysis is also not useful for big companies that have multiple sources of income from entirely different industries. Because of the complexity of the big company, relevant benchmarks won't be available.

2. Analysis based on a small subset of ratios might not be reliable because one set of financial ratios might indicate a certain level of performance, but another set of ratios on the same company might indicate that that performance level is not sustainable.

3. Ratios calculated from financial reports built on differing accounting standards may not be immediately comparable. (Accounting treatments differ in inventory evaluation, appreciation, and off-balance sheet items).

9. Non-Financial Performance Indicators (NFPIs)

While the profit is the main objective of any commercial organization, CSFs, KPIs, and non-financial performance indicators (NFPIs) should also be considered to measure the performance of the company. Non-financial performance indicators include indicators like customer satisfaction, quality, etc. These NFPIs differ from business to business, industry to industry; however, these can be grouped into two main types;

- Productivity indicators
- Quality indicators

Productivity Indicators: These indicators measure the labor efficiency or resource utilization efficiency of the organization.

Production-volume ratio

The production/volume ratio compares how much was made compared to the budget or plan.

Production-volume ratio = (Actual output measured in standard hours/ Budgeted production hours) *100

A Production-volume ratio less than 100 means production is less than planned and vice versa.

Efficiency ratio

It measures the output in comparison to the inputs

Efficiency ratio = (Actual output measured in standard hours/ Actual production hours worked)*100

Capacity ratio

The capacity ratio tells you how many hours of work have been possible during a certain time period.

Capacity ratio = (Actual production hours worked/Budgeted production hours) *100

Quality

Monitoring Quality through Non-Financial Performance Indicators (NFPIs)

Poor quality goods and services may cost consumers their reputation and competitiveness. Businesses must establish quality and monitor performance using internal and external indicators to maintain and enhance standards.

Operations, customer happiness, and staff performance depend on Non-Financial Performance Indicators (NFPIs), whereas financial measurements measure profitability and efficiency. These indicators provide a more complete picture of organizational success, particularly in areas where financial statistics may not disclose concerns.

Examples of Quality-Related NFPIs

Internal Perspective (Operational Quality)

- Wastage levels – measuring inefficiencies and material losses in production.
- Labor turnover – assessing staff retention and satisfaction.
- Staff absences – monitoring employee well-being.
- Development plans – reviewing staff training and professional growth.
- Job satisfaction – gauging employee engagement and morale.
- Overtime working – may indicate understaffing or poor planning.
- Product improvements – tracking continuous quality enhancement efforts.

• Sales from new products – reflecting innovation and acceptance as well as investment in innovation and future quality.

• Cleanliness– indicators of operational discipline and safety.

• Meeting staff needs – evaluating internal support and communication.

External Perspective (Customer-Focused Quality)

• Customer complaints – direct feedback on quality issues.

• Speed of delivery – timeliness in fulfilling customer orders.

• Accuracy of delivery – ensuring correct products and quantities are delivered.

• Number of returns – a signal of product faults or customer dissatisfaction.

• Repeat sales – indicating customer loyalty and satisfaction.

• New customers – a measure of market reach and reputation.

• Growth in sales – a general indicator of customer demand and perceived value.

• Meeting government targets on emissions – reflecting environmental responsibility, which can affect public perception and compliance.

Limitations of Non-Financial Performance Indicators (NFPIs)

Non-Financial Performance Indicators (NFPIs) are being widely used; however, putting them into practice can be hard in a number of ways.

1. Resource-Intensive Implementation

Setting up and keeping a full system of NFPIs can take a lot of time and resources for collecting data, training staff, and keeping an eye on things all the time.

2. Complexity and Usability Issues

An NFPI system covers a lot of ground, making it hard for managers to use, which could cause people to get confused or make bad choices.

3. Lack of Standardization

Unlike financial performance measures, there is no universally accepted set of NFPIs. Their usage and implementation are highly subjective.

4. Limited Benchmarking and Comparability

Because NFPI systems are personalized, it is hard to compare them to other systems.

10. The Balanced Scorecard by Kaplan and Norton (1993)

It integrates financial and non-financial performance measures to create a balanced approach to measuring performance. Balanced scorecard examines an organization's performance from four interrelated perspectives:

The Four Perspectives

1. **Financial Perspective**: Focus on creating value for shareholders. Performance measures being used are Return on Capital Employed (ROCE), Return on Shareholders' Equity (ROSE), Profitability, and revenue growth.

2. **Customer Perspective**: (Understanding and satisfying customer needs). Measures include customer satisfaction level, customer retention & loyalty, sales to new vs existing customers.

3. **Internal Process Perspective**: It measures operational efficiency. Measures include unit cost analysis, production quality metrics, cycle time or process reliability

4. **Learning and Growth Perspective**: (Innovation, staff development, and continuous improvement). Measures include revenue generated from new products, Investment in staff training and development, and R&D expenditure

Advantages and Disadvantages of Balanced Scorecard

Advantages:

By combining various elements, it enhances comprehension and minimizes the risk of overlooking significant factors. It addresses both short-term and long-term performance. Its difficulty in manipulation contributes to its reliability.

Disadvantages:

It may demand significant resources, involve complex calculations, be challenging to implement, hard to understand, lack standardization and comparability, and be subjective.

11. Benchmarking

Benchmarking: A Strategic Management Tool

Benchmarking is the process of comparing competencies with best practices, including those outside the organization's industry. This evaluation helps assess performance, learn from others, and pursue ongoing improvement.

Purpose

It helps the organization

• to determine their actions, motivations, and performance levels

• to analyze industry benchmarks and practices of competitors and top firms

• to fully dedicate themselves to achieving best practices as a mark of excellence

Types and Levels of Benchmarking

Benchmarking varies by comparison target and can be categorized as follows:

Internal Benchmarking:

Examines the performance of different departments or functions within an organization to identify internal best practices.

• **Competitive Benchmarking**:

Involves comparison with direct competitors within the same industry.

• **Functional Benchmarking**:

Examines processes across organizations within comparable functional areas, irrespective of industry.

• **Strategic Benchmarking**:

Emphasizes overall business results like market share and strategic positioning.

The Benchmarking Process

A benchmarking process involves four key stages:

1. **Planning**

- Select the activity or process
- Involve relevant staff members
- Identify key stages and performance indicators (inputs, outputs, outcomes)
- Establish benchmarks against a standard of best practice

2. **Analysis**

- Assess the performance gap between current practices and best practices
- Explore reasons for underperformance
- Generate improvement ideas, potentially including new methods or technologies

3. **Action**

- Develop and implement a plan to achieve performance improvements
- Allocate appropriate resources and assign responsibilities
- Ensure that improvement efforts are aligned with overall business goals

4. **Review**

- Monitor progress against benchmarks
- Review the relevance and effectiveness of performance measures
- Adjust targets and actions based on new insights

Sources of Benchmarking Information

In practice, benchmarking relies on a range of internal and external data sources. The most valuable insights often come from:

- Trade associations
- Industry forums
- Collaborative networks and inter-firm comparison programs

Organizations are encouraged to compare themselves with best practices wherever it is found, regardless of industry or geography, to drive meaningful improvement.

Chapter 17: Performance measurement in specific situations

Chapter 17: Performance Measurement

1. There are many kinds of businesses according to their activity.

Major types can be

- Manufacturing businesses
- Services providers
- Non-profit organizations
- Government organizations/public sector organizations

These organizations have different types of goals regarding their nature of business. For instance, the manufacturing sector might want to have the lowest price of their product, while public sector organizations need to optimize consumer benefits with the lowest possible cost. Like that each type of organization has its own types of problems or constraints, and each faces different challenges in performance and cost measurement, i.e, it's hard to calculate the cost of a service provided.

1.1 Measuring success by division

1.2 Measuring managerial performance

1.2.1 Managerial Performance Evaluation

Judging a manager's effectiveness purely by their department's overall results can be misleading. Performance outcomes are often shaped by external forces that managers cannot influence, which makes a straightforward comparison between departments problematic.

For instance, one manager might be tasked with running operations in a highly saturated market with unfavorable working conditions, where progress is naturally limited. In contrast, another might lead a unit in a stable industry with minimal competition, where positive results are more easily achieved.

Given such disparities, assessing managers based solely on division-wide outcomes risks overlooking the true quality of their leadership.

1.3 Two Key Approaches to Fair Evaluation

1.3.1 Set Tailored, Strategic Objectives

A more accurate way to assess managerial effectiveness is through the use of personalized performance targets. Each manager should be assigned goals that are not only specific to their role but also aligned with broader organizational aims.

For example, while a firm may seek an annual revenue increase of 5%, maintaining current sales might be a more appropriate target for a unit operating in a challenging business environment. The key is to ensure that these objectives are both ambitious and realistically attainable.

When goals are mutually agreed upon by both managers and executive leadership, it builds transparency and promotes motivation. Furthermore, reaching these targets can be tied to financial rewards, reinforcing performance-driven accountability.

1.3.2 Focus on Controllable Financial Outcomes

Another effective method involves using financial indicators that reflect only those areas a manager can influence. Budgets should clearly distinguish between variables under the manager's control—such as staffing costs or department-specific revenues—and those shaped by external forces.

By focusing on "controllable profit," organizations can gain clearer insight into how well a manager allocates resources and manages day-to-day operations, regardless of outside market fluctuations. This system also protects managers from being unfairly penalized for unpredictable events like economic downturns or shifts in consumer behavior.

1.4 Taking responsibility

The type of center a manager is in charge of will also affect how they measure performance:

1.4.1 Responsibilities

Performance can be evaluated based on responsibilities across various centers. For cost centers, a manager's primary role is to minimize production costs. Their performance can be assessed through changes in total cost and metrics that gauge cost efficiency and output. Revenue centers are evaluated on their ability to generate sales revenue and maintain customer satisfaction. Profit centers combine costs and income, allowing for broader financial analysis through gross profit margins, net profit margins, and return on investment. Investment centers focus on generating profits and making long-term capital decisions, making metrics like ROI and asset management crucial for their evaluation.

1.4.2 Rate of return on investment (ROI)

This is a similar measure to ROCE (return on capital employed). However, it is a bit different in here. It is used to judge how well a department made its investment.

ROI = (Controllable profit / Capital employed controllable) x 100

Controllable profit is earnings after depreciation but before taxes. If a profit figure is given, but there is no other data available, then the profit is taken as controllable profit. Controllable Capital is total assets minus current liabilities.

1.4.3 ROI as performance measure

It is a widely recognized method for evaluating divisional performance, particularly in investment centers. While it offers several advantages, it also presents notable limitations.

Strengths of ROI:

- ROI is a well-established metric, commonly used across industries for performance comparison.
- As it is used widely and expressed in percentage, ROI enables performance comparisons between divisions of varying sizes.
- It relies on data that is readily available within financial reports.
- The calculation is straightforward, making it easy to communicate and understand.

Limitations of ROI:

- ROI is based on historical accounting data, which can be affected by evaluation methods used, like depreciation methods, inflation, or other reporting decisions.
- Managers might manipulate figures to improve ROI in the short term, such as delaying necessary expenditures or avoiding new investments.
- Discourages investment: A project that generates returns lower than the division's current ROI—but still above the firm's cost of capital—might be rejected, leading to missed growth opportunities.
- Misleading comparisons: ROI can create misleading impressions when used to compare divisions with different asset bases or risk profiles.

1.4.4 Residual Income (RI)

Conceptually, residual income is the income that keeps coming in after you've put time and effort into something at first. Here, it is the excessive income you earn over the minimum rate of return (i.e, cost of capital) on operating assets or invested capital. The return on investment (ROI) is a percentage or rate, while the residual income (RI) is a dollar amount.

Residual Income = Net Income - (Cost of Capital * Invested Capital).

Or

Residual Income = Net Income - (Minimum Required Rate of Return * Operating Assets).

Strengths of RI:

- Unlike ROI, RI encourages managers to pursue any investment that exceeds the cost of capital, supporting long-term growth.
- RI delivers a clear monetary value of additional income, which may be more tangible than a percentage.
- Since it incorporates a charge for the use of capital, RI supports decision-making that aligns with wealth creation.

Limitations of RI:

- Because it is an absolute figure, it can be difficult to compare divisions of different sizes or investment levels.
- RI depends heavily on accurately determining the cost of capital, which can vary over time and may be subjective.
- It is more difficult to calculate and interpret than ROI, which can limit its adoption in some organizations.

1.5 Manufacturing industry

Manufacturing companies can use the measures we discussed in the last chapter to rate the work of managers and divisions. As an example:

1. Financial indicators of profitability, liquidity, and risk

2. NFPIs

3. Variance analysis

4. Labor turnover and related ratios

We need to use appropriate measures for different costing systems. For instance;

1.5.1 Contracts costing (for long-term projects)

For a large project that extends across multiple accounting periods, contract costing is a suitable method for monitoring and managing expenses. This costing is mostly used in projects like construction, engineering, and consultancy, where projects tend to be complex and lengthy.

Given the significant value and length of these contracts, it is crucial to manage costs effectively. This involves regularly comparing budgeted (planned) figures with actual figures to track progress:

- Excess expenses
- Project timeline delays

1.5.1.1 Essential Metrics in Contract Management

- Comparison of approved contract value to actual costs incurred
- Level of rework or remedial efforts needed after completion
- Profitability evaluations based on certifications from professionals like architects or quantity surveyors

Alongside financial data, it is essential to track operational efficiency indicators.

- Time when workers or machinery are not active
- Waste of materials • Levels of inventory • Use of equipment and facilities

A structured four-step approach is employed to evaluate a project's financial performance and compare it with budgeted expectations, allowing for the determination of attributable profit on a long-term contract.

Step 1: Calculate the overall value of the contract. Determine the contract price.

Step 2: Calculate the Overall Completion Cost. Estimate the total expenses needed to complete the project.

Step 3: Determine the Anticipated Overall Profit or Loss. Deduct the total estimated costs from the total contract value. If a loss is anticipated, the entire loss should be acknowledged right away, irrespective of the progress made on the work.

Step 4: Distribute Profit According to Advancement. Profit can be determined using one of two methods:

1. Certified work value to date divided by total contract value, multiplied by expected total profit. (This assesses progress according to the ratio of certified work).

2. Costs incurred to date divided by total estimated costs, multiplied by expected total profit. This approach recognizes profit based on cost progress instead of output.

1.5.2 Job costing: (keeping track of one job at a time)

When work is done on a job-by-job basis, job costing is employed. Every work is seen as a distinct cost unit. Businesses that do short-term, one-of-a-kind jobs, like repair services, printing companies or consulting organizations, often use this strategy.

Although smaller in scale than long-term contracts, job costing still demands close monitoring of costs and time. Success is usually measured by how well resources are used and how efficiently work is completed.

1.5.2.1 Performance Measures in Job Costing:

• Cost efficiency: Staying within budgeted costs for labor, materials, and overhead.

• Managing time: Making sure that deadlines are met without any unnecessary delays.

For instance, by field:

• Accountancy firms: the number of billable hours compared to the overall number of hours worked.

• Auto repair shops: The average age or turnover of the inventory they have on hand.

• Printing services: Cost for every page that is printed.

1.5.3 Process Costing: (For production that happens again and over again)

Companies that make screws and bolts, make chemicals, or make food employ process pricing since they make things all the time and can't tell them apart.

In this system, items go through a number of steps, and each step has its own price. The main goals are to keep things running smoothly, cut down wastages, and keep prices down across the system.

1.5.3.1 Key Performance Indicators, or KPIs, are

• Loss levels that are out of the ordinary or not normal.

• Lost production time.

• Production cycle time: Finding out how long it takes to finish each step of the process.

Managers often compare actual production and expenses to find issues early and fix them.

1.5.4 Batch Costing: (Keeping Costs in Check by the Batch)

Batch costing is in between task costing and process costing. People utilize it when they make things in groups, such as clothes or baked goods. Each batch is handled as one cost unit, which makes it simpler to handle vast amounts of things without having to keep track of each one separately.

Since batch costing shares features with both job and process costing, the success measures from either system can be applied, depending on the specific business and production style.

1.5.4.1 Examples of Success Measures in Batch Production:

- Clothing: Level of fabric waste per batch.
- Furniture: Volume of stock held.
- Electronics firms: Frequency and severity of quality control issues.

1.6 The Service Industry

The methods we assess success change as economies change. In many developed countries, the service sector has risen quickly while the manufacturing sector has shrunk. Today, the economy is mostly made up of businesses like banking, aviation, transportation, hotels, consultancy, and retail. Core management ideas like Key Performance Indicators (KPIs) and Critical Success Factors (CSFs) are still useful in service-based firms, but they need to be used more carefully and in context to each industry type.

In service sectors, performance is usually looked at in two basic ways:

1.6.1 Financial performance in the service industry

Companies that provide services use both standard and customized financial indicators. Standard accounting ratios like liquidity, profitability, and activity ratios are still helpful, but they need to be looked at in the context of the sector and the fact that service delivery is focused on people.

1.6.1.1 Common Financial KPIs in the Service Sector:

- Revenue per service unit (e.g., per room, client, seat, consultation)

- Revenue per partner/principal (in legal or consulting firms)
- Staff costs as a percentage of revenue
- Rent costs relative to sales
- Training cost as a share of sales
- Gross and net profit margins
- Current and quick ratios
- Market share and year-on-year growth in market share

However, since service delivery is deeply human and variable, financial data alone rarely tells the full story. That's why we need to keep a close eye on the quality of service as well.

1.6.2 Quality of Service: A Success Factor That Doesn't Cost Money

Customer experience and perceived quality are very important in service firms. The problem is that the quality of service is frequently hard to measure, depends on the situation, and is subjective. So, measuring quality has to be methodical and cover a lot of ground.

1.6.2.1 Example: Health and wellness center

The operations manager of a health and wellness facility is in charge of several different areas, such as spa treatments, fitness training, nutrition consultation, front desk services, and marketing. Clients typically utilize more than one of these services, which makes it hard to figure out which department is responsible for shared overhead expenditures. It's usually easy to see how much money a company makes directly, but a lot of indirect costs aren't allocated to any one unit. Because of this, staff bonuses are generally based on the center's overall financial success instead of the output of each department.

This encourages teamwork and keeps managers focused on the big picture.

1.6.2.2 Internal quality management

Service firms put internal control systems right into their operations and don't wait for customers to complain about quality. Professional service businesses may look at the skills and availability of their personnel as a way to judge how well their service is.

Sometimes, the quality of the service is measured after it has been delivered by looking at things like how happy the customer is, how many complaints there are, and how many people succeed.

Strong financial outcomes are not the only thing that matters for success in the service industry. Service firms need to find a balance between making money and always providing great service.

1.7 Non-Profit and Public Sector organizations

It is important yet hard to measure how well charities, schools, and government institutions that serve the public are doing. These organizations do not work to profit, so standard financial indicators do not adequately show their performance.

1.7.1 Issues in assessing performance

Two main challenges exist:

- Identifying and measuring objectives
- Measuring and identifying outputs

1.7.1.1 Identifying and measuring objectives

Non-profit organizations and governmental organizations differ in their objectives. For example:

Charities strive to offer the best assistance possible despite having limited donations or grants. Government agencies in health and education aim to provide essential public services while adhering to fixed budgets. Despite their differences, these institutions often have common objectives like providing high-quality services efficiently within their resource constraints.

1.7.1.2 Recognizing quantifiable inputs and outputs

Unlike private businesses, non-profit and public organizations do not usually make physical goods with clear financial value. How can we judge a hospital's effects or a school's usefulness? Even though performance goals are set, they are often subjective and open to interpretation.

1.7.2 Value for Money (VFM) Framework

Many such organizations use the Value for Money (VFM) model to measure their output performance. It gives a whole picture of how well things work..

The Value for Money (VFM) framework is built on three key principles, called the Three Es—economy, Efficiency, and effectiveness.

Economics examines if the organization obtains resources—like supplies, services, or equipment—at the most favorable cost while maintaining quality. It involves being financially prudent while upholding reasonable standards.

Efficiency assesses the effectiveness of resource utilization. Is converting time, money, and staff efforts into outputs as efficiently as possible? This principle examines the flow of resources within the system.

Effectiveness examines if the organization is successfully reaching its intended objectives. Being resourceful is insufficient; what truly matters is the alignment of outcomes with the organization's mission.

The VFM approach goes beyond merely assessing expenditure. The emphasis is on the effective use of resources to achieve significant outcomes.

1.7.2.1 Example: Implementing the 3Es in a University Context: Finding the right balance between cost and quality for books, training, and equipment. Inexpensive resources may reduce costs but negatively impact education.

Effectiveness Resource utilization: frequency of student book borrowing, IT facility usage, and staff time allocation.

Efficiency Outcomes of success include exam results, graduation rates, and employment statistics for recent graduates.

Chapter 18: Spreadsheets

1. Getting Started with Spreadsheets

Spreadsheets are digital tools designed to store, calculate, and organize data. Whether you're managing a budget, tracking inventory, or analyzing trends, spreadsheets like Excel or Google Sheets are powerful and flexible solutions.

At the core of every spreadsheet are rows, columns, and cells—each cell can hold numbers, text, or formulas. One of the most useful features? Formulas that automatically calculate results as your data changes.

1.1 Entering Formulas: The Basics

A formula tells the spreadsheet to perform a calculation. In most spreadsheet programs, every formula begins with an equal sign (=). This signals to the software that you're entering a command—not just text or numbers.

Formula Elements Include:

Cell references: Like B3 or F10, pointing to specific data.

Operators: Such as +, -, *, / (add, subtract, multiply, divide).

Functions: Pre-built tools like SUM, AVERAGE, and MAX.

Example:

=(B3 + C6) * 0.75

This adds the values in cells B3 and C6, then multiplies the result by 0.75.

1.1.1 Order of Operations

Just like in math, spreadsheets follow the BODMAS rule:

Brackets

Orders (exponents)

Division and Multiplication

Addition and Subtraction

Always use brackets to make your intentions clear:

=(A2 + A4) / 2

1.1.2 How to Enter a Formula Step-by-Step

Click on the cell where you want the result to appear.

Type the equal sign =.

Input the formula manually, or click the cells to add them into the formula.

Press Enter, and the answer will appear in the cell.

(The full formula will still be visible in the formula bar).

1.1.3 Common Functions for Quick Calculations

Here are some helpful built-in functions used across spreadsheet tools:

Function Purpose Example

SUM Adds values in a range =SUM(D3:D8)

AVERAGE Finds the average =AVERAGE(A1:A5)

MAX Returns the highest value =MAX(C2:C10)

MIN Returns the lowest value =MIN(E1:E4)

These functions save time and reduce errors, especially with long lists of data.

1.2 Real-Life Spreadsheet Applications

Spreadsheets aren't just for numbers—they're tools for solving problems, testing ideas, and making decisions.

1.2.1 Scenario 1: "What If" Analysis

Suppose you're planning a product launch. You can set up a formula where changes to estimated sales will automatically update projected revenue.

=Units_Sold * Price_Per_Unit

Adjust the number of units, and instantly see the financial impact. This is great for questions like:

"What if sales fall by 15%?" or "What if we raise prices?"

1.2.2 Scenario 2: Budgeting and Cash Flow

Spreadsheets are often used to prepare budgets, where different categories of spending are totaled and compared to available income.

=SUM(F5:F11) → Total Expenses

=B2 - F12 → Net Cash Flow

=F13 + G12 → Closing Balance

This helps monitor your financial health and plan for the future without recalculating everything manually.

1.2.3 Scenario 3: Performance Reporting

Companies often use spreadsheets to track performance across months or years—like comparing profit margins or sales trends. One sheet may contain raw data, while another calculates ratios or visualizes trends with graphs.

=Profit / Revenue

This might calculate a profit margin, and show it as a percentage.

1.2.4 Understanding Variance Analysis

Variance analysis is used to compare actual outcomes with planned targets. For example:

If your budget expected marketing costs to be $4,000 but the actual spend was $5,200, you'd have a negative variance of $1,200.

Formulas like this are commonly used:

=Actual - Budgeted

It helps managers understand whether costs, sales, or other metrics are on track—and why.

1.3 Strengths and Weaknesses of Spreadsheets

1.3.1 Advantages:

Easy to learn and widely accessible

Great for handling small to medium datasets

Built-in tools for calculations, graphs, and formatting

Useful for simulations, planning, and analysis

1.3.2 Limitations:

Can be error-prone if not carefully managed

Not ideal for storing large amounts of raw data

Limited collaboration and version control

Vulnerable to accidental deletion or incorrect input

For large-scale data handling, a database may be more suitable.

1.4 Example: Expected Value Calculation

Let's say a student wants to calculate the expected return from different investment scenarios:

Investment Probability Return

A 0.3 200

B 0.4 300

C 0.3 500

The expected value formula:

=(0.3*200) + (0.4*300) + (0.3*500)

Spreadsheets make this kind of analysis simple and dynamic.

Don't miss out!

Visit the website below and you can sign up to receive emails whenever Dr. M. Imran Ahsan publishes a new book. There's no charge and no obligation.

https://books2read.com/r/B-A-SVILE-RVUTG

BOOKS 2 READ

Connecting independent readers to independent writers.

Did you love *ACCA F2: Management Accounting*? Then you should read *ACCA: Business & Technology*[1] by M. Imran Ahsan!

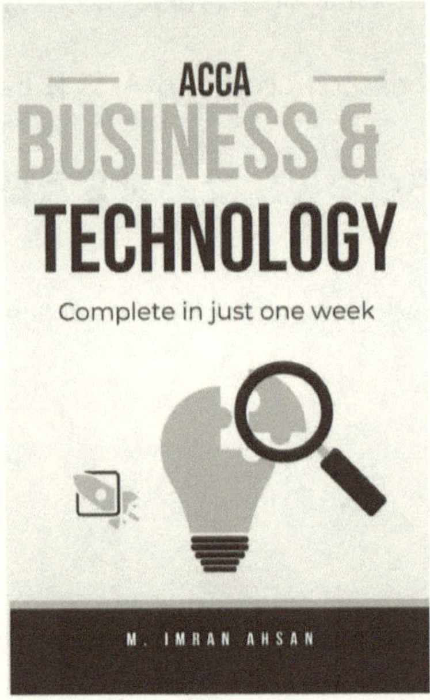

[2]

Here is a comprehensive guide to the ACCA Business and Technology course; you will find all the information you need to succeed.

Is "Business Technology: Mastering ACCA's Business and Technology" anything that interests you?

Brief Synopsis: Take a close look at businesses to learn about their inner workings, key players, and environment. We eliminate any complexity and ensure you have no problem learning these fundamental notions by offering simple examples and clear explanations.

"Business Technology: Mastering ACCA's Business and Technology Subject" goes above and beyond what is often found in textbooks. You may use it to your advantage in your ACCA studies since it simplifies complex concepts, provides real-world examples, and offers practical strategies.

---

1. https://books2read.com/u/3y9J6l

2. https://books2read.com/u/3y9J6l

Preparation is critical to succeed in the ACCA Business and Technology course. "Business Technology: Mastering ACCA's Business and Technology Subject" is an essential resource for anybody seeking to acquire knowledge, understanding, and skill in this field. Rest assured, you are fully prepared to crush ACCA!

Also by Dr. M. Imran Ahsan

ACCA

ACCA F2: Management Accounting

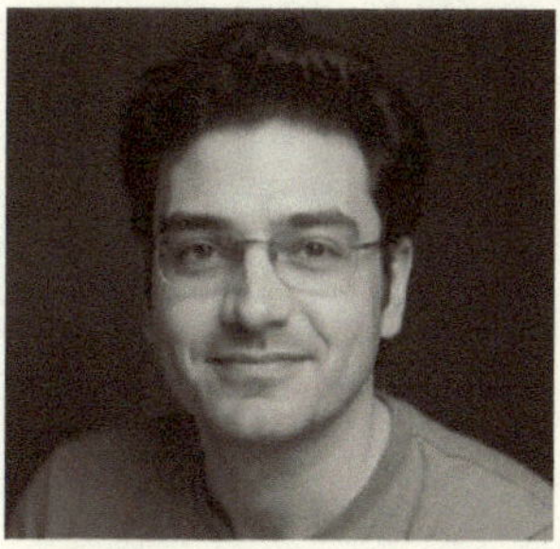

About the Author

Instructor | CFA & ACCA Specialist | Financial Economics Expert. **Dr. Imran Ahsan** is a celebrated instructor specializing in **CFA, ACCA, and Financial Economics**. Known for his engaging teaching style and ability to simplify complex concepts, he has helped hundreds of aspiring finance professionals excel in their exams and careers. With a strong blend of academic expertise and practical industry knowledge, Dr. Ahsan is passionate about empowering students to build lasting skills in finance, investment, and economics.

www.ingramcontent.com/pod-product-compliance
Lightning Source LLC
LaVergne TN
LVHW090408210926
848480LV00002B/501